I0485855

Essays from
The Arthritis Trust of America Website

http://www.arthritistrust.org
Anthony di Fabio, Editor

Published by Arthritis Trust of America
Copyright August 11, 2015

Life Robbing Poison Approved by the United States Government
by
Anthony di Fabio

I'm about to get you more angry than you've been in a long, long time.

So you believe, like so many of us did, that our government looks out for us, that doctors and dentists are knowledgeable and would not do us harm, that fluoride is a certain means for avoiding cavities, and that Federal and State public health employees have the facts to back up their authoritative instructions.

Well, if you believe all of that then don't read this article! You'll be very uncomfortable.

There are numerous ways by which the lie of the use — and over use — of fluroide enters our life. I'm about to tell you the way it entered mine — and then I'll tell you more truth!

I was city manager of a small town in Tennessee, reporting chiefly to a board of city commissioners that was elected by its citizens. According to the city's constitution, as approved by the state of Tennessee, the city manager was the executive branch of government and the commissioners were the legislative branch. A local lawyer was hired from time to time to act as the judicial branch, primarily handling speeding complaints.

How Poisoning a Town Starts

A young nurse from one of the State of Tennessee offices asked to speak before our City Commissioners for the purpose of requesting that the city add fluoride to the water supply.

Of course, anyone who wishes it could speak before our City Commissioners, and so the young nurse was invited to do so.

Her pitch consisted primarily of a request for building healthier teeth by our young ones — who can resist such an appeal? — And to point out that surrounding communities and much larger cities throughout the nation already had fluoridation added to their municipal water supplies.

The City Commissioners turned to me and asked my opinion. Being somewhat naive and sans any research data, I agreed with the nurse, and so together we innocently, and stupidly added fluoride to the City of Fairview's (Tennessee) water supply and that addition continues to this date, despite the fact that the citizens of the City of Fairview, TN have never had an opportunity to know the pros and cons of fluoridation or to vote for or against the issue. My reasoning was based on the false idea that there existed excellent science behind the use of fluoride in potable water.

Not so, I later learned!

The commissioners enacted the ordinance to add fluoride to the municipal water system and from then on, if a citizen wanted to remove it from their drinking water they had to install in their home their own reverse osmosis water purifier as ordinary filters would not take out either fluoride or chlorine, the later chemical already laced throughout our water system.

Many years later, and no longer a city commissioner, I learned the truth about fluoride. I wrote a long article containing my proof of the damage that fluoride routinely did to adults and children, and I mailed a copy to every then new member of the city commission.

My data was totally ignored and therefore, for the past forty years I've held myself responsible for needlessly poisoning thousands of citizens.

There's no way I've found to reverse a recommendation that had stemmed from the authoritative body, the state, the Tennessee Department of Health.

There's a moral, here. Bureaucratic knowledge always trumps scientific knowledge and truth!

Excerpt from:

Hileman B. (1988). "Fluoridation of water. Questions about health risks and benefits remain after more than 40 years." *Chemical and Engineering News.* August 1, 1988, 26-42. (See article)

"Although *skeletal fluorosis* has been studied intensely in other countries for more than 40 years, virtually no research has been done in the U.S. to determine how many people are afflicted with the earlier stages of the disease, particularly the preclinical stages. **Because some of the clinical symptoms mimic arthritis, the first two clinical phases of skeletal fluorosis could be easily misdiagnosed.** Skeletal fluorosis is not even discussed in most medical texts under the effects of fluoride; indeed, a number of texts say the condition is almost nonexistent in the U.S. Even if a doctor is aware of the disease, the early stages are difficult to diagnose."

Few cases in Canada or the United States will be found to be as dramatic as that recorded here from Southwest China, . . .

Dental surgeon, Geoffrey E. Smith says, "My 12-year-old granddaughter, Jade-Emma, has 'mottled' teeth, and my wife suffers from osteoporosis.

"Jade's disfigured teeth were caused by fluoride, and there is now a growing body of evidence suggesting that fluoride can be a factor in the development of osteoporosis.

"Is the dental wonder of the 1950s set to become the medical blunder of the 21st century?

"Such a thought is particularly frustrating for me since I belong to the profession — dentistry — which has, for the past 40 years, claimed that fluoride was essential for sound teeth and 'good' for bones[45]."

Back to my serious mistake: The city commissioners and I, as then City Manager, unknowingly exposed hundreds of Fairview citizens to Arthrosis, vertebral and hip fracture, osteosarcoma (cancer), infertility, birth defects, bone damage, damage to the immune system, fluorosis, fluoride neurotoxicity, and many other poorly diagnosed conditions, as fluoride affects every human system, often by inhibiting enzymes which are essential for the functioning of every human system.

No citizen of Fairview had knowledge of the pros and cons and no citizen was allowed to vote up or down.

Besides the damaging of human tissue by 1 ppm of fluoride added to our public water systems, the health problem is also one of massive overconsumption of fluoride. We are being bombarded with fluoride from all our dental products and also many industrial sources.

Physicians and nurses, of course, are authoritative figures, especially in the minds of those who do not specialize in health care. If doctors, nurses, or public health officials say that a drug is good for us, we tend to believe them, and we don't question their credentials or source of information. Had we known that we were dooming thousands of people to lesser, or even damaging, health, we might have questioned further. For example, if the City Commissioners wish to purchase a new truck, each of them holds himself out as somewhat knowledgeable in mechanics, and each would question data brought in by someone that they deemed to have invalid information, or contrary information.

Likewise, when building a ballpark for the City's youth, each commissioner would feel that they had valuable knowledge to contribute.

But question a medical authority or public health official?

Hardly!

Who Benefits By Fluoridation?

So who does benefit by the addition of Fluoride to Public Water Systems?

Municipalities may use either Sodium Fluoride plus lime or HydroFluosilic Acid.

The only ones definitely known to benefit from fluoridation are chemical companies and fluoridation equipment firms. Fluoride is one of the most common and also one of the most caustic of industrial chemicals. "Hydrofluoric acid is used to refine high-octane gasoline, to make fluorocarbons and chlorfluorocarbons for freezers and air conditioners, and to manufacture computer screens, fluorescent light bulbs, semiconductors, plastics, herbicides, and fluoride toothpaste. It also has the ability to burn flesh to the bone, destroy eyes, and sear lungs so that victims drown in their own body fluid. What's worse is that hydrofluoric acid boils at 680 deg rees F. On a warm day, released hydrofluoric acid forms a low, dense cloud that can remain hazardous 6 miles from its origin.

"Even though industry takes extreme safety precautions, accidents still happen. In 1987, a crane operator at Texas City's Marathon Oil refinery dropped a 90-ton heating unit on a tank of hydrofluoric acid, releasing 5000 gallons of the stuff. Approximately 5,800 people were evacuated, and 1,037 required hospital treatment. Many of the people exposed still have difficulty breathing. Since 1986, thirty-three such incidents have involved evacuation, injuries, or death.

"Hydrofluoric acid is made in three U.S. towns, Geismar, Louisiana; La Porte, Texas; and Calvert City, Texas — and five Mexican ones. More than 21 million gallons are produced and shipped each year. Given its caustic nature and dangerously low boiling point, one can understand why Energy Safety Council, an advocacy group based in Illinois, wants to replace it with sulfuric acid. Almost half of the U.S. refineries use sulfuric acid as a refining catalyst already[32]."

It has been said that Fluoride, or hydrofluosilic acid, used in Public Community water supplies is chiefly a waste byproduct of the aluminum industry, and those companies benefit immensely by having us add their toxic waste product to our water system. If we didn't, they'd have an environmental disposal problem which would increase the cost of aluminum. We, however, very nicely solve the problem for them by paying them for it and then adding it to our drinking water, thereby diluting the poison, and spreading the dangerous pollutant throughout the land via our waste water.

Anne Anderson, R.P.N. and Richard G. Foulkes, B.A., M.D.[33] say that 99.9% of the fluoride added to community drinking waters will not be drunk, but flushed down the sewage system, and that the effect will be to deposit, for example, roughly 150 tons of fluoride into the North Pacific's Bow River and environment each year. This effect of spreading toxic substances throughout our environment, through sewage and river systems and ground table waters is repeated and multiplied from every municipality that fluoridates drinking water for the wrongly presumed decrease of human cavities.

"Often overlooked, and deliberately obscured, is the effect of fluoride pollution that comes about as a result of fluoride waste disposal, not only from industry" but also from community sewage disposal[33]. While there are many factors that affect decreasing fish returns, such as natural cycles, changes in ocean temperature and currents, overfishing, destruction of spawning grounds by poor logging practices, building activities, dams and pollution, obviously the dumping of toxic poison into our streams, lakes and oceans is a major part of the declining fish problem.

The Presumed Scientific Basis for Adding Fluoride to Public Water Systems

Initial Studies Invalid

In 1930, Dr. Trendley Dean, "the father of fluoridation," was responsible for developing the hypothesis that fluoridation was safe and would protect teeth from cavities. He was also the person who established the first trial of fluoridation of the water supply in Grand Rapids, Michigan in 1945. Since that time, he has twice confessed in court that statistics from the early studies, allegedly supporting the use of fluoridation in community water systems, were invalid[1]. (See *City of Oroville vs. Public Utilities*, California 1955 and *Chicago Citizens vs. City of Chicago*, 1960.)

The very earliest studies not supporting the use of fluoridation were published in 1953 in the *Journal of the American Dental Association*[18] and in 1955 in the *American Dental Association*1[9.]

In the first, a comparative study of tooth decay in 12-14 year olds in six Arizona cities, no reduction in decay and filled or missing teeth could be observed due to fluoridation[20].

The second compared teeth of residents of Cameron, Texas (with 4/10th parts per million [ppm] of naturally present fluoride) and those of Bartlett,

5

Texas (with 8 ppm of fluoride). The incidence of tooth decay was found to be no different between Cameron and Bartlett residents.

1979 Injunction Against Fluoridation

Pennsylvania Supreme Court Judge John P. Flaherty, on July 31, 1979, after meticulous study of the scientific data presented before him, wrote, to the Mayor of Auckland, New Zealand, saying, "you are correct that I entered an injunction against the fluoridation of the public water supply for a large portion of Allegheny County. . . . In my view, the evidence is quite convincing that the addition of sodium fluoride to the public water supply at one part per million is extremely deleterious to the human body, and a review of the evidence will disclose that there was no convincing evidence to the contrary[1]."

Richard G. Foulkes, B.A., M.D., former Special Consultant to the Minister of Health, Province of British Columbia, and author of a 1973 report, *Health Security for British Columbians*, that convinced Candadians to require Fluoride additions to public water systems, says, "Today, [Judge] Flaherty could make the same judgement of the evidence concerning the effectiveness of fluoridation in the reduction of dental caries, . . . "

Why a Former Consultant to the Minister of Health
Changed His Support for Fluoridation

Originally, in 1973, Richard Foulkes, B.A., M.D., commissioned to "study and report on the health care system of the province and to make recommendations. . . ., wrote in his report, "We have studied the data and recommendations submitted to us by the Division of Preventive Dentistry, Health Branch, the College of Dental Surgeons of British Columbia and others referring to the effectiveness and potential hazards of the fluoridation of piped water supplies. We have concluded that the artificial fluoridation of community water supplies is both effective and safe.

"Therefore, we recommend . . . that discussion begin immediately to prepare legislation . . . to make fluoridation of major water supplies mandatory in the Province . . . .[1]"

What Dr. Foulkes studied, and recommended in his 1973 *Health Security for British Columbians* was typical of studies and recommendations then occurring around the globe, regarding adding fluoride to public water systems. The government studies by honest, professional and knowledgeable doctors and scientists unknowingly began with incomplete and falsified data.

Dr. Foulkes, author of the 2000-page report that convinced Canada to add fluoride to their municipal water systems, has since rocked the Canadian establishment when he recently recanted and said:

• No reference was made to the fact that Dr. Trendley Dean's data supporting fluoridation was based on statistics that were invalid.

• There was no reference to Philip R.N. Sutton's critique in 1959 of five studies carried out at Newburgh, Grand Rapids, Evanston and Brantford that had begun in 1940's, relating fluoride concentration to dental caries, and which had served as the original justification for fluoridation in the United

States, Britain, Canada, Australia, New Zealand and several other English-speaking countries. Only three of these studies had controls for the full period of the study, and Philip Sutton had criticized them for poor experimental design, poor or negligible statistical analysis and failure to take into account large variations in caries found in the control towns.

• The studies that had been reported prior to 1972 on the toxic effects of fluoride did not find their way into [Dr. Foulkes'] hands, or his advisors. These studies had revealed tumor formation in mice (1952, 1956), genetic damage to plants (1966) and fruit flies (1970, 1971).

• A report by Dyson Rose and John R. Marier for the Research Council of Canada in 1971, entitled *Enviromental Fluoride* reviewed the hazards of fluoride in its various distribution including water supplies, and was again updated in 1977. Dr. Foulkes says, "If *all* information then extant had been examined, it should have been obvious that there was a need for caution and further studies, including study of those areas of potential non-lethal effects of chronic accumulation on populations exposed to lifetime ingestion [of fluoride] . . . our 1973 recommendation should have gone against that of the 'establishment and submitted that fluoridation of community water supplies for the purpose of causing a reduction in tooth decay was on shaky ground and was far from being proved with regard to safety. . . . In light of what is currently found in reputable journals with peer review mechanisms and in various Government documents and correspondence, I now hold a different view. That is that the fluoridation of community water supplies can no longer be held to be either safe or effective in the reduction of dental caries . . . Therefore, the practice should be abandoned or 'put on hold' until all available information is evaluated by persons who are competent in the principles of research and who have no vested interest in those institutions and professional organizations that are currently involved in the thrust[1]."

• The World Health Organization (WHO 1970) and the National Academy of Science (NAS 1971) both expressed concerns about the safety of fluoride.

Summary of Studies Since 1973

A summary of scientific studies made since 1973 conclude that the prescribed or "optimal" level of 1 ppm (1 mg/l) of fluoride, presumed to reduce incidence of decayed, missing or filled teeth can no longer be considered true.

Scientist D. Ziegelbecker[2] in 1981 found no correlation between the level of fluoride in water and dental caries. Other studies performed in Japan in 1972 also destroyed the basic hypothesis that supported the case for adding fluoride to community water systems[1].

Mark Disendorf[3] studied the relationship to decayed, missing or filled teeth between fluoridated and non-fluoridated areas in [8] developed countries over 30 years and showed reductions in tooth decay in both Fluoride and Non-fluoride areas that could not be attributed to Fluoride.

According to Yiamouyiannis, in an analysis of U.S. data provided by the National Institute of Dental Research (NIDR) covering 40,000 children, there was no showing of reduced decay rate between Fluoride and Non-Fluoride regions[1].

In new Zealand, J. Colquhoun[4] demonstrated that reductions in dental caries were taking place before the fluoridation of water supplies and the introduction of fluoride toothpastes.

Pro-fluoridation professionals conducted a study presuming to show a difference between Fluoride and Non-fluoride populations, and came up with a difference of 17% to 20% respectively, which is a difference of 1 tooth surface on the average[5]. A similar study[7] in an aging community showed the same small difference without mentioning the extremely high risks encountered by the elderly which will be discussed in this report later.

A ten-year study of Canadian children (British Columbia) came to the conclusion that fluoridation of community water supplies was "yesterday's technology[6]."

The studies on presence of decayed, missing and filled teeth are "subjective" and easy to manipulate, and there is strong evidence that this was originally done in New Zealand and areas such as Scotland where Fluoridation has at last been discontinued[1].

A Pharmacist Speaks Out

The registered pharmacist, Robert O. Dustrude, R.Ph. of Wausau, WI wrote to the Criteria and Standard Divsion of Drinking Water, Environmental Protection Agency, in Washington, D.C., saying:

"My first approach is as a pharmacist who became interested in the fluoridation issue several years ago. My research of the literature has disclosed that fluoride is a protoplasmic poison as described in the reference book *Clinical Toxicology of Commercial Products*. The same reference book discloses that fluoride salts have a toxicity rating between 4 and 5 (very toxic to extremely toxic). Aside from the literature, I remember when I first started working in drug stores that we used to sell sodium fluoride powder as an effective cockroach poison. I have often asked myself: 'Why on earth would any sane person want to add that stuff to our drinking water?'

"Just about everything that I dispense in filling prescriptions has passed the rigors of controlled, double-blind studies before it becomes part of our medical armamentarium. No such studies exist for fluoride, meaning there is no scientific evidence substantiating the claims made for it. Why should this substance be exempt from the standards that apply to other medicines? On the other hand, according to Dr. Hans Mollenburgh in *Fluoride: The Freedom Fight*, a double-blind test showed that fluoridated water caused side-effects.

"Another consideration is the fact that sodium fluoride requires a prescription. I cannot sell the tablets or drops from any shelves without a valid prescription being presented by my customers. Incongrously, laymen who don't know the difference between a halogen and a halide, can "prescribe" fluoride for our drinking water in concentrations that would otherwise require a prescription. For example, at 1 ppm there would be 1 mg of fluoride in

8

1000 ml of drinking water, a volume easily ingested considering all avenues (e.g., drinking water, soups, Kool-aid, etc.)

"This leads to another issue, the doctor-patient relationship. I know of cases where doctors, using their knowledge of their patients' conditions (arthritis and pre-disposition to cancer), have advised those patients to avoid fluoride. This advice is all but impossible to heed when the drinking water is fluoridated. I submit that it is more logical and ethical to leave the doctor-patient relationship intact by having fluoride available, if at all, only by prescription, instead of forcing it literally and figuratively down our throats.

"I would like to approach the issue not as a pharmacist, but as a concerned, outraged citizen. Even if artificial fluoridation was beneficial, there can be no excuse for the arrogant, heavy-handed, arbitary way in which that procedure is accomplished. I reside in the town of Rib Mountain, a township which has recently installed its own water and sewer system. Before long, the sanitary commission, without any expertise or qualifications, proposed fluoridating our water. At a subsequent meeting, a representative from the Wisconsin Division of Health gave a talk on the virtues of fluoride. Inasmuch as dental caries is not a contagious, communical disease, his attendance was not only inappropriate, but he gave probably the most mendacious presentation I have ever heard. The agenda for this meeting was posted only the legal 24-hours ahead of time, not allowing me time to bring in a professor acquaintance of mine to present his testimony on fluoride toxicity. The sanitary commission then, in what was obviously a predetermined decision, voted to install fluoridation without holding a referendum or otherwise allowing the citizenry a chance to examine both sides of the issue. An attorney friend still insists that the above action was in violation of Wisconsin's open-meeing law, but the local district attorney decided not to prosecute.

"Inasmuch as fluoride is readily available by prescription, and in mouth washes, toothpastes, etc. thus making artificial fluoridation passe, I urge your committee to undertake whatever action you are authorized to do to remove this known poison from our drinking water[8]."

Safety of Fluoridation Questioned

Dental Fluorosis

Dental Fluorosis is the discoloration and pitting, even crumbling of teeth, and overgrowth and weakening of bone.

"While evidence of a link with cancer is relatively new, the link between fluoride and brittle bones is well established . . . . Despite solid evidence to the contrary, fluoride is still prescribed as a treatment for osteoporosis.[11]"

There is now sufficient information in scientific studies to demonstrate that 1 ppm, or higher, of fluoride in community drinking water is neither safe for health nor effective in preventing cavities. At this "optimal" level," dental and skeletal fluorosis (discoloration and pitting, even crumbling, of teeth and overgrowth and weakening of bone) have been identified. . . . [4]" About 30% of children in fluoridated areas suffer from fluorosis compared to 4.25% in low fluoride areas[4].

Although most of the studies concentrate on "cosmetic impairment," that is, the appearance of the teeth, Colquhoun[4] says that "The claim that only tooth cells are damaged by fluoride is extremely implausible on scientific grounds. There is evidence of general harm[4]," [to the body].

Apparently there is also an increase in fluorosis in tropical countries, as I.D. Brouwer and others[13] reported in its incidence in Senegal where WHO standard of 1.2 ppm was adopted. Richard G. Foulkes, B.A., M.D. says, "The hot climate and poor nutritional status of the inhabitants result in high ingestion of the dangerous substance.

"Dental and skeletal fluorosis is seen, also, at low doses in those with kidney disease and can be anticipated to be a more frequent occurence in the developed countries as the total fluoride increases from all sources including: industrial air emissions, water, fluoridated dental and other medicinal agents, foods and even teflon cooking utensils[1]." (See "Dietary Fluoride Intake in the U.S.A. Revisited," *Fluoride*, Vol. 24, No. 1, 1991 for the ever-present distribution of Fluoride).

Hip Fractures

Hip Fractures have occurred with increasing frequency among women, especially post-menopausal, since the addition of fluoride to drinking water. M. Bely, M.D. says, that it is commonly recognized that about 10% of bone tissue is reorganized each year. As bone tissue breaks down, other cells rebuild it. "It is a generally accepted fact, that . . . fluoride causes enlargement of the whole bone mass . . . Authors agree that the [newly] formed bone is inferior to normal, the matrix is irregular, the collagen structure of the newly formed bone tissue differs from normal, and the mineralization is enhanced. . . . so fluoride exerts its effects not only on the newly generated (newly formed) bone tissue, but also changes the collagen structure of the preexisting bone too[9]."

The incidence of hip fractures in 246 patients 65 years of age or older was compared in three communities in Utah, one with and two without water fluoridated to 1 ppm, over a seven year period. Christa Danielson, M.D., Joseph L. Lyon, M.D., Marlene Egger, Ph.D. and Gerald K. Goodenough, M.D. concluded from this study that "We found a small but significant increase in the risk of hip fracture in both men and women exposed to artificial fluoridation at 1 ppm, suggesting that low levels of fluoride may increase the risk of hip fracture in the elderly[10]." The relative risk of hip fracture in the higher fluoride group, over the lower fluoride group, was 27% greater for women, and 41% greater for men. John R. Lee, M.D. concluded from the Utah study that "Fluoride is toxic to bones and increases risk of fracture at all levels of exposure including fluoridation at 1 ppm. Regardless of any other consideration, this is reason enough to discontinue fluoridation immediately[40]."

There have been four additional studies in recent years that demonstrate an increased incidence of hip fractures for elderly people who live in fluoridated areas[11]. Jacobsen (USA), Cooper (UK) and Colquhoun (New

10

Zealand) all state that increased fracture of the hip (proximal femur) has occurred since the advent of fluoridation[12]. Colquhoun says, "I find it astonishing therefore that, at a time when women's hip fractures in New Zealand are reaching epidemic proportions, health boards are still claiming that fluoridated water is perfectly safe[12]."

According to John R. Lee, M.D., there have been "seven studies showing a positive correlation of fluoridation with increased hip fracture incidence and not one acceptable study showing the contrary[41]."

Red Blood Cells

According to Richard G. Foulkes, B.A., M.D., quoting D.S. Kumari[14], "Severe skeletal fluorosis occurs in India where, in some villages, the residents are exposed to drinking water with a fluoride content of 7.2 to 10.7 ppm. It has been found that the fluoride is accumulated in bone and that this accumulated fluoride is associated with an adverse effect on red blood cells[1]."

Cancer

In an alarming report from the New Jersey Health Department, dated 11/8/92, it was shown that osteosarcoma was found in males under age 20 to be 50% higher in New Jersey municipalities serviced with artificially fluoridated drinking water, than their non-fluoridated counterparts[3].

"In the three most heavily fluoridated communities, an almost sevenfold increase in osteosarcoma was found in young males between 10 years and 19 years of age." John Lee, M.D., said, 'I can think of no other agent with this degree of risk which is mandated by the Public Health Service to be added to our food or water'[3]."

John Yiamouyiannis, Ph.D., says[7,] "In 1963, Drs. Herskowitz and Norton from St. Louis University showed that increasing levels of fluoride increased the incidence of melanotic tumors in fruit flies. In 1965, Drs. Taylor and Taylor from the University of Texas at Austin found that fluoride in the drinking water at levels of one-half to one part per million increased tumor growth rate in mice by 15-25%. In 1984, Drs. Tsutsue and co-workers from the Nippon Dental university were able to transform normal cells into cancer cells merely by exposure of the normal cells to fluoride.

"It is generally agreed that the ability of a substance to cause genetic damage is a warning of its possible cancer-causing effects. Fluoride has been shown to cause genetic damage by researchers from Texas A & M University, the University of Missouri, Columbia University, and the National Institute of Environmental health Sciences — as well as by researchers from the Central laboratory for Mutagenicity Testing (W. Germany), the Russian Research Institute for Industrial Health and Occupational Diseases, the Pomerian Medical Academy (Poland), the Kunming Institute of Zoology (People's Republic of China), the Nippon Dental University, Tokyo (Japan), and others. The University of Missouri study showed that as little as one part per million fluoride in the drinking water resulted in genetic damage.

"In 1977, epidemiological studies by Dr. Dean Burk, former head of the

Cytochemistry Section of the National Cancer Institute, and a second scientist (Yiamouyiannis)were the subject of full-scale Congressional Hearings. Our studies showed that fluoridation was linked to about 10,000 cancer deaths yearly. During the hearings, U.S. Public Health Service officials (the U.S. Public Health Service is the world's leading promoter of fluoridation) claimed that our results were due to changes in the age, race and sex composition of the populations examined. We were able to show that these officials had made mathematical errors and had left out 80-90% of the data. When these errors and omissions were corrected their very own method confirmed that 10,000 excess cancer deaths yearly were linked to water fluoridation. (In three out of four court cases tried since 1977, the courts ruled that the preponderance of the evidence indicates that fluoridation results in an increase in cancer death rate.)

"The Congressional Hearings also revealed that U.S. Public Health Service officials sent their erroneous and omissive data to scientists in Britain who were told by U.S. Public Health Service to publish it as if it were their own and to pretend that they had come up with the same results independently.

"As a result of these hearings, Congress mandated that U.S. Public Health Service conduct animal studies to determine if they could find whether or not fluoride caused cancer under laboratory conditions. These tests were designed to determine whether or not water fluoridation results in an increase in human cancer risk. They were conducted by the National Toxicology Program (NTP) under the auspices of the U.S. Public Health Service. Special attention was given to oral, liver, and bone cancers[15]. Scheduled for completion by 1980, it was not until 1990 that the results were reluctantly released.

"Analysis of the results in rats shows that (a) precancerous changes occurred in oral squamous cells as a result of increasing levels of fluoride in the drinking water. (Late last year, I obtained through the Freedom of Information Act, 'carcinogenicity studies with sodium fluoride performed by Proctor and Gamble' which had been submitted to, but covered up by, the U.S. Public Health Service for 4 years. Dose-dependent increases were observed in every parameter tested, including squamous cell metaplasias. These results appeared in the February 22, 1990 issue of the *Medical Tribune*.) (b) there was an increase in the incidence of tumors and cancers in oral squamous cells as a result of increasing levels of fluoride in the drinking water, (c) a rare form of cancer (osteosarcoma) occurred only in animals with fluoride in the drinking water, and (d) there was an increase in the incidence of thyroid follicular cell tumors as a result of increasing levels of fluoride in the drinking water. Analysis of the results in mice shows that (e) a rare form of liver cancer (hepatocholangiocarcinoma) occurred only in animals with fluoride in the drinking water.

"In the National Toxicology Program (NTP) study, higher doses of fluoride were given to compensate for (1) the limited number of animals used, (2) the relatively short time of their exposure to fluoride, and (3) the fact that

'On a body weight basis, man is generally more vulnerable than the experimental animal, probably by a factor of 6-12' [16]. The doses of fluoride that were linked to cancer in this study were only 1/10th to 1/50th of the amount used to produce cancer by benzene.

"In-depth analysis of the National Toxicology Program (NTP) study shows that the cancer-causing potential of fluoride is not limited to one type of cancer. Furthermore, the types of cancer caused by fluoride in rats and mice may be entirely different than the types of cancer caused by that same substance in humans. Thus, if fluoride had caused cancer in the tails of all the rats and mice, this would be compelling evidence that fluoride was carcinogenic. However, you wouldn't do a follow-up study in humans to see if fluoride caused cancer in human tails. The main point is that fluoride is a carcinogen and that the Burk-Yiamouyiannis study showing a link between fluoridation and cancer has been confirmed."

". . . Dr. William Marcus, chief toxicologist for the Environmental Protection Agency's (EPA) drinking water program and Robert Carton, Ph.D., an environmental scientist in the EPA's Office of Toxic Substances, and local president of the National Federation of Employees, . . . publicly accused the Public Health Service (PHS) of underplaying the dangers of fluoride[11]."

Dr. Carton said that EPA's 1985 review was "a shoddy job, bordering on scientific fraud. You could call it a coverup[27]."

When Dr. Marcus charged that "In almost all instances, the Battelle board certified pathologists's findings [on the carcinogenicity of fluoride] were down-graded[1]" by NTP, so that the use of fluoridation would be politically upheld, he was commanded by his EPA superiors not to speak out. He was in danger of being fired for telling scientific truth, but fortunately Dr. Marcus was not . . . alone in his forthcoming court suit against the EPA, as The National Federation of Federal Employees was said to be entering a suit against EPA[1].

The Battelle report that NTP, and the EPA attempted to distort, or downgrade, for political reasons, according to Dr. Lee, ". . . indicated that the animals were awash with illness and abnormalities of all kinds including kidney disease, liver disease, blood diseases, tumors, and cancer. In particular, the fluoridated groups showed thyroid adenomas, dysplasias of the oral and nasal mucosa, liver cancer of a very special rare type (hepatocholangiocarcinoma), and the osteosarcomas of which one appeared in a mid-range male rat and four appeared in high-range male rats. Female rats exhibited dose-related osteosclerosis and all fluoridated rodents developed dental fluorosis. It is important to know that the bone fluoride level of the 'high range' rats was no higher than that which occurs in human bones after 15-20 years in fluoridated communities. Since fluoride is cumulative in bone, the so-called 'high range' rats had achieved in 2 years only what human bones achieve in 15-20 years. [That] is, the tissue level of fluoride was *no different* than what humans will experience[1]."

John R. Lee, M.D., an internationally recognized authority on fluoridation stated "that the strength of the fluoride-cancer link study by NTP is greater than that which resulted in the banning of Alar, Red Dye #3, or Cyclamate[26]."

Neurotoxicity: Effects on the Brain

According to Dr. John Yiamouyiannis, there is an ongoing profound increase in Alzheimer's disease, migraine, and other neuropsychiatric disorders. The ingress of fluoride into the brain can be influenced by altered permeability of the blood-brain barrier; the inihibition of acetylcholinesterase activity by fluoride has been reported to be 61% by as little as 1 ppm; and the adverse effects of long-term fluoride exposure include headaches, ringing in the ears, depression, confusion, drowsiness, visual disturbances, severe fatigue, and loss of memory[23].

Court Suits

Besides the threat of two possible suits against the EPA, there was a class action suit by 35-40 dentists against the American Dental Association (ADA), its committees and affiliated organizations in the Superior Court of the District of Columbia for the ADA's "acting contrary to the ethical precepts in a number of areas, [including] the promotion of fluoridation, the pressuring of the EDP to raise the Maximum Containment Level (MCL) [from 1 ppm to 4 ppm], and failure to distribute to its members and to the general public, literature regarding the significant possibility of adverse effects of fluoridation[9] and the use of dental amalgam [which is another unhealthy practice.][1]."

"Dr. David Kennedy, one of these dentists, says: 'I think it is criminal to expose large groups of the population to toxic substances without any evidence of safety. The proponents of toxic dentistry claim that you can't prove the agent caused a specific problem. . . . It is not our responsibility to prove that a poison is not a poison. It is the responsiblity of the person who applies the poison to prove that it is harmless. . . .[11]"

In Canada, a suit was filed by a mother and her 7 year-old child, against the Calgary Board of Health and others for dental fluorosis associated with the use of fluoride drops and tablets[1].

Dominic Smith died of over-dose of fluoride caused by a broken water pump that allowed the water level to decrease while the fluoride injector continued to add fluoride to the water supply. Thirty other villagers also became sick with symptoms similar to Smith's. People suffered nausea, vomiting, diarrhea and fatigue and some also had neurological symptoms such as tingling hands and arms. As these symptoms appeared, people drank more of the water to satisfy an increasing thirst.

Dominic's sister, too, nearly died.

"Officials of Middletown, MD warned residents by radio in November, 1993 not to drink or cook with city water due to high fluoride levels. Malfunctioning fluoridation equipment caused excessive levels of 70 parts per million (ppm) in the distribution system. This is 70 times the normal level and almost 18 times the level considered safe by EPA.

"Based on other fluoridation accidents, the 70 ppm of fluoride is sufficient to cause vomiting, diarrhea, skin rashes, fever, and other effects. In 1986, a fluoridation accident in New Haven (North Branford), Connecticut, resulted in the public receiving water with 51 ppm fluroide for twelve hours. A health survey, conducted four days later on 312 persons, determined that 55 of those experienced symptoms of fluroide poisoning which lasted from 1-60 hours[44]."

Robert Carnton, Ph.D., scientist and editor of the newsletter *The Fluoride Report*, pointed out that toxic spills of fluoride in drinking water are never publicized by flurodiation promotion agencies, the Public Health Service, the National Institute for Dental Research and the Center for Disease Control[44]."

A partial list of such accidents includes:

• Poplarville, MS, August 1993: 40 poisoned; 15 sought treatment at hospital[44].

• Galesburg, IL, August 1993: Delivery tank leaked 15-20 gallons on city street[44].

• Chicago, IL, July 1993: 3 dialysis patients died; 5 additional patients allergic (toxic) reaction[44].

• Kodiak, AK, May 1993: Residents were warned by phone and public radio of high fluoride levels, and danger becomes higher with boiling of water, concentrating fluoride further[44].

• Sarnia, Ontario, January 1993; Fluoride at 13 ppm. Fail-safe system had failed to shut down[44].

• Marin County, California; Pump malfunction allowed too much fluoride in the Bon Tempe treatment plant, so bad water diverted to Phoenix Lake, elevating lake surface by more than two inches, forcing some water over the spillway[44].

• Danvers, IL, June 1992; Pump malfunctioned; flushed water through fire hydrants onto city streets[44].

• Hoopper Bay, AK; May 1992; 1 death, 260 poisoned, 1 airlifted to hospital in critical condition. First diagnoses speculated that residents had the "flu." Widow of deceased sued for $3 million[44].

• Rice Lake, WI, February 1982; Residents vomiting; Centers for Disease Control stated that 150 water consumers potentially at risk. Pump overfed fluoride for two days, thought to have reached 20 ppm[44].

• Benton Harbor, MI, December 1991; Faulty pump allowed about 900 gallons of hydrofluosilicic acid to leak into a chemical storage building at the water plant. So corrosive that it ate through more than two inches of concrete[44].

• Calgary, Alberta, Canada, September 1991: Leak of seven liters of fluoride sent two water treatment personnel to hospital for oxygen after breathing fluoride fumes[44].

• Burlington, NC, September 1991; 4,000 gallons of a 6,000 gallon fiberglass fluoride tank ruptured[44].

• Portage, MI, July 1991; About 40 children with abdominal pains, sickness, vomiting and diarrhea at an arts and crafts show at school. One of the city's pumps had failed. Fluoride levels reached 92 ppm[44].

• St. Louis, MO, November 1990; 500 gallons of hydrofluosilic acid leaked from ruptured pipe[44].

• Westby, WI, October 1990; 4 families suffered a week of diarrhea, upset stomach and burning throats. Malfunctioning equipment caused fluoride to surge to 150 ppm. Fluoride eroded copper pipes in area homes[44].

• Schenectady, NY, January 1988; 2,000 gallon spill completely destroyed fluoridation facility[44].

• New Haven (North Branford), CT, March 1986; Of the 312 persons interviewed 18% had symptoms of abdominal cramping, nausea, headache, diarrhea, vomiting, diaphoresis (profuse sweating), and fever. There were rashes and irritation from bathing and washing dishes. Fluoride peaked at 51 ppm. It leached copper pipes[44].

• Annapolis, MD, November 1979; 1 death in a dialysis patient, other dialysis patients suffered a cardiac arrest (resuscitated), nausea, hypotension, chest pain, diarrhea, itching, flushing, vomiting (blood tinged), difficulty breathing, profuse sweating, weakness, numbness and stomach cramping. Those not on dialysis reported nausea, headache, cramps, diarrhea and dizziness[44].

Wife of the dialysis patient who died sued and settled out of court. Pepsi Cola sued for $1.6 million for damage to product. Waterworks personnel also sued, then demoted and had payroll deductions[44].

Even though state and county health officials learned of the spill nine days after it occurred, no public announcement was made and the City Council was not told of the situation for six more days[44].

So, in addition to increasing perception of liability for adding fluoride to municipal water systems based on acceptance of faulty scientific analysis, and authoritarian pronouncements from those who have never studied the literature and are not themselves scientists, there is also a constant threat of litigation from catastrophic incidents. However, the persistent threat to each person consuming a steady diet of fluoride in their public drinking water looms the larger.

Silicon implants were said to be safe, until, many years later, thousands of women were sickened or disfigured by the effects of leaking silicon. This resulted in multi-billion dollar litigation that has been consistently won in the plaintiff's favor, and even threatens to bankrupt insurance companies.

"In the 1920's, senior public health officials and the American Public Health Association *endorsed lead gasoline as a 'Gift of God and perfectly safe'*[31]. As everyone now knows lead in gasoline was a dangerous and persistent poison.

It is not too difficult to envision a like situation with fluoride where, because of the unknowledgeable and religious conviction of public health department employees, fluoride public water supplementation has become nation-wide spread. Court suits usually begin here and there, scattered, and as objective judges study all the evidence, they rule in favor of plaintiffs. Then the filing of suits widen, until at last the public is faced with truth — and also multi-billion dollar damages that must come from each citizen's pocketbook.

According to William Campbell Douglass, M.D.[29], "A study from Britain reported that the difference between a safe dose of fluoride and a harmful dose is 'impressively small'. Danish scientists concurred in a report in which they said: 'There is no magic borderland' between a safe and a toxic dose.

"The most shocking report comes from a former chief dental officer in Auckland, Australia: 'When you are indoctrinated with a particular belief for a lifetime, it is hard to break out. But I examined the figures in my own city of Auckland and found that decay was less in the non-fluoridated than the fluoridated parts.

"'The figures that had been given to the public had been shockingly doctored. . . . . I pointed out these discrepencies to a conference of senior dental officers of the New Zealand Department of Health. There was simply a stony silence[29]."

What Cost Savings?

One argument in favor of fluoridating the public water supply, is that parents will have less cost in repairing their children's cavities. This has already been debunked in proper scientific studies at every level. However, let's look at potential cost savings.

According to Ralph S. Blois[20], The National Preventive Dentistry Demonstration Program (sponsored by the American Fund for Dental Health, a pro-fluoride group) conducted a study of 30,000 school-age children. The study ran from 1977 through 1987, and was the largest ever conducted. Some of the children were on sealants, some on fluoride water, some on toothpastes, and so on, and some received the whole range of "protection."

Cost of 'medication' was $55 per child per year with a resulting saving of only two tooth surfaces over a four year span. Equivalent children, who were non-fluoride children, had one fewer tooth surface decay over the four year span at a cost of $1 per child per year. "To cut through the garbage, what it says is that in four years the test showed that children having fluoride had saved only 2 tooth surfaces (at a cost of $55X4 = $220) while non-fluoridated children saved only one tooth surface (cost $4). For Pete's sake — fluoride claims to produce one less decay in four years than non-fluoride. **That is not at all statistically signficant.** Yet nobody seems to have picked up on this.

"Of those children who had fluoride mouth wash — the study laments the poor performance of mouth washes. Here over 4 years, the amount of tooth surfaces saved was less than one. The report states, 'On the basis of our results, we can't make any strong argument that fluoride mouth rinse programs are effective enough to be recommended and in fluoridated communities they are not merited at all'[20]."

We were promised, with the addition of fluoride to public water systems, that tooth decay would decrease by 60 percent. Later studies revised this figure to somewhere between 20 and 40 percent. New evidence from New Zealand and Canada suggest that **with the use of fluoride, tooth decay is higher**[11].

Argumentation in favor of fluoridating municipal water supplies usually starts out with "'How could anyone be against water fluoridation? It is the most cost-effective public health measure in history. It costs 50 cents per year to protect a child from what is, perhaps, the most common disease in the world, and the benefits last a lifetime.'

"This quotation was taken from an editorial 'Let's Get With It,' written by Richard J. Mielke, D.M.D. in the Washington state Dental Association *News* of April 1993 to praise its members' support of a Bill [which lost] to empower Public Utility Districts to fluoridate, an effort that failed a second time in April 1993. This statement is similar to that found in *Fluoridation Facts*, the official pamphlet of the American Dental Association (ADA). It is based on the amount paid per year on behalf of each person in the population served by a water district to purchase fluoride chemicals. This is an average of 35-40 cents in the ADA document[36]."

Assuming that fluoride addition to municipal water supplies is both safe and effective — which scientific evidence says it is not — then exactly what are the savings?

Richard G. Foulkes, B.A., M.D. has detailed the presumed savings by comparing the cost of supplying fluoride tablets for children as opposed to the tax load placed on communities to fluoridate the water in Tables 1 and 2 on the cover of this article. According to these calculations, on average, *"for every $1,000 spent by the taxpayer for fluoride chemicals, less than 50 cents goes toward purchase of fluoride for children.* Apparently, according to Tables 1 and 2, the ten-year lifetime cost to supply an individual child with fluoride tablets, for the purpose of preventing teeth caries, is somewhere between $12 and $18. The remainder [of fluoride] expenditures is used to purchase a pollutant such as industrial grade sodium floride or hydrofluosilicic acid to flush through the community water system into the environment[36]."

To place Foulkes' analysis in further perspective, In Tacoma, WA, **$125,000 for chemicals provides $10 for dubious protection of all its children for one year.**

Considering the true cost of fluoridation, one wonders if children's caries are the primary reason for political hue and cry in favor of fluoridating city municipalities, or is it a means of disposing of industrial waste at taxpayer's expense, and also a way around the enforcement of pollution laws? David B. Hill, P.Eng., Professor of Computer Science at the University of Calgary, said, "The current estimated annual running costs of water fluoridation in Calgary are $230,000 a year just for the chemicals, and 99.9% of this will not be drunk, but will be flushed straight down the city sewers. The effect will be to deposit roughly 150 tons of fluoride into the Bow River and environment each year. The Reynolds Aluminum Company of Canada Ltd. in Baie-Comeau, Quebec, is only legally allowed to discharge 36.5 tons of fluoride into the St. Lawrence River each year . . . under pollution control regulations[36]."

Summary

Assuming that fluoride added to public water systems was both safe and effective, it obviously is far, far from a cost effective way of preventing caries.

Assuming that 1 ppm of fluoride added to public water systems was safe and that it did reduce caries, **"Fluoridating the water supply makes a fundamentally simplistic assumption: that all the people drinking it, no matter what their size, age or state of health, require the same fluoride level[11]."**

No respectable scientist, biologist, or medical doctor would agree with this premise.

"Fluoride also accumulates in the body from a great number of natural sources[11]"

Respectable scientists recognize that other sources of fluoride are tea, industrial air emissions, foodstuffs grown, manufactured or cooked in fluoridated areas, and even teflon cooking utensils.

An over-accumulation (even assuming the alleged safety of 1 ppm) is clearly damaging to health.

"Dentists routinely recommend fluoride tablets for children, never testing to see whether fluoride levels are actually low and without being trained to recognize existing fluoride damage[11]."

According to a Danish study of 56 children regularly taking fluoride tablets, "almost half showed dental fluorosis to some degree[21]." These tablets can also kill, according to reports on the case of a 3-year-old boy who collapsed and died after consuming the equivalent of 16 mg/kg body weight of fluoride tablets[22].

In 1991 tests conducted by Dr. Peter Mansfiled discovered that 1 in 4 people were in danger of overconsuming fluoride[11].

"The great problem with overconsumption of fluoride is that only around half of that ingested is excreted by the body in healthy adults.

"Children, diabetics or those with kidney problems may retain up to two-thirds of the fluoride they take in[11]."

According to Gibson's research, "It is, . . . , more likely that fluoride affects cellular metabolism at all concentrations, but that in some [human] systems this effect is not detectable until doses in excess of 10 micrograms per millilitre are reached, . . . The present series of experiments clearly demonstrate effects of fluoride as low as 0.5 micrograms per millilitre[11]."

According to Richard G. Foulkes, B.A., M.A., "There may have been some grounds in 1973 for accepting the hypothesis that fluoridated water is associated with reduction in dental caries and that water artificially fluoridated to the 'optimal' level was safe.

"Public Health officials at all levels pushed actively for fluoridation. The Dental and Medical associations had moved from opposition to a position of support. The literature supporting the opposite view was difficult to obtain.

But, . . . , there was evidence sufficient to suggest caution.

"The situation appears different in 1992 and on. The fluoridation of water supplies as a viable concept is at the point of collapse. The effectiveness of fluoride, especially as an additive to community water supplies, to reduce dental caries is dubious. The idea that this well-known industrial toxin is safe at 1 ppm in the drinking water has been struck a blow; perhaps a mortal one.

"[Pennsylvania] Justice Flaherty . . . continued in his letter [to New Zealand]: 'Prior to my hearing this case, I gave the matter of fluoridation little, if any, thought. But, I received quite an education and **noted that the proponents of fluoridation do nothing more than impune the objectivity of those who oppose fluoridation**. I seriously believe that few responsible people have objectively reviewed the evidence'.

"Canada, the USA, and the few countries left that have not discontinued the fluoridation of community water supplies should join those countries who have discontinued the process or who never did fluoridate. A list of such countries includes West Germany, the Netherlands, Belgium, Finland, Sweden, Norway, Denmark, Japan[1]," and France[45].

Dr. Geoffrey Smith asks, "If artificial fluroidation is so effective, then why have scientifically advanced countries [such as the above] totally rejected the measure? There is absolutely no credible evidence that children's teeth in those countries are any worse than those in Australia, Canada, Ireland, new Zealand and the United States[45]."

True Causes of Declining Dental Caries

"If one were to argue that swallowing fluoridated water leads eventually to higher fluoride levels in dental enamel, one would then have to explain away the fact that dental enamel fluoride concentration in children from fluoridated communities in the U.S. is no different than the fluoride concentration in teeth of children from non-fluoridated communities."

More than likely, the true causes for decrease in dental caries are the following factors, given by Dr. Lee.

• Better nutrition

• Less sugar intake (e.g., use of artificial sweetners in kids' diets).

• Better dental hygiene (tooth brushing)

• Rising immunity to *Strepoccocus mutans*, the plaque germ responsible for the conversion of simple dietary starches into acids that dissolve enamel

• General use of antibiotics bacteriostatic or bacteriocidal to *Strepoccocus mutans*.

• Use of fluoridated toothpaste. This latter factor does not vindicate water fluoridation. The concentration in toothpaste (which is applied directly to dental enamel) is 1000-1500 ppm whereas drinking water (which passes the teeth into the gut and then excreted in urine) contains only 1 ppm fluoride. The higher concentration in toothpaste is sufficient to kill or seriously impair the enzyme processes of *Strepoccocus mutans* plaque germs, whereas the low concentration in drinking water is simply ineffective[42].

More than likely safer substitues are available for the same teeth brushing purpose, that will serve to kill *Strepoccocus mutans*.

Gerard P. Judd, Ph.D.[46] summarizes the actual and indicated dangers from forceful feeding of fluoride as follows:

• Slightly poorer teeth (more Decay, Missing Teeth, Fillings), with egg-shell white fluorosis and brittleness[46]. According to Professor Cornelius Steelink, Department of Chemistry at the University of Arizona, who headed up a subcommitte for study of addition of fluoride to the Tucson, AZ water supply, their study showed that ". . . the more fluoride a child drank, the more cavities appeared in the teeth[47]."

• More brittle bones in the aged[46];

• Destruction of at least 60 out of 63 enzymes, including cytochrome C, cholinesterase and others handling oxygen[46];

• Genetic change, both in the sperm and other cells[46];

• Dramatic heart death increase in Antiogo, Wisconsin, where a long-term study was made[46];

• Down's Syndrome increase of 250%[46];

• Probable major cause of Sudden Infant Death Sydrome (SIDS) and Chronic Fatigue Syndrome (CFS), since allergic (toxic) symptoms the same[46];

• Infant mortality increase: for Washington, D.C. Blacks 4 times, for Whites 3 times (48 years of fluoridation) and for the average U.S. population 1.4 times[46];

• Infant birth defects increased 3 times in Chile during its experiment with fluoridation[46];

• 39% increase in cancers overall, with 80% for rectal cancer in the U.S. after 33 years[46];

• Fluoride accumulates about 50% daily in the bones and soft tissue[46];

• Miscarriages and spontaneous abortions increase[46];

• 50 side effects: arthritis, immobility, blindness, bladder and urinary tract effect, blood loss in kidneys, uterus, and vagina, bone pain, bruises, cancer increases, Chizzola macula, collapsing legs, diarrhea, dizziness, dry mouth; 8 allergies proven by double blind tests by Moolenburgh using 12 physicians and 60 patients, Down's Syndrome increase with 70% cataracts, epileptic seizures, fatigue, weakness, loss in strength, fluorosis, genetic chromosome change, severe headaches, large heart death increase, hemorrhages in the skin, incoherence, inner ear disorder, intestinal cramps, distention and constipation, itching, mental depression, mental concentration inability, nasal disease, nausea, nystagmus (involunatry movement of eyes), pain in muscles, intestines, bowels, head, spine, and stomach, polyuria, scotoma, seziures, spastic bowels, stomach bloat, cramps and gas, stomatitis (lip cracks), tendon-ligament calcification, thyroid calcification, tinnitus, ulcers in the mouth, skin eruption around the mouth, vision blurring, vomiting and weight loss[46].

• Possibly Alzheimers, Multiple Sclerosis (MS) and other viral disease are made worse due to antibody destruction[46].

How to Avoid Fluorosis

Know Truth

According to Foulkes, "Many of us know that senior scientists working for the U.S. Environmental Protection Agency have been trying for more than a decade to persuade their superiors to lower the Maximum Contaminant Level (MCL) for fluoride to levels that would prevent dental fluorosis (0.1-0.2 ppm) only to be overruled by successive Surgeons General and [to wrongly] have the level increased to 4 ppm 'to prevent cirppling skeletal fluorosis'[31]."

Robert J. Carton, Ph.D. was an environmental scientist with the U.S. Army, and from September 1972 until May 1992, he spent 15 years in the Office of Toxic Substances with the EPA, managing risk assessments. For two years he was responsible for writing regulations under the Federal Water Pollution Control Act. He was also program manager for compliance of new pollution sources with the National Environmental Policy Act[34].

According to Robert J. Carton, Ph.D., who testified under sworn testimony to the court in Manitowoc, Wisconsin during litigation on the city's fluoridation of water, the EPA officials conducted scientific fraud when they raised the standards from 1 Recommended Maximum Contaminant Level (RMCL) for fluoridated drinking water, to 4 RMCL. Carton[35] testified that:

• The fluoride in drinking water standard, . . . , published by the EPA in the *Federal Register* on Nov. 14, 1985, is a classic case of political interference with science.

• The regulation is a fraudulent statement by the Federal government that 4 mg/l of fluoride in drinking water is safe with an adequate margin.

• There is evidence that critical information in the scientific and technical support documents used to develop the standard were falsified by the Department of Health and Human Services and the EPA to protect a long-standing public health policy.

• EPA professionals were never asked to conduct a thorough, independent analysis of the [scientific] fluoride literature. Instead, their credentials were used to give the appearance of scientific credibility. They were used to support the predetermined conclusion that 4 mg/l of fluoride in drinking water was safe.

• The EPA management ignored the requirements of the law to protect sensitive individuals such as children, diabetics or people with kidney impairment. Contrary to law, they made the criteria for considering health data so stringent that reasonable concerns for safety were eliminated. Data showing positive correlation between fluoride exposure and genetic effects in almost all laboratory tests were discounted.

• EPA management based its standard on only one health effect: crippling skeletal fluorosis. They ignored data showing that healthy individuals were at risk of developing crippling skeletal fluorosis if these individuals happened to drink large quantities of water at the presumed "safe" level of 4 mg/l. EPA's own data showed that some people drink as much as 5.5 liters per day. If these people ingested this amount of water containing 4 mg/l of fluoride, they would receive a daily dose of 22 mg. This exceeds the minimum dose necessary to cause crippling skeletal fluorosis, or "20 mg/day for 20 years" as stated by the EPA and Public Health Service.

• Most unsettling is the fact that the EPA and the National Academy of Sciences cannot document the scientific basis for the 20 mg/day threshold established by the EPA. In a recent series of letters between the National Academy of Sciences, Ms. Darlene Sherrel, and Sen. Graham of Florida, the National Academy of Sciences was forced to admit that it could *not* document the deriviation of the chronic effect level for crippling skeletal fluorosis, which the single health effect upon which the fluoride in drinking water standard is based. The threshold is probably lower.

• There is evidence, ignored by the EPA, in a study by Dr. Geoffrey Smith, that exposure to fluoride at 1 mg/l in drinking water over a long period of time may calcify ligaments and tendons, causing arthritic pains, and may be responsible for the alarming increase in cases of repetitive stress injury.

• EPA management relied upon a report from the Surgeon General which they knew was false. This report claimed to represent conclusions of an expert panel (on which the EPA was present as an observer) when, in fact, the concerns of this panel for the effects of fluoride on the bones of children, for its effects on the heart, for dental fluorosis, and for the overall lack of scientific data on the effects of fluoride in U.S. drinking water *were deleted*. These changes were made in the final report without the knowledge or approval of the expert panel.

• The EPA accepted the falsified report from the Surgeon General's office and asked a contractor to turn this into an "assessment." The contractor dutifully collected only literature that supported the report. The report was submitted for public comment, but was never altered to incorporate the volumes of information sent in by world class experts. Any opinions contrary to the report were dismissed. The result is actually a "Draft" stamped "Final."

• The apparent cover-up of fluoride risks within EPA prompted the EPA professionals' union, Local 2050 of the National Federation of Federal Employees, to attempt to file an amicus brief in support of the Natural Resources Defense Council, who sued EPA in 1986 over the fluoride standard.

• EPA has also attempted to silence scientists who do not follow the party line. In 1992, EPA fired William L. Marcus, Ph.D. from his job as senior toxicologist in the Office of Drinking Water, EPA. Judge David A. Clarke, Jr., declared in his decision on this case on December 3, 1992, that "the reasons given for Dr. Marcus' firing were a pretext . . . his employment was terminated because he publicly questioned and opposed EPA's fluoride policy." Judge Clark ordered Dr. Marcus to be reinstated and provided with back pay, fringe benefits and interest, attorneys fees, and paid $50,000 in compensatory damages. It was said that every time Dr. Marcus testified it cost the polluting companies a couple of million dollars. It was reported to have cost Dow $8 million when he testified against this chemical giant[43].

• Despite knowledge by the EPA that dental fluorosis is considered a visible sign that potentially destructive effects of fluoride are also occurring in bone, and even though aware that the report of the Surgeon General's expert panel had been altered, nevertheless they followed the altered version and declared in 1985 that dental fluorosis was not an adverse health effect.

• Transcripts obtained of the closed-door testimony by the expert panel, obtained under the Freedom of Information Act, showed that the panel had in fact voted to declare dental fluorosis an adverse health effect. Their declaration was doctored by unknown individuals to achieve a political end.

There's an obvious political problem that must be solved, which is to get the Environmental Protection Agency, and other public agencies, to do the job for which our taxes pay. Even more basic, is that one can join the growing throng of those who are now aware that **scientific studies, worldwide, demonstrate that fluoridation is damaging to health.**

One example of the persistence of advocates of fluoridation was demonstrated in Eugene, Oregon[34]:

• In 1956, the folks of Eugene were asked to approve water fluoridation. The civic leaders felt it was important and all the pressure and persistence we've come to know from the fluoridation lobby was brought to bear. The folks of Eugene said "no."

• The issue was placed on the ballot again in 1958. Despite the protagonism by the civic leaders the folks voted "no" a second time.

• The next time, in a 1964 election, the proponents of the poison won and the city of Eugene fluoridated its water.

• By September 28, 1965 another election was forced by those who objected to dripping the toxic chemical into the water supply and they voted fluoride out, once and for all — or so they thought.

• A year later the power of the fluoride lobby had the issue back on the ballot a fifth time. In a heated and close race, the fluoridation advocates won and the city water again felt the drip, drip, drip of fluoride compounds.

• The people of Eugene rose up even more determined and petitions circulated for another referendum on the issue. On June 28, 1977 fluoridation was repealed by a vote of 9,804 to 5,580.

• Despite the almost two to one defeat, the city council declared they would be back with another ballot on the matter during the 1978 general election. However, the people had spoken and today the city of Eugene is fluoride free.

• City water treatment superintendent Mitch Postle told *Search for Health* that he removed the fluoridation equipment in 1978 and he's "glad."

• Although the question of poisoning Eugene's water supply has come up repeatedly, it is still not accepted by Eugene's voting population.

• What seems to have been constantly overlooked by those advocating the poisoning of the water supply is that if folks want fluoride for their kid's teeth, they can always buy floride pills.

"On March 17, 1991, in Washington, D.C., . . . the Parent Teacher's Association (PTA) took a major step away from its long-held (1952) position in support of fluoridation of the water supplies. . . . . PTA will seek to have its membership educated about the risks and benefits of aggregate fluoride exposure, and the appropriate use and ingestion of products containing fluoride."

A proposed bill that would have allowed public utilities in Washington state to fluoridate water was defeated in the Senate Energy and Utilities Committee in February 1992, by a coalition of those interested in safe and clean water[24].

In support of removing fluoridation from municipal systems, H.J. Roberts, M.D., says, ". . . elected officials who lack an adequate scientific and medical background must exercise *extreme* prudence and caution when voting on public water fluoridation, or continuing to do so.

"This issue transcends the important matter of freedom of choice. It involves exposing citizens to a toxic substance under the challenged guise of preventing dental caries. The problem is compounded by the absence of truly informed consent, and the [already] excessive fluoride intake by many persons in non-fluoridated areas.

"Elected individuals and their commissions also ought to anticipate criminal charges for 'practicing [medicine] without a license' if suit were to be brought by constituents for the fluoride-associated or — aggravated medical disorders. . . .[23]"

The late Dr. George Waldbott[11] listed the following symptoms, stating that their severity and duration will depend on an individual's age, nutritional status, environment, kidney function and susceptibility to allergies, and he also suggested various immediate fixes.

Symptoms
• Chronic fatigue not relieved by extra sleep or rest
• Headaches
• Dryness of throat and excessive water consumption
• Frequent need to urinate
• Aches and stiffness in muscles/bones
• Muscular weakness and spasms
• Gastrointestinal disturbances, including diarrhoea and constipation
• Pinkish-red or bluish-red spots on the skin, which fade after around a week
• Skin rash or itching after bathing
• Dizziness
• Visual disturbances

"The first sign of general systemic poisoning by fluoride is usually a mottled tooth, which turns gray and develops brown or black spots. The blemish is permanent and grows worse as exposure continues. After a time the molars begin to decay, then the gums and the mouth evniroment are affected. After mottling comes a bewildering variety of bodily aberrations, seldom diagnosed correctily because most physicians know almost nothing about chronic fluoride poisoning and thereefore they don't look for it[28]."

Suggestions

• If you are displaying what you believe are symptoms, have your fluoride levels tested.

• If you live in a fluoridated area, your only option is to use solely bottled water; or fit a reverse-osmosis water purifier in your home. You may also purchase a service which will deliver bottled mineral water and supply a dispenser.

• Reduce your intake of tea and soft drinks. Drink herbal tea made with non-fluoridated water instead. [Tea contains considerable fluoride, and soft drinks may have been made with city water that is fluoridated.]

• Switch to a non-fluoridated toothpaste. Never let children use "adult" fluoride toothpaste.

• Check your nutritional status. A poor diet will only increase your susceptibility to symptoms of fluoride poisoning. Adequate levels of magnesium, zinc and iron will help your body counter the effects of fluoride.

• Watch your consumption of prepared foods, particularly frozen vegetables.

• Never use fluoridated water for baby formula (another good argument for breastfeeding.)

2007 Developments

According to the November 2007 *Townsend Letter* (page 23), 500 Physicians, Dentists, Scientists and Environmentalists urged the U.S. Congress to stop water fluoridation until Congressional hearings are conducted. "Signers include a Nobel Prize winner, three members of the prestigious 2006 National Research Council (NRC) panel that reported on fluoride's toxicology, two officers in the Union representing professionals at the Environmental Protection Agency (EPA) headquarters, the President of the International Society of Doctors for the Environment and hundreds of medical, dental, academic, scientific, and environmental professionals."

For more information covering recent discoveries visit http://www.fluorideaction.net or http://fluoride.mercola.com/

Are you angry yet?

You certainly should be!!

In an intrerview with Andrew W. Saul, very knowledgeable Robert J. Carton, Ph.D. said, the "EPA has more than enough evidence to shut down fluoridation right now.

"Fluoridation, presents unacceptable risks to public health, and the government cannot prove its claims of safety. It is clear that fluoride is mutagenic, and that it may well cause cancer. EPA has attempted to silence scientists who do not follow the party line."And with that, he is just warming up. "Fluoridation," he adds, "constitutes unlawful medical research. It is banned in most of Europe; European Union human rights legislation makes it illegal." (http://www.rvi.net/~fluoride/000247.htm)

References

1. Richard G. Foulkes, B.A., M.D., "Fluoridation of Community Water Supplies 1992 Update," *Townsend Letter for Doctors*, 911 Tyler St. , Port Townsend, WA, 98368-6541 June 1992, p. 450.

2. D. Ziegelbecker, *Fluoride* 14; 1981, p. 123-128.

3. Mark Disendorf, *Nature*, Vol. 322; July 1986, p. 10.

4. J. Colquhoun, *Fluoride*, No. 3, July 1990, p. 23.

5. *Journal PH Dent*, Vol. 49; No. 5; 1989; includes studies by Kumar and Newbrun in *Dent* Vol. 49; No. 4; 1989.

6. Allen Gray, *J. Canad Dent. Assn.*, No. 10; 1987.

7. R.J. Hunt, *Jour PH Dent*, Vol. 49; No. 3; 1989.

8. Robert O. Dustrude, R.Ph., *Health Freedom News*, 212 W. Foothill Blvd., Monrovia, CA 91016, January 1993, p. 36.

9. M. Bely, M.D., Arthrosis, *The Journal of the Academy of Rheumatoid Disease*, Vol. 1, No. 3, The Arthritis Trust of America/The Rheumatoid Disease Foundation, 7376 Walker Road, Fairview, TN 37062-8141, 1987, p. 41.

10. Christa Danielson, M.D., Joseph L. Lyon, M.D., Marlene Egger, Ph.D., Gerald K. Goodenough, M.D., Fluoridation Abstract, *JAMA*, 1992; 268: 746-748; from "Hip Fractures & Fluoridation in Utah's Elderly," *Townsend Letter for Doctors*, Op. Cit., April 1993, p. 374.

11. Fiona Bawdon, "Fluoride," *WDDTY Dental Handbook*, 1993, p. 15-18.

12. Jacobsen, *JAMA* 264; 500-502; 1990; Cooper, J. *Epidem ad Comm Health* 44; 17-19;1990 and *JAMA* Vol. 266; No. 4; July 24, 1991 (letter); Colquhoun, *New Zeal Med J* 14 Aug. 1991.

13. I.D. Brouwer, et. al. *Lancet*, Jan. 30, 1988.

14. D.S. Kumari, *Biochemistry International*, Vol. 23, No. 4, March 1991.

15. Experimental Pathology Laboratories, Inc., *Quality Assessment Narrative*: Rats, p. 13; Mice, p. 18.

16. Drinking Water and Health (National Academy of Sciences, Washington, D.C., 1977) p. 52-3.

17. John Yiamouyiannis, Ph.D., "Update on Fluoride and Cancer," *Townsend Letter for Doctors*, December 1990, p. 865.

18. *Journal of the American Dental Association*, Vol. 47, pp. 159-179, 1953.

19. *American Dental Association*, Vol. 50, pp. 272-277, 1955.

20. JFS, "Letters to the Editors," *Health Freedom News*, Op. Cit., April 1993, p. 43.

21. M.J. Larsen et. al. *Community Dent Oral Epidemiol*, 1989.

22. *National Fluoridation*, vol. XXXIX, No. 1.

23. H.J. Roberts, M.D.,"Re: Toxicology of Fluoride," *Townsend Letter for Doctors*, Op.Cit., July 1992, p. 623.

24. Betty Fowler, "Proposed Fluoridation Bill Defeated in Washington State," *Townsend Letter for Doctors*, Op., Cit., August/September 1992, p. 697.

25. "National PTA Reverses Its Endorsement of Fluoridated Water," *Townsend Letter for Doctors*, Op., Cit., February/March 1992, p. 147.

26. Betty Fowler, "Don't Applaud Fluoride Use for Cavities," *Townsend Letter for Doctors*, Op., Cit., May 1990, p. 286.

27. "Fluoride Linked to Bone Cancer in Fed Study," *Townsend Letter for Doctors*, Op., Cit., April 1990, p. 162; from the *Medical Tribune*.

28. "Safe Water Coalition of Washington State," *Townsend Letter for Doctors*, Op., Cit., June 1989, p. 291.

29. William Campbell Douglass, "Fluoridation Losing its Bite," *Second Opinion*, December 1992, p. 3.

30. "Fluoride Linked to Bone Cancer in New Government Study," *Health Freedom News*, Op. Cit., March 1993, p. 21; see *A Brief Report on the Association of Drinking Water Fluoridation and the Incidence of Osteosarcoma Among Young Males*, Perry D. Cohn, Ph.D., produced by the New Jersey Department of Environmental Protection and Energy and the New Jersey Department of Health, November 8, 1992.

31. Richard G. Foulkes, B.A., M.D., "'Open Letter' in Response to Dr. John Millar's Address to Kamloops City Council, December 15, 1992," *Townsend Letter for Doctors*, Op., Cit., May 1993, p. 459

32. Citizens for Alternative Health Care, "Hydrofluoric Acid," *Townsend Letter for Doctors*, Op., Cit., July 1993, p. 696.

33. Anne Anderson, R.P.N., Richard G. Foulkes, B.A., M.D., "Re: Fluoride Pollution," *Townsend Letter for Doctors*, Ibid, p. 734.

34. "Fluoridation Drama in Eugene, Oregon," *Health Freedom* News, Op.Cit., August 1993, p. 11.

35. Robert J. Carton, Ph.D., "Fluoridation: Scientific Fraud Alleged," *Health Freedom* News, Op.Cit., August 1993, p. 9.

36. Richard G. Foulkes, B.A., M.D., "The 'Cost' of Fluoridation," *Townsend Letter for Doctors*, Op., Cit., November 1993, p. 1086.

37. Levy, S.M., Muchow, G., "Provider Compliance with Recommended Dietary Supplement Protocol," *Am. Jour. P.H.*, Vol. 82, No. 2; Table 1, Feb. 1992.

38. Marquis, C., "New Fluoride Supplement Recommendations," *B.C. Med Jour*, Vol. 35, No. January 9, 1993.

39. Hill, D.R., Discussion paper presented to public forum sponsored by The Chemical Institute of Canada, Calgary, Sept. 29, 1992.

40. John R. Lee, M.D., "Fluoridation and Osteoporosis: The Facts," *Health Freedom News*, Op.Cit., January 1994, p. 26.

41. John R. Lee, M.D., "Fluoridation and Hip Fracture According to the National Research Council Report: Health Effects of Ingested Fluoride," *Townsend Letter for Doctors*, Op., Cit., May 1994, p.487.

42. John R. Lee, M.D., "Does Fluoridation Work?" *Health Freedom News*, Op.Cit., June 1994, p. 13.

43. "Whistle Blower Reinstated," National Council Improved Health flyer, received 1994, source unknown.

44. "Middletown, Maryland Latest City to Receive Toxic Spill of Fluoride in Their Drinking Water," *Townsend Letter for Doctors*, Op. Cit., October 1994, p. 1124.

45. Geoffrey E. Smith, LDS, RCS, "Fluoride: Dental Wonder or Medical Blunder?" *Explore!*, Numbers 5 & 6, 1994, p. 60.

46. Gerard P. Judd, Ph.D., "Evidence Against Fluoride Continues to Mount," *Health Freedom News*, November/December 1994, p. 29.

47. Cornelius Steelink, "Tooth Decay & Fluroide," *Townsend Letter for Doctors*, Op. Cit., October 1994, p. 1128.

The Good Guys Bacteria — Lactobacillus acidophilus & Bifido bacterium
by
Anthony di Fabio

Introduction

I've been told that there are ten times more bacteria in and on our bodies than the number of cells that make up our body. Some of these are good guys and some are not.

Sometimes we get overwhelmed by the bad guys, as we all know. Louis Pasteur was right about that. Germs can cause misery and sometimes death!

One of the major discoveries during modern times was that some germs can change both shape and function, depending upon the environment that surrounds them: more acide, more alkaline, more this or that and wham! we have apparently a different organism.

Microbiologists have known this fact for many years but apparently the facts have yet to filter down to medical schools and hence to graduate medical doctors.

What we eat and our state of emotions can, indeed, affect the surrounding environment of microorgansims!

This article is about two of the good guys, *Lactobacillus acidophilus* and *Bifido bacterium.*

The subject of intestinal microflora is of importance to everyone for two major reasons: (1) it is essential for good health to have a good colony of synergistically (working together and reinforcing one another) behaving microflora; and (2) it is essential for metabolization of some of the medicines we recommend when halting the progress of various Diseases

There are more bacteria in the world today than all the humans ever born. There are more bacteria than all the mammals that have ever been born. The head of one pin may contain one trillion or more of them! Bacteria, as will be seen, exist under the most varying, most extreme, most hostile conditions on our planet. They are pervasive!

Clearly bacteria are the dominant life form on planet Earth!

As man's lifeline evolved from simple, one-celled origins, and became an interacting group of single-celled bacteria, and thence onward where each cell specialized to help the whole survive, we carried along with us a special set of cells that helped to digest food, produce certain key vitamins, maintain balance of acidity/alkalinity, and a host of other good features many of which are not yet known.

The single cell — whether classified as plant or animal — is a wonderous and complex machine, not at all fully understood by the wisest men.

As with all life-forms, bacteria strive to survive, and they do this by reproducing themselves again and again and again. Where was one bacteria, there are now two, then four, then eight, then sixteen, thirty-two, sixty-four, one hundred and twenty-eight — and they double each period of time, so long as nourishment is available to permit growth, and so long as space is there to grow in, and so long as no predators gobble them up or kill them. At room temperature bacteria on our food stuff will double in number every ten minutes, I've heard.

An individual bacterium is unimportant to the species' survival, the group (species') is all-important.

Yet an individual bacterium differs in ways that are too subtle to notice until the environment becomes hostile to the species. Perhaps one bacterium out of a trillion has the fascinating ability to survive in conditions that are inimical to most. A penicillin environment, for example, may kill all but one in a trillion, but that last goes on to double and redouble, until finally the a new species has different characteristics, different abilities — and most of the surviving progeny can survive in the changed environment. The use of penicillin — usually a dangerous environment for bacteria — is an excellent example. Use it to get well, and most bacteria die. Sooner or later there is spread amongst us progeny of that single or small colony of bacteria that are naturally resistant to pencillin.

Some bacteria can live in the absence of oxygen, and some require oxygen. Some live on sulfurs and hydrogen at the deeps of the sea, near turmoiling and broiling volcanic vents. Certain bacteria grow well on oil, and others on otherwise deadly poisons. Some must float nicely in conjunction with other miniscule life-forms in the ever-changing and billowing white clouds.

Some bacteria produce deadly toxins, and others produce life-giving (to humans) vitamins.

You can't kill all of the microrganisms in your food, unless you boil your water at 126 degrees Centigrade (258.8 degrees Fahrenheit), under some pressure (autoclaving) for 96 hours. As water under standard pressure conditions boils at 100 degrees Centigrade (212 degrees Fahrenheit), such persistent determination to kill all microorganisms will also destroy your food.

Some can live to 190 degrees Centigrade (324 degrees Fahrenheit) below zero.

Despite Howard Hughes' billions and his alleged fanatic attempts to shield himself from bacteria, he was surrounded in a sea of them. Only his immunological system, such as it might have been, waged the actual warfare, not his reputed ineffectual "non-contact" procedures.

If world governments sling holocaust bombs at each other, bacteria will still be alive and well!

A bacterium, called Radiodurans, thrives inside operating nuclear reactors. These bacteria have the highest levels of Super Oxide Dismutase and Catalase and some other antioxidant enzymes than any others measured[2].

According to Gerald Domingue, M.D.[3], in a talk presented in part at the 75th Annual Meeting of American Society for Microbiology and subsequently published by *Microbia*, in his article "Naked Bacteria in Human Blood," many common and disease-producing bacteria, under the influence of many antibiotics, do not die, but rather are stripped of their walls so that they are no longer recognizable by our immune system. Our immune system uses the invader's cell walls to recognize a foreign invasion. If the cell wall is missing, our immune system assumes there is no invasion!

Some of these "Cell-Wall-Deficient Bacteria" can revert to and reduce themselves down to a filterable virus size — among the smallest known forms of virus.

Amazingly, it has been shown that these viral particles and the incomplete bacteria — Cell-Wall Deficient Bacteria — can and often do restructure themselves again. Since the bacteria has restructured itself to include a cell wall, it is once again recognized as an invader by our immune system. So now our systems react and it appears as though another full-fledged disease is at hand, "another infection" that must be treated with more antibiotics, which then strips off the walls to produce bacteria that go unrecognized again, and so on, ad infinitum. . . . . .!

Consequences of this unexploited and little known phenomena are possibly vast. Sadly, very little has been done in established medicine to test for and to design treatment strategies for this fantastic survival ability of bacteria. Lida Mattman, Ph.D., formerly of Wayne University,[4] trained numerous Ph.D. candidates in this new field of microbiology, but few of her graduates carry on with the work. She trained one laboratory to test for Cell Wall Deficient Bacteria, but the people with the training are long gone from that laboratory.

Quite clearly, microorganisms are the dominate species on planet earth!

According to Dr. Ken Rifkin[5], "The average human body contains approximately three and a half pounds of bacteria some of which perform essential functions AND others which promote disease." [This is about 11 trillion organisms: Ed.] "When the equilibrium of 'friendly' and pathogenic bacteria is disturbed through the ingestion of chemical additives (think medicines), birth control pills, antibiotics, alcohol, pesticides, food additives and even stress — disease producing bacteria will multiply within the intestinal tract."

In an article in *Health World,* Brad Everett[6] says that *Giardia lamblia* is the most widespread intestinal parasite in the United States. It is estimated to affect 7.4% of our population. It is a flagellate organism that moves through its liquid environment by moving its whip-like tail. *Giardia* can be spread through contaminated food and water, sexual and household contacts. It may even be contracted from household pets.

"*Entamoeba histolytica* is the second most common intestinal parasite in this country, affecting 3% of the population and causing amoebic dysentery. An amoeba is a single-celled or a cellular organism that moves by forming a 'pseuopod' or *fake foot*, with its protoplasm. It is a particular problem for travelers, homsexuals, and residents in mental institutions.

"Both of these organisms have similar life cycles. When ingested, protective cysts survive passage through the stomach. As the organisms are moved into the more dehydrated regions of the bowel, cyst formation is triggered by the decreasing amount of fluid. Cyst formation is essential for the survival of these organisms."

Both *Giardia lamblia* and *Entamoeba histolytica* are amoebae, not bacteria, and while they number in the hundreds — nay, thousands of millions — they are nowhere near as numerous as are bacteria. They do, however, help to make up the colony of "bad guys" intestinal microflora — along with bacteria, mycoplasmas, yeasts/fungi, and other assorted and odd living companions. (Mycoplasmas are the smallest free-living bacterial form, but have no cell-wall.)

Some intestinal organisms live within us as parasites, sapping our life-blood, or cellular life. Some live on dead matter that we shed daily or ingest and these are called saprophytes. Some are commensal with us — they "dine at the same table." Some take over our cellular machinery, using it for their own advantage.

You want to be completely free of bacteria and related micro-organisms?

Go to the moon before man's presence is there in any great numbers!

For man shall literally shed them wherever s/he goes, and they shall adapt and multiply!

Various pharmaceutical companies sell different strains of *Lactobaccilus acidophilus* or *Bifido bacterium* or other organisms in order to help replace our valuable microflora. While one strain may be better for producing certain vitamins or effects than another, the wise choice is to colonize with a variety of "good-guys". It's like diversifying your excess earnings into money market, blue-chip stocks, commodities, foreign money markets and real estate. If one goes bad (or weakens), the other markets may be stronger, and compensate for losses. Similarly, a variety of different strains of "good-guys" bacteria in colonies in the intestinal tract may have one or several of the strains placed under undue stress, but the others pick up the synergistic biological load, all to protect you — and their species!.

The following article came from such a source without identification and was passed on to me from our Chairman Emeritus John M. Baron, D.O. It is, in our opinion, an excellent article.

"The Role of Microorganisms in the Intestinal Tract

"<u>Introduction</u> Numerous factors influence the interactions among intestinal microorganisms as well as those between microorganisms and their hosts. The cumulative effects of these interactions control the composition and metabolic activity of the intestinal microflora. An optimum 'balance' in microbial population has been associated with good nutrition and health. There is increasing evidence indicating that certain microorganisms can help maintain such a favorable microbial profile[11].

32

The microorganisms most associated with this 'balance' are Lactobacilli and bifidobacteria.

"Intestinal Flora Competition among microorganisms in the large intestine is a major consideration since the highest numbers of bacteria occur here.

"Bifidobacteria are the predominant organisms in the large intestine of breast-fed infants, accounting for about 99% of the cultivatable flora. Lactobacilli, Enteterocci, and Coliforms comprise about 1% of the flora.

"Bifidobacteria are a major component in the large intestine of adolescents and adults, while Lactobacilli, Enterococci, and Coliforms are a smaller component of the flora[12]. Bifidobacteria are reduced significantly in the stools of old people, but Clostridia, Streptococci, and Coliforms are increased[12].

"Lactobacilli are the predominant organisms in the small intestine. Lactobacilli have important metabolic activities, although they may occur in smaller numbers than Bifido bacteria in the upper and lower intestines combined.

"The Role of Lactobaccilli in the Intestinal Tract

"A. Antibiotic Production

"Inhibits the pathogenic flora by production of the following antibiotics [The author recommends verification by contacting the references.]

Lactolin (*L. plantarum*)
Lactobrevin (*L. brevis*)
Bulgarican (*L. bulgaricus*)
Acidophilin (*L. acidophilus*)
Lactocidin (*L. acidophilus*)
Acidolin (*L. acidophilus*)
Lactolin (*L. acidophilus*)[2,12,13]

"The strains vary in their ability to produce these substances and cultural conditions will influence the amount produced[13].

"In vitro [lab conditions: Ed] inhibitory activity has been reported against the following intestinal pathogens:

Salmonellae
Shigellae
Staphylococci
Proteus
Kelbsiella
Pseudomonads
Enteropathogenic Escherichia coli
Bacilli
Clostridium perfringens
Vibrio

"B. Organic Acid Production

"Lactobacilli produce lactic acid. Organic acetic and lactic acids which are produced by lactic acid bacteria will inhibit the growth of many bacteria, especially pathogenic gram-negative types[7]. *Lactobacillus acidophilus* produces DL-lactic acid which is metabolized to a limited

33

extent[12].

"C. Lower pH and Oxidation Reduction

"Inhibition of pathogens by Lactobacilli is attributed to the lowering of the pH values by the liberation of acids, resulting in antimicrobial action (altering oxidation-reduction potential)[13].

"D. Competitive Antagonists

"Lactobacilli may outcompete other bacteria for nutrients and occupy the sites, making them unavailable to other microorganisms[13].

"In particular, Lactobacilli consume certain B-vitamins and biotin, decreasing their availability for other organisms[14].

"E. Bile Deconjugation

"The role of Lactobacilli in the deconjugating of bile acids was studied. The results indicated that Lactobacilli can liberate (deconjugate) free bile acids in the intestinal tract and can exert an influence on the balance of bacteria present[13]. [Deconjugation is the chemical process of separating the two amino acids taurine and glycine from bile acids, the bile then being recycled for reuse: Ed.]

"The Role of Bifidobacteria in the Intestinal Tract

"A. Antibiotic Production

"The antibacterial nature of *B. bifidium* against a number of pathogenic organisms like *E. coli*, *Salmonella sp.*, *Shigella sp.*, and *Bacillius sp.* suggests that *B. bifidium* might produce certain antibacterial substances[7].

"The oral administration of a freeze-dried culture of *B. bifidium* in conjunction with lactulose has been reported to eradicate enteropathogenic *E. coli* strains in infants and children[12].

"B. Organic Acid Production

"Bifidobacteria produces both acetic and lactic acids, but produces more acetic acid. Acetic acid has a stronger antagonistic effect against gram-negative bacteria than lactic acid[12]. Bifidobacteria ferment carbohydrates to L(+)-lactic acid and acetic acid in a molar ratio of 2:3, producing small amounts of formic acid, succinic acid, and ethanol[10]). L(+)-lactic acid is more easily metabolized.

"C. Lower pH

"Bifidogenic factors (e.g. lactulose) added to the diet induce the growth of Bifidobacteria, decreasing the pH in the large intestine[12].

"D. Competitive Antagonistics

"Bifidobacteria prevent the colonization of the intestine by invading pathogens by competition for nutrients and attachment sites to the epithelial surfaces[12].

"Strains of Bifidobacteria may partially or completely inhibit the reduction of nitrates by other organisms through beneficial competition with other intestinal bacteria[12].

"E. Bile Deconjugation

"Bifidobacterium have a certain resistance to bile acids. The growth of Bifidobacteria has been demonstrated in MRS-broth with up to 2% ox-gall

[4]. Bifidobacteria continue to grow after the addition of 2% bile salts. This proves that Bifidobacteria survive passage through the gastrointestinal tract[9].

"F. Detoxification

"The roles of *B. bifidium* and lactulose in the detoxification of subjects with chronic liver disease has been studied. The results showed that *B. bifidium* with lactulose may assist in re-establishing the normal intestinal flora which is usually disturbed in chronic liver cirrhosis. This is accomplished by a reduction of ammonia and free phenols in the blood[12].

"**Summary**

"Certain microorganisms such as *Lactobacillus acidophilus* and Bifidobacterium species can help to maintain a favorable intestinal microflora which has been associated with good nutrition and health.

"Bifidobacterium are the predominant organisms in the large intestine of breast-fed infants. They decrease into adulthood and diminish with old age.

"Although Lactobacilli occur in smaller numbers than Bifidobacteria overall, they have important metabolic properties, especially in the small intestine where they predominate.

"When taken in combination, a more complete, favorable intestinal microflora is achieved. The regular ingestion of Bifidobacteria with Lactobacilli will suppress harmful bacteria in the intestines by producing antibiotics and acetic and lactic acids which lower the intestinal pH, by competing for attachment sites, and through bile deconjugation.

"**The Role of Lactobacilli in the Upper Intestinal Tract**

"A. Antibiotic production — inhibits antibacterial substances.

"B. Organic acid production — acetic and lactic acids inhibit pathogenic gram-negative bacteria.

"C. Lactobacilli lower the pH and have an oxidation reduction potential which activates the acids, making them particularly antimicrobial.

"D. As competitive antagonists, Lactobacilli outcompetes other bacteria for attachment sites.

"E. Lactobacilli liberate free bile acid, thereby influencing the balance of existing bacteria.

"**The Role of Bifidobacteria in the Lower Intestinal Tract**

"A. Antibiotic production — *B. bifidium* in conjunction with lactulose eradicate enteropathogenic *E. coli*.

"B. Compared to Lactobacilli, Bifidobacteria produce more acetic acid which has a stronger antagonistic effect against gram-negative bacteria than lactic acid.

"C. Bifidogenic factors (i.e. lactulose) induce the growth of Bifidobacteria, thereby decreasing the pH in the large intestine.

"D. As competitive antagonists, Bifidobacteria prevent the colonization of the intestine by invading pathogens.

"E. Bifido resist bile acids and survive passage through the gastrointestinal tract.

"F. Compensational <u>detoxification</u> has been reported in subjects with chronic liver disease.

In *The Art of Getting Well*[1] we mention that it is best to use with our recommended medicines *Lactobacillus acidophilus*. We were told by a research pharmacologist at a well-known university that Metronidazole would not metabolize via the human enzyme system, but rather required such an organism to be metabolized. It now appears that for good health, one should use a varied strain of *Lactobacillus acidophilus* as well as *Bifido bacterium*. (See *The Art of Getting Well, Arthritis: Little Known Treatments, Arthritis: Osteoarthritis and Rheumatoid Disease Including Rheumatoid Arthritis* (Amazon.com. Also available on Kindle, book stores and Arthritis Trust of America.)

We also cautioned that many of these organisms are sensitive to temperatures around or greater than 23.3 degrees Centigrade [74 degrees Farhenheit] and that it is vitally important when obtaining your product to insure that from manufacture (from a reliable company) through packaging, shipment and sales to you the organisms are temperature controlled. Sometimes they will come via overnight shipment, and sometimes, when shipment time is longer, they come packed in dry ice.

It is equally important that you place them in your refrigerator, and keep them there when not in use.

The Bifido Factor overlooked in our books *The Art of Getting Well* (Also in *Arthritis: Little Known Treatments, Arthritis: Osteoarthritis and Rheumatoid Disease Including Rheumatoid Arthritis*, is said to be the first line of immune defense for infants and children, according to an article titled "Bifido Factor" and earlier published for distribution by Natran, Inc. 2382 Townsgate Rd, Westlake Village, CA 91361. With their permission we have reproduced their article:

"What is [Bifido Bacteria]?

"It is a micro-organism essential to the health of infants and small children called 'BIFIDO-BACTERIA.' This is the predominant strain of 'friendly' bacteria found naturally in the gastro-intestinal tract of healthy breast-fed infants.

"As breast-fed infants are weaned, the bifidobacteria are gradually replaced by acidophilus. This transaction usually occurs around the age of seven.

"Why is it so important?

"Breast-fed infants were found to be far less susceptible to infection than bottle-fed babies and the bifidobacteria in the colon plays a vital role in the baby's resistance to infection. When present in the intestines in large quantity, this bacteria creates an environment hostile to pathogens.

"Research indicates that bifidobacteria inhibit growth of common pathogenic and toxin-producing bacteria including *E. coli* and Salmonella (which can cause severe cramping). It was also recently revealed that viruses will settle more readily in colons deficient in bifidobacteria.

"Clinical Research

"In a Guatemalan study, out of 210 babies born in a village, 109 were breast-fed. Only 4 of the breast-fed babies developed Shigella infection, which causes severe diarrhea. This rate was much lower than the infection rate of the entire population.

"The authors of this study concluded that the bifidobacteria in breast-fed infants allowed resistance to Shigella infection or caused the elimination of it when contracted. In the same study it was noted that children who were breast-fed had an extremely low incidence of intestinal infections.

Other studies show the reduction or absence of putrefactive bacteria (such as disease-causing Bacteroides, Veillonella, Clostridum, Proteus and others) in the stools of breast-fed infants.

"All of the above-mentioned studies show that bifidobacteria aid in bettering the nutrition of infants and thus indirectly contribute to a greater resistance to infection. Bifidobacteria also help produce B vitamins and Vitamin K.

"Breast-feeding Alone May Not be Enough

"Breast-feeding alone does not seem to be sufficient to introduce bifidobacteria into the infant's colon. In a University of Pennsylvania Hospital study it was found that of 61 urban breast-fed babies, only 20% had an adequate number of bifidobacteria present. A similar study conducted at a suburban hospital found 66% of the breast-fed babies tested had large numbers of bifidobacteria.

"No scientific reason had been found to explain this contrast but environmental factors are suspected. The health of the mother and the nature of her surroundings may adversely affect her ability to transmit these vital microorganisms to her child.

"Contamination of Mother's Milk

"In another study conducted by the University of Nebraska, fresh mother's milk collected in sterile containers was studied. The milk was found to be infected with Salmonella (causes intestinal cramping among other things), streptococcus and herpes virus. Therefore, pasteurization of the mother's milk was recommended to minimize the spreading of infection through the milk banks.

"What Can Be Done About It?

"1. Bifidobacteria should be included in the diets of both bottle-fed and breast-fed babies.

"2. Expectant mothers should increase their reserves by daily supplementation. . . .

"3. Nursing mothers should also raise their bifidus levels by daily supplementation.

"Adults May Require It Too

"A small percentage of adults do better on BIFIDUS supplementation than on acidophilus.

"Bifidobacteria have been found effective in treating patients with liver disease. A significant decrease in certain toxic waste products (free serum phenol, free amino nitrogen and blood ammonia) which may cause nausea, vomiting, decreased appetite and other reactions when present in excessive quantities in the blood. The authors of this study concluded that bifidobacteria contributed greatly to patient recovery.

"**Usage**
"Infants and small children (to 7 years).
1/8 to 1/4 teaspoon in 4 oz. unchilled water once daily between meals
"Adults:
1/2 teaspoon in 8 oz. unchilled water twice daily between meals.

For further information, Contact Natren Co.

Natasha Trenev, President of Natren, reports on a finding so scandalous that it is of concern here. She reports her findings in *Townsend Letter for Doctors*, November 18, 1988[18].

She says that the majority of products sold under the name of *Lactobacillus acidophilus* are actually *L. casei*, a product used for making cheese, and provided to cheese-making customers. She asked a professional organization (NNFA) to set standards on acidophilus. They assayed twenty-two products labeled as acidophilus, and the findings were so scandalous that the results were never published. Forty or so of the so-called acidophilus products were found to be *L. casei* (Rhamnosus sub-species) and not *Lactobaccilus acidophilus*.

Apparently this deception came from one corporation. When the product (acidophilus) began to become known and popular, they feared to lose their market. Their solution to the problem was to introduce "a cocktail mix of microorganisms including *S. faecium*, *L. acidophilus*, *L. bifidus* (*L. bifidus* re-classified in 1974 to bifido-bacteria, per *Bergy's Manual of Determinative Bacteriology*, 8th Edition), *L. casei* and *L. bulgaricus*. The product mix would vary slightly with each private label customer, however, *S. faecium* would always be a part of the mix."

Natasha Trenev says that (1) Customers are buying acidophilus but getting something else, (2) the only apparent reasons for using *S. faecium* is because it is "easy and inexpensive to produce and withstands moisture and heat abuse, whereas *L. acidolphilus* and *Bifidobacteria* cannot. Heat and moisture destroy *L. acidophilus* and *Bifidobacteria*."

If you mix organisms together, the stronger will dominate, and that means that *S. faecium* will reign supreme.

Trenev adds: "I have checked with various manufacturers and suppliers in the industry and found that:

1. No American-based supplier of friendly bacteria cultures will sell *S. faecium* for human consumption. *S. faecium* is sold exclusively for animal feed in the United States.

2. All *S. faecium* mixed cultured products currently sold in Canada and the United States are made by [the same firm that supplies *L. casei*, sold as *L. Acidophilus*]"

38

Ray C. Wunderlich, Jr., M.D.[19] (in William H. Lee's R.Ph., Ph.D. pamphlet, *The Friendly Bacteria)* has written a "Foreward" which contains this statement: "One is continually surprised, too, at the beneficial role of 'friendly bacteria' in improving the health of patients. We suspect that a disturbance of the micro-biological flora runs rampant among the patients that we see. Some of my patients have severe, incapacitating, putrefactive flatus unless they include lactobacilli among their daily supplements."

Friendly Bacteria, is well worth reading. It shows how these friendly organisms can be helpful in Osteoporosis, cholesterol problems, with antibiotic action, with lactose intolerance, nutrient deficiencies, anxiety, cancer, skin problems, liver detoxification, diarrhea, children's needs and other uses [such as part of the treatment and prevention of Candidiasis.

"Lactic bacteria supplements are available in different forms, including tablets, capsules and freeze-dried preparations. It is estimated that a dose of at least 10[to the 8th power] (one billion) of live bacteria delivered to the appropriate site — the large intestine for *Bifidobacterium bifidium*, the small intestine for *Lactobacillus acidophilus* — is required for efficacy. . . .

"Acidophilus capsules are not advantageous, because moisture is trapped within them in the manufacturing process, and; this moisture accelerates the life cycle of the bacteria, causing them to continue metabolism and feeding. By the time the capsule is consumed by the purchaser, the bacteria often have exhausted the food supply and starved to death.

"Purchasing supplements of guaranteed specified potency from a reputable manufacturer and taking them according to the indications given . . . gives the best chance of getting the benefits."

It is my belief, based on readings, physicians, and personal experience, that these bacteria should be used constantly by all patients, as an important wellness supplement. Gus J. Prosch, Jr., M.D. claimed that out of all the brands he's tried, he's only been satisfied with Klaire laboratories [1995]. He also asserted that the proper way to use the powdered *Lactobacillus acidophilus* is to swish it around in the mouth, gargle it, and then swallow it.[21]

Consider: the average person has 11 trillion bacteria making up 3-1/2 pounds in the intestinal tract. A billion or so bacteria washed down with water isn't a very large percentage of the total, and either we must supplement quite heavily at first, or for a long, long time, or both, depending upon our condition, metabolism, diet, and so on. In other words, don't expect immediate results, although it will be very nice if you get it.

The following treatment recommendations have been provided by the courtesy of Natren, Inc. There may be other organisms and treatment protocols desired by your physician.

A Treatment Protocol for *Bifidobacteria* and *Lactibacillus Acidophilus* as Used by Some Physicians

[As the proper dosage depends upon your condition and your doctor, these have been left off. The protocols were provided by Natren, producers of Bifido Factor and Superdophilus. Other brands may also be viable and useful: Your physician may prefer a different brand. Natren recommendations are included here as an example, only. Ed.]

Bifido bacteria Recommended Uses for Adults
<u>Maintenance Dose:</u>
___ 1/8 tsp; ___ 1/4 tsp; 1/2 tsp; ___ times daily. Mix with 8 oz. of unchilled filtered or spring water. Always take at least 45 minutes before meals. Never to be mixed with juices, milk or other beverages.

<u>Therapeutic Dose:</u>
___ 1/2 tsp; ___ 1 tsp; ___ times daily. Mix with 8 oz. of unchilled filtered or spring water. Always take at least 45 minutes before meals. Never to be mixed with juices, milk or other beverages.

<u>Liver Detoxification:</u>
1 (one) tsp 3 times daily at least 45 minutes before meals. Mix in 8 oz. of unchilled filtered or spring water. Never to be mixed with juices or other beverages.

<u>Oral Application (*Candida albicans*):</u>
1 tsp of **Bifido Factor** combined with 1 tsp **Superdophilus** in 8 oz. of unchilled filtered or spring water taken three times daily at least 45 minutes before meals. Never mix with juice, milk, or other beverages. In addition, use Biotin ___ mcg; ___ times after meals; Linseed or Primrose oil ___ capsules ___ times daily. Continue dosage until complete improvement is attained, then reduce to 1/2 tsp of **Bifido Factor** combined with 1/2 tsp of **Superdophilus** three times daily at least 45 minutes before meals. Never mix with juice, milk, or other beverages.

<u>For vaginal/rectal application, use the Superdophilus Applicator Pack, available from your health care professional.</u>

Recommended Uses for Babies and Children Up to Seven Years Old:
<u>Maintenance Dose:</u>
___ 1/8 tsp; ___ 1/4 tsp; ___ times daily. Mix with 4 oz. of unchilled filtered or spring water.

<u>Diaper Rash and Minor Skin Infections:</u>
1 (one) rounded tsp **Bifido Factor**. Mix with enough lukewarm fresh milk to form a paste. Spread evenly onto the rash or infected area. Leave on until dry, then remove with a clean damp cloth. Continue oral maintenance dose.

Recommended Uses for Pregnant Women and Nursing Mothers:
<u>Maintenance Dose:</u>
___ 1/8 tsp; ___ 1/4 tsp; ___ 1/2 tsp; ___ times daily. Mix with 8 oz. of unchilled filtered or spring water. Always take at least 45 minutes before meals. Never to be mixed with juices, milk or other beverages.

<u>Therapeutic Dose:</u>
___ 1/2 tsp; ___ 1 tsp; ___ times daily. Mix with 8 oz. of unchilled filtered or spring water. Always take at least 45 minutes before meals. Never to be mixed with juices, milk or other beverages.

Bifido Factor is a pure strain of *Bifidobacteria* which is essential to the well-being of the immune system in infants, small children, and adults with toxic livers.

. . . Clinical studies show that environmental factors such as pollution, food chemical additives, alcohol, and smoking contribute to the destruction of the *Bifidobacteria in* mothers' milk.

There is an unknown daily consumption of antibiotics in dairy products, meats, and poultry which contribute to the eradication of the friendly and healthful bacteria in adults and nursing mothers.

Bifido Factor is a single strain *Bifidobacteria*, uniquely formulated and produced in such a way that, when taken orally, becomes a potent natural antibiotic.

Certain adults (with chronic gastronintestinal problems since birth) show better improvements when using **Bifido Factor** initially, After the administration of **Bifido Factor** for a few months, however, the individual may be switched to **Superdophilus** alone, or a combination of both products can be administered together because they are compatible.

For certain individuals who have a dairy (lactose) intolerance, the following is recommended. This supplementary schedule is designed to enable the individual to "recreate" the proper flora in the intestines which will produce lactase, an enzyme which digests the lactose present in dairy products. By taking very small amounts of **Bifido Factor**, the individual should not have a reaction.

Lactose Intolerance: Intial use: 1/16 tsp 2 times daily of **Bifido Factor** (follow instructions under Maintenance Dose). After 3-5 days depending on response to initial use, increase to 1/8 tsp 2 times daily. Again, after 3-5 days proceed to increase amount taken until meeting Maintenance level and/or Therapeutic Level. After 6-8 weeks proceed with full **Superdophilus** schedule.

Note: For persons with casein (protein) or fat intolerance, do not use **Bifido Factor**, unless directed by a health care professional.

Bifidobacteria (1) inhibits the growth of common disease-causing bacteria such as *E. coli*, *Salmonella*, etc.; significantly reduces blood ammonia levels; works as a potent natural antibiotic; detoxifies the liver in adults by removing (a) free phenols and (b) free alpha-amino nitrogen; greatly improves liver function, therefore enhances tolerance of proteins.

Lactobacillus acidophilus **Recommended Uses:**

Maintenance dose:
___ 1/8 tsp; ___ 1/4 tsp; ___ 1/2 tsp; ___ times daily. Mix in 8 oz. of unchilled filtered or spring water. Always take at least 45 minutes before meals. Never to be mixed with juices, milk, or other beverages.

Therapeutic:
___ 1/2 tsp; ___ 1 tsp; ___ times daily. Mix in 8 oz. of unchilled filtered or spring water. Always take at least 45 minutes before meals. Never to be mixed with juices, milk, or other beverages.

Oral Application (*Candida albicans*):
1 tsp of **Superdophilus** combined with 1 tsp of **Bifido Factor** in 8 oz. of unchilled filtered or spring water: 3 times daily, at least 45 minutes before meals. Never to be mixed with juices or milk. In addition, use Biotin

___ mcg; ___ times daily after meals; Linseed or Primrose oil ___ capsules ___ times daily after meals; ___ garlic capsules ___ times daily.

Continue dosage until complete improvement is attained. Then, reduce to 1/2 tsp. of **Superdophilus** mixed with 1/2 tsp of **Bifido Factor**, 3 times daily at least 45 minutes before meals. never to be mixed with juices or milk, or other beverages.

Local Application Against Yeast Infection (**Superdophilus** Implant)::

2 tablespoons full of plain yogurt (full fat); 1 rounded tablespoon full of **Superdophilus**. [Mix two (2) separate mixtures of the above recipe.] Fill individually, a vaginal applicator and a rectal syringe* and insert accordingly each night before going to bed. Follow this regime for ten days.

(*Use the Natren Superdophilus Candida kit, available from your docter, for vaginal and rectal application.)

Superdophilus Douche:

Plain lowfat yogurt diluted with warm water (50/50). Stir briskly forming a smooth texture. Add 1 teaspoon of **Superdophilus**, mix well and let stand, covered with a paper towel until slightly sour to taste, approximately 30 to 45 minutes. Use as a douche to remove excess insert mixture from previous night. Follow this regime for 10 days.

Constipation/Diarrhea:

1 tbsp; 3 times daily. For chronic constipation, use this amount until first normal elimination occurs. After which, reduce dosage to 1 tsp; 3 times daily. Resume maintenance dose after the problem becomes normal; 1 tsp daily, at least 45 minutes before meals in 8 oz. of unchilled filtered or spring water. Never to be mixed with juices or milk, or other beverages.

Lactose Intolerance**:

Initial use: 1/16 tsp 2 times daily of **Bifido Factor**. (Follow instructions under Maintenance Dose above). After 3-5 days depending on response to initial use, increase to 1/8 tsp 2 times daily. Again after 3-5 days, proceed to increase amount taken until meeting Maintenance level and/or Therapeutic Level. After 6-8 weeks proceed with full **Superdophilus** schedule.

(**See full supplement schedule with **Bifido Factor** protocol above.)

Superdophilus Facial Mask (Normal/Dry Skin):

1 heaping teaspoon of **Superdophilus** mixed with enough whole milk to make a thin paste. Spread over face and neck area. Pat extra on blemished area. Keep on area until dry. Remove with water.

For Normal to Oily Skin: Follow same directions given above, except substitute whole milk with skim milk. After dry, remove with clean damp cloth or plain water. Rub lightly in circular motion until you have removed the mask. Splash with cool water and pat dry with a clean towel. Use no lotions, creams, or makeup for 10 to 15 minutes.

Superdophilus Facial Mask (Normal/Oily Skin):

Same as above except substitute whole milk or skim milk. After mask has thoroughly dried (20 minutes to 1 hour) remove with a clean dampened washcloth or warm water. Rub lightly in circular motions until you have removed all of the mask. Follow with splash of cool water and pat dry with a clean towel. Do not apply creams, lotions, or makeup for 10 to 15 minutes.

For Problem Skin (Acne/Blemishes):

Follow directions for facial mask for normal/oily skin. However, for optimum results, always use in conjunction with oral application in the following manner:

1 tsp **Superdophilus** with 1 tsp **Bifido Factor** in 8 oz. of unfiltered or spring water 3 times daily, 45 minutes before meals. Never mix with juices or milk. Continue using for ___ months.

It has been long understood that overall system immunity has improved via the absorption mechanism when the intestinal tract is rendered more efficient.

In turn, intestinal absorption as well as digestion and detoxification of the intestines are promoted by the presence and action of friendly lactobacilli, principally, *L. acidophilus*. Poor nutrition, illness, chlorine, fluorine and pesticide-laden tap water, the use of alcohol and drugs have historically produced fatal effects on *L. acidophilus*.

In recent years, the use of antibiotics and medicine, the unknown consumption of antibiotics in dairy products, meats, poultry, etc. and the effects of industrial and chemical pollution in our food and atmosphere have had even more lethal results. Furthermore, the high stress in today's life, cigarette smoking, alcohol, and diets that are high in sugar, fats, and hidden food chemicals that are consumed daily contribute to the eradication of the friendly healthful *L. acidophilus* bacteria in our intestines. Therefore, in the absence of *L. acidophilus*, the intestines become the fertile ground for growth of unfriendly putrefactive bacteria. This, in turn, leaves the intestines without any protection and thus become open to numerous kinds of infection and digestive distress.

Superdophilus is a single strain *Lactobaccilus acidophilus* DDS-1 uniquely formulated to produce a potent, natural antibiotic.

Supplementation of **Superdophilus** should always <u>follow</u> use of broad spectrum antibiotics. Any gastroenteritis or diarrhea discomfort requires the use of **Superdophilus** both during and immediately following the cause.

As the body eliminates quantities of bacteria, both healthy and pathogenic, on a daily basis, when supplementation stops, a gradual decrease in the number of healthy bacteria occurs.

Therefore, **Superdophilus** should be used as a daily, long-term supplement, to ensure <u>continued</u> beneficial nutritional and general health effects.

Lactobaccilus acidophilus produces natural antibiotic agents that can inhibit 27 bacteria, 11 of them known as pathogens; helps many skin disorders; helps reduce cholesterol levels in the blood; is a vehicle for detoxification programs; inhibits the growth of toxic producing micro-organisms in the intestines; produces enzymes which help the digestion of food; produces enzymes necessary for development of <u>lactase</u> which "digests" lactose (milk sugar); produces B vitamins that aid food digestion and are <u>especially</u> needed <u>when</u> under stress and nerve dysfunction; and helps to establish normal pH balance throughout the gastrointestinal and urinary tracts.

Sources of *Lactobaccillus acidophilus* and/or *Bifido bacterium*

The Arthritis Trust of America/The Rheumatoid Disease Foundation is not associated with any manufacturer nor do we make any commission from any sale. There are undoubtedly other good sources that we do not know about. Check with your doctor.

A Possible New Discovery

While this article has mentioned chiefly *Lactobaccilus acidophilus* and *Bifido bacteria*, there are probably thousands of unknown "friendly" bacteria in the intestinal tract. Some probably exist in very small numbers, or act synergistically with others, providing for the health of other "good guys", and these little fellows, in turn, may assist us.

Almost any scenario is imaginable, but that's all it is — imagination!

Because of the possibility of more than just the two friendly organisms discussed in this paper, I wanted to bring to your attention claims made about the usefulness of *Bacillus laterosporus* and *Bacillus sphaericus*.

Many folks take Yogurt for its helpful *Lactobacillus bulgaricus*, which, incidentally, feeds *Lactobacillus acidophilus* and *Bifidobacteria*. To use *Lactobacillus bulgaricus* in this manner requires, of course, having some of the latter organisms internally[20].

References

1. Anthony di Fabio, *The Art of Getting Well*, The Arthritis Trust of America, 7111 Sweetgum Road, Fairview, TN, 1988. [Also see *Arthritis: Little Known Treatments* and *Arthritis: Osteoarthritis and Rheumatoid Disease Including Rheumatoid Arthritis*, Amazon.com, bookstores and at Arthritis Trust.org]

2. Ed McCabe, *Oxygen Therapies*, Energy Publications, 99-RD1, Morrisville, NY 13408, p. 165.

3.Gerald Domingue, M.D., "Naked Bacteria in Human Blood," Enterobacteriaceae Roundtable, New York, New York, 1975, and subsequently published by *Microbia*, Annee 1976, Tome 2, No. 2.

4. Lida Mattman, Ph.D., *Cell Wall Deficient Forms*, Chemical Rubber Company CRC Press, Cleveland, OH 1974; *Cell Wall Deficient Forms, Stealth Pathogens*, 2nd Edition, CRC, Press, Inc., 2000 Corporate Blvd., N.W., Boca Raton, FL 33431, ISBN 0-8493-4405-0; *Cell Wall Deficient Forms, Stealth Pathogens*, 3rd Edition, CRC, Press, Inc., 2000 Corporate Blvd., N.W., Boca Raton, FL 33431; ISBN 0-8493-8767-1.

5. Dr. Ken Rifkin5 "What Are 3-1/2 Pounds of Bacteria Doing in Our Bodies", *Health Consciousness*, Vol IX, No. 6, p 33-34, December 1988.

6. Brad Everett, "Intestinal Parasites Can Create Chronic Health

Problems," *Health World*, May-June 1989.

7. Anand RK, et. al.: Antibacterial Activity Associated with Bifidobacterium Bifidus. *J. Cultured Dairy Prod* Nov:608 (1984).

8. Babel FJ (1977) and Shahani KM (1980): *Nutritional and Healthful Aspects of Cultured Dairy Foods.*

9. Hansen R: Bifidobacteria Have Come to Stay. *N. European Diary J* 3:8 (1985).

10. *Chr. Hansen's Laboratorium*, Copenhagen, Denmark.

11. Gut Ecology and Health Implications. *Nat Dairy Council Digest* 50(3):13-17 (1979).

12. Rasic JL: The Role of Dairy Foods Containing Bifido and Acidophilus in nutrition and Health? *N European Dairy J* 4:1-10 (1983).

13. Sandine WE: Roles of Lactobacillus in the Intestinal Tract. *J Food Protection* 42(3):259-62 (1979)

14. Savaiano DA, et. al.: Lactose Malabsorption in Yogurt and Sweet Acidophilus Milk. *Am J Clin Nutr* 40(6):1219-20."

15. Poupard, J.A., Husain, I., Norris, R.F.; June 1972 Biology of Bifidobacteria. *Bacteriological Review*, Vol. 37, No. 2, p. 136-165.

16. Angel, E.N., Friend, B.A., Long, A.C., Shahani, K.M.; Bacterial Content of Raw and Processed Human Milk. *Journal of Food Protection*, Vol. 45, No. 6, p. 533-536.

17. Vi Congresso Internazionale Di *Microbiologia.* - 1953; Riasunti Delle Communcazioni Zisezioni 17-22: p. 799-1028."

18. Natasha Trenev, *Townsend Letter for Doctors*, November 18, 1988.

19. William H. Lee, R.Ph., Ph.D, *The Friendly Bacteria*, Keats Publishing, Inc., New Canaan, Ct., (Ray C. Wunderlich, Jr., M.D., "Forward.")

20. Jule Klotter, briefer, "Science News in Brief, Intestinal Bacteria," *Townsend Letter for Doctors*, August/September 1994, pp. 962.

21. Personal interview.

Selection Criteria For Probiotic Supplements

By Dr. S. K. Dash

Permission to publish granted by UAS Laboratories

UAS LABS, 555 N. 72nd Avenue, Wausau, WI 54401

All probiotic products are not alike and do not have similar nutritional and therapeutic values. The name "probiotic" does not mean anything unless it contains the right strain, in the right amount, in the right formulation and in the right condition (viable) for the intended use. It must also be stored and shipped correctly.

For this reason one needs to know the strain, its viability, implantation criteria, and other features and health benefits.

Strain Selection

Lactic acid bacteria have a long history of safe use in dairy products. However, some probiotic supplements now contain bacteria, which have no record of safe use in humans or even animals. There are instances of probiotic supplements containing soil bacteria that are not normal inhabitants of the human gastrointestinal tract. These cultures may potentially be pathogenic. It is imperative to select bacteria for incorporation in probiotic supplements that are on the GRAS (Generally Recognized As Safe) list. For example, *Lactobacillus acidophilus* species and some *Bifidobacterium* species are considered GRAS. Safe, proven cultures are your first and most important criteria for selection.

Any new bacterial culture that has no history of prior safe use in humans should be subject to toxicological studies prior to incorporation in any probiotic supplements. We want to know that the culture is benefiting, not harming the host.

The bacterial strains used in a superior probiotic supplement should play an important role in:

·   Colonization within the intestinal, respiratory and urogenital tracts
·   Cholesterol metabolism
·   Inhibiting the carcinogenesis, directly or indirectly, by stimulation of the immune system
·   The metabolism of lactose, the absorption of calcium and the synthesis of vitamins
·   Reduction of yeast and vaginal infection
·   Constipation and diarrheal diseases
·   Gastritis and ulcers
·   Acne and skin problems

Additionally, the culture should adhere to the intestinal walls and proliferate. The probiotic strain must be proven to survive stomach acids in live human subjects. And of course, it should produce natural antibiotics, lactic acid and hydrogen peroxide and inhibit pathogenic bacteria such as:

Bacillus subtilis	*Serratia marcescens*
Bacillus cereus	*Proteus vulgaris*
Bacillus stearothermophilus	*Lactobacillus casei*
Escherichia coli	*Streptococcus faecalis*
Salmonella typhosa	*Salmonella schottmuelleri*
Streptococcus faecalis var liquifaciens	
Shigella dysenteriae	*Streptococcus lactis*
Shigella paradysenteriae	*Psuedomonas aeruginosa*
Lactobacillus lactis	*Psuedomonas fluorescens*
Lactobacillus plantarum	*Staphylococcus aureus*
Lactobacillus leichmannii Vibrio comma	
Klebsiella pneumoniae	*Sarcina lutea*

(Source: US Patent #3,689,640 In Vitro Antibacterial Activity of DDS-1 *Lactobacillus acidophilus*.)

Not all strains of *Lactobacillus acidophilus* and other probiotics are acid-resistant. Selecting acid-resistant strains of *L. acidophilus* and other probiotics is the key to the success of the probiotic supplement. It is important to remember that enteric coating of bacteria is a poor and unproven substitute for actual acid resistance. Stay away from enteric-coated cultures for a few reasons. One is that no studies show that they work. In nature these cultures are not enteric coated. The process of coating these live cultures with a protective layer may in fact kill them or reduce their viability. If these cultures are supposed to get into the intestinal tract on their own and be acid resilient, the whole process of enteric coating is suspect.

Probiotic Supplements with Multiple Bacteria

Some probiotic supplements now contain several different cultures; many of these bacterial cultures have no safe-use history in human health and nutrition. These bacteria may be antagonistic to each other and may alter the gut flora in an undesirable way. So it should not be believed that if one bacterium is good, numerous cultures combined together are even better. To the contrary, a few select cultures have been proven beneficial and almost all the others are yet to be proven.

L. acidophilus and *Bifidobacterium* species are normal inhabitants of the human gastrointestinal tract and are GRAS (Generally Recognized as Safe). Probiotic formulations containing these beneficial bacteria along with prebiotic fructooligosaccharides (FOS) are considered safe and offer many health benefits described earlier.

Manufacturing

The manufacturing process used to produce microorganisms for use in probiotic supplements plays an important role in the viability of the culture. The medium, the temperature and other associated factors influence the viability and identity of the microorganisms. If the probiotic supplements do not contain the same microorganisms with the same viability, they will not offer the same, consistent, good results. Also make sure that the probiotic culture has not itself been contaminated with other harmful bacteria during manufacturing process and packaging. Make sure the company manufacturing the product has a strong history of providing proven safe cultures (do not let yourself be a guinea pig).

Viability

The viability of probiotics is not only strain-dependent but is also influenced strongly by their physiological and chemical environment. For example probiotics in liquids including milk and yogurt do not normally survive longer than a few weeks.

Exposure of probiotics to oxygen decreases the stability of probiotic bacteria. For this reason, eliminating oxygen from and including nitrogen into probiotic supplement bottles can enhance the stability of probiotics.

Guarantee/Assay

In order to know more about the keeping qualities of a probiotic product, it is important to know that the supplement is tested for viable microorganisms at the time of manufacturing and at the expiration date. This quality control procedure is important to the manufacturer as well as the consumer.

The viable cells are guaranteed as CFU (colony forming units) per gram at the time of probiotic supplement packaging. If the supplement does not list viable cells, or does not list the amount in CFU form, it is not valid. Consumption of probiotic supplements with two to five billion CFU per day is necessary to have any chance of offering significant beneficial effects.

Storage, Handling and Shipping

Refrigerated storage of probiotic supplements (-40 degrees F) is recommended to maintain the viability of the microorganisms. This means even before the bottle is opened! Just like with yogurt, cheese and other refrigerated cultures. Probiotic supplements, if not kept refrigerated, may spoil and lose potency rapidly.

Probiotic supplements should be shipped in insulated containers via airfreight to avoid exposure to heat. Viability will not decline with short exposure to heat during shipping. Some companies package probiotic supplements in nitrogen-flushed bottles to maintain viability of the microorganisms during shipping and handling. It is certainly a good idea for these supplements to contain higher potency (higher CFU) than guaranteed on the label. This ensures that at a minimum, you get more than you pay for.

Glass Bottle vs. Plastic Bottle

Probiotics are "anaerobic" organisms, meaning they live in the absence of oxygen. Therefore, exposure to air is undesirable. This makes glass a preferred container over plastic, which is somewhat porous. Probiotics packaged in plastic bottles can lose potency during prolonged storage.

Dairy vs. Non-Dairy

Some Candida specialists recommend that individuals who are allergic to dairy products should consume non-dairy probiotic supplements for better results. This of course makes sense. If an individual has dairy sensitivities, suffers from yeast infections and so forth, it is a good idea to minimize exposure to dairy and dairy-based products.

Prebiotic/Probiotic Combination

Combinations of prebiotics with probiotics offer better opportunities to the probiotic strains to grow. They can then multiply faster in the gastrointestinal tract as prebiotics selectively feed probiotics. Since yeast and pathogenic cultures are absent, and the probiotic product has its own supply of prebiotics, this is an excellent choice for yeast sufferers.

Capsule, Tablet, Powder or Liquid?

Capsules are a preferred form of supplementation over powder. Some individuals find it difficult to measure exact dosages with the powder. In addition, each time the powder bottle is opened, the contents are exposed to atmospheric contamination. The powder is oxidized, and is exposed to humidity as well as to some potential contaminants. The spoon used to measure the powder may also add to the contamination if it is not sterile, as well as adding moisture to the powder. For these reasons, deterioration of powder tends to be more rapid when compared to capsules and tablets. However, there is versatility with powder when using with mixes for children or even for esoteric Candida treatments (beyond the normal oral routes).

· Capsules add another layer of insulation against the potential for contamination, moisture and oxygen related damage, etc. Consumers and health professionals alike prefer capsules due to convenience and viability.

· Chewable Tablets are a good choice for children, elderly patients who have difficulty swallowing and even those seeking to benefit the upper digestive tract. This may be for halitosis, (bad breath) for the esophagus (GIRD) or similar problems. Chewable acidophilus (bifidus does not lend itself to viable tablet manufacturing) is vegetarian (vegan). Those wishing to avoid gelatin capsules

48

may choose tablets as a convenient alternative.

· Liquid Probiotics do not normally survive longer than just a few weeks. Another disadvantage is that microorganisms in liquid medium can mutate and change. If it is in a liquid, do not rely on it.

How, When and Why to Use Probiotic Supplements:
A Quick Summary

A number of factors are responsible for the lack of friendly cultures in our intestinal tract. Beneficial microflora are reduced by excessive use of antibiotics, chlorinated/fluoridated water, food preservatives, junk foods, and pollution in our environment. Seventy percent of the women in America and as high as forty percent of the men will suffer from yeast infections. Probiotics are almost always greatly lacking in the presence of a yeast infection and those who have sufficient quantities of beneficial microflora are not as susceptible to yeast infections. Studies at the VA Hospital of Minneapolis show that even amongst normal persons (with no obvious signs of poor health) there are virtually no probiotics in the gastrointestinal tract.

Health professionals recommend probiotic supplements for Candidiasis (yeast infection), digestive disorders (including diarrhea and constipation), gastritis, lactose intolerance, gas, heartburn, irritable bowel syndrome, (including colitis and Crohn's disease) immune dysfunctions and as a follow up to antibiotic therapy. Under these conditions higher amounts of the probiotic supplements should be used.

For this reason, it is advisable that one should take a proven probiotic supplement daily. Probiotic supplements containing *L. acidophilus, Bifidobacterium* species and FOS with two to five billion live cells (2-5 x 10^9 CFU) should be taken daily just before breakfast or between meals for maintenance. Remember, if the probiotic supplements are not refrigerated and viable, they will offer no health benefits. Also, if these supplements are not taken in sufficient quantities, they will produce no results.

Remember that although probiotics play a key role in good health, they are not intended to be a substitute for a good healthy diet and active lifestyle. All these things work best together and the synergism of one helps the other! Use of probiotics or any other supplements for therapeutic reasons should be taken with the advice of a health professional who has knowledge and expertise in probiotics and other supplements.

References:
1. Donahue, D.C. et al, "Safety of Probiotic Bacteria, Lactic Acid Bacteria". 1998, p 369-383

2. Fuller, Roy. History and Development of Probiotics. *Probiotics* – The Scientific Basis 1992, p 1-8

3. Dash, S. K. How to Select an Acidophilus Supplement. *The Garden Within* 1989, p 12-18.4.Havenaar, R. et al. Selection of Strains for Probiotic Use. *Probiotics – The Scientific Basis*. 1992, p 210-224.

The Miracle of Hydrogen Peroxide Therapy

Anthony di Fabio and Charles H.Farr, M.D., Ph.D. and
Gordon Josephs, D.O., MD(H)

Hydrogen peroxide therapy is one of the oldest treatments in America. It is also a very effective treatment against infections while being very much ignored by mainstream medicine. I must report on this promising therapy, as so many physicians and patients have given me good tidings from its use. What is probably not so well known by the general public, and many practicing physicians, is that hydrogen peroxide has been used for more than a century, the abstracts of articles and research reports published from 1966 through 1988 alone reaches 2" high when printed on 8-1/2"X11" paper.

A number of alternative medical clinics in the United States and Mexico use hydrogen peroxide therapy as well as other treatment modalities on a routine basis, usually given by intravenous injection (IV).

Before scoffing, keep in mind that one of the very first lines of defense against any and all microorganisms recognized as invaders by our immunological system are macrophages and leucocytes, one of which uses hydrogen peroxide to oxidize the foreigners; and that vitamin C is effective principally by its ability to promote hydrogen peroxide use against foreign invaders including parasites, viruses, bacteria, yeast/fungus; and that all body tissues contain catalase and that hydrogen peroxide in the presence of catalase is reduced to oxygen and water. So, there is strong reason to believe that added hydrogen peroxide, used properly, may be both effective against certain organisms and safe.

Hydrogen peroxide is an essential metabolite, meaning that it is necessary to life's process according to William Campbell Douglass, M.D.

As we age, our immunological system weakens, which permits organisms of opportunity to spread, thereby breeding colonies of organisms whose presence is anathema to good health. Killing these organisms should permit at least temporary respite from microbial warfare, and give your system time to heal.

According to William Campbell Douglass, M.D.[2], not only is H2O2 (Hydrogen Peroxide) involved in phagocytosis (killing and absorption of foreign germs), but also "it acts like insulin in that it aids the transport of sugar through the body." It is also at least as important, or perhaps more so, than thyroid for heat generation because it creates "intraceullar thermogenesis, a warming of your cells which is absolutely essential to life's processes."

Various alterntive medical physicians also use hydrogen peroxide therapy for various ailments. Physicians have independently discovered such treatments to be effective against some types of cancer, leukemia, arthritis, coronary heart disease, arterial circulation disorders, colitis, gum diseases, and assorted children's diseases.

The First International Conference of Bio-oxidative Medicine was held February 17-19, 1989 in Dallas/Ft. Worth, TX. Physicians presented papers on the efficacy and safety of hydrogen peroxide infusions. Since that date the non-profit International Bio-Oxidative Medicine Foundation[1] grew rapidly. It attracted many physicians who had also presented many scholarly works based on their treatment of patients.

While Chelation Therapy is an extremely useful treatment and preventive measure for at least 80% of peripheral circulation problems, it apparently cannot clean out hardened plaque in arteries, like the large heart arteries and the aorta[3].

According to Douglas, the Baylor University Medical Center may "have gone a long way toward proving that H2O2 dripped into the leg and carotid vessels of patients known to have severe arteriosclerosis will clear those arteries of disease. When these patients died, autopsies were done to compare arteries that had been treated with H2O2 with those not treated. They reported: 'The elution [separation] of lipids from the arterial wall by dilute hydrogen peroxide has been accomplished. . . .' In simple English that means the plaque buildup was removed by injecting H2O2 into the blood vessels. . . . "That was over 20 years ago[2]."

Dr. Douglass added that, "The investigators also reported that the improvement is not temporary."

While H2O2 has been used to good advantage for hardening of the arteries, temporal arteritis, shingles, chronic obstructive pulmonary disease, the yeast syndrome, various viral infections, including AIDS, certain forms of cancer, dental gum diseases, colds (35% H2O2 in cold humidifier), growing better food, purifying water without chlorine complications, increasing thyroid activity, arthritis, depression, emphysema, lupus erythematosis, multiple sclerosis, . . ., a list of claims made would exceed our space limitations.

[After the death of its founder, Charles Farr, M.D., PhD., the International Bio-Oxidative Foundation possibly no longer exists.. As with any new, effective treatment protocol, the FDA sat down hard on this one also, more than likely because it detracted from profits of large pharmaceutical companies.]

A word of caution: while many reputable physicians and researchers have made legitimate claims on the safety and efficacy of H2O2 , it is my opinion that there are a lot of scam artists using or selling H2O2 , and so one must be careful[12]. I believe that you can relie on the past work of the International Bio-Oxidative Medicine Foundation, ECHOS and Charles Farr, M.D., Ph.D..

There are also many important forgotten facts in the past medical literature. For example, William Campbell Douglass, M.D. reports on "Dr. Edward C. Rosenow, author of 450 published medical papers and associate at the Mayo Clinic for over 60 years . . . proved [more than] 70 years ago (1914) that bacteria could be found consistently in the lymph nodes that drain joints (*J.A.M.A.*, April 11, 1914). He was probably the first scientist to postulate that H2O2 would help arthritis because of its ability to supply oxygen to oxygen-hating organisms causing arthritis (*Streptococcus viridans*)."

Charles H. Farr, M.D., Ph.D., said, "Perhaps we have become myopic about biological oxidation! The majority of investigational studies seem to concentrate on the damaging effects of biological oxidation and the production of free radicals. Hydrogen peroxide is usually treated as a[n] intermediate or by-product of metabolism and considered of minor significance in metabolic pathways except as it relates to biochemical disruption, tissue or cellular damage.

"We feel the physiological effects of bio-oxidation and, in particular hydrogen peroxide, should be investigated with a new prospect.

"From the 2,500 or more references on hydrogen peroxide we have collected and reviewed we have come to appreciate this physiological product as a[n] extremely important molecule in metabolism. Hydrogen peroxide is produced by all cells of the body for many different physiological reasons. The granulocytes produce $H2O2$ as a first line of defense against bacteria, yeast, virus, parasites, macrophages, and most fungi. It is involved in any metabolic pathway which utilize oxidases, peroxidases, cyclo-oxygenase, lipoxygenase, myeloperoxidase, catalase and probably many other enzymes. Hydrogen peroxide is naturally involved in protein, carbohydrate and fat metabolism, immunity, vitamin and mineral metabolism or any other system you might wish to explore.

"Our studies demonstrate a positive metabolic effect to intravenous infusion of $H2O2$. Its ability to oxidize almost any physiological or pathological substance, in addition to producing increased tissue and cellular oxygen tensions, has proven it to have therapeutic value.

"We feel the evidence presented should stimulate a new appreciation in the study of the potential therapeutic application of bio-oxidative mechanisms."

Two Means of Administration

There are two ways to administer hydrogen peroxide for medical purposes. Both means require a pure grade of hydrogen peroxide which is something different than one can purchase at the drug store for topical treatment of sores and wounds. The 3% drugstore hydrogen peroxide also contains tin and phosphate compounds that are dangerous to consume either by means of IV (intravenous) or orally.

I must caution at the outset that Dr. Farr and some other physicians[11] do not approve of use of $H2O2$ for oral treatment, as so many treatment modalities describe[11].

Dr. Farr, and some other physicians, feel that free-radicals are produced in the stomach when $H2O2$ is administered orally, and these free-radicals are not safe. Combinations of fatty acids which are likely to be in the stomach in the presence of iron and ascorbate may reduce hydrogen peroxide to hydroxyl and superoxide free radicals. These may have a deleterious effect upon the gastric and duodonal mucosa, with an increase of glandular stomach erosion, duodonal hyperplasia (abnormal increase in number of cells), adenoma and carcinoma, although in rats there seems to be inconsistencies in the studies related to carcinogenesis using 0.8% concentration for ten weeks versus 1% concentration for 32 weeks, the former indicating carcinogensis, the latter not so.

Since some clinics are using both intravenous and oral techniques with patients successfully, or to some good advantage, apparently not all possible research is in on the subject of oral versus IV administration.

I have twice tried the oral method, and have failed to continue onward, because of a terrible, revolting nausea. Some folks react similarly, others don't, and some persevere despite all.

As stated earlier, Dr. Farr's research demonstrates that hydrogen peroxide stimulates oxidative enzymes which increases the metabolic rate. Intravenous use rapidly relieves allergenic reactions, influenzal symptoms, chronic systemic candidiasis, acute viral reactions as a result of the oxidation of antigenic substances and regulation of immune system functions.

To prepare the IV (intravenous) solutions, Dr. Farr begins with 30% H_2O_2 of USP food or cosmetic grade. **Thirty percent H_2O_2 is a powerful oxidizer and should be handled with extreme caution.**

The 30% solution is diluted with equal amounts of sterile distilled water to make a 15% stock solution. The stock solution is passed through a Millipore 0.22mm medium flow filter for sterilization and removal of particulate matter. The stock solution is stored in 100 ml sterile containers and kept refrigerated for future use.

His infusion solutions are then prepared using sterile 5% dextrose in water. The addition of 1/4 ml sterile of the 15% H_2O_2 stock solution to each 100 ml of carrier solution produces a 0.0375% concentration that is finally used for the intravenous infusions.

Dr. Farr further warns that "caution must be exercised that nothing is added to the H_2O_2 solution because of its tremendous oxidizing power. Even ascorbic acid (Vitamin C) is rapidly oxidized to the mono-dehydroascorbate radical, an unstable compound which degrades into numerous other chemical fragments. . . . Vitamins, minerals, peptides, enzymes, amino acids, heparin, EDTA, or other injectable materials should never be mixed with the H_2O_2 solution."

By far the widest use for hydrogen peroxide, whether wisely or not, seems to be that of oral use, where a 35% "food grade" is diluted to a 3% concentration by use of 1 ounce of 35% H_2O_2 to 11 ounces of distilled water. The 3% concentration is then used by quantities of drops in distilled water, increasing the dosages and number of oral treatments daily throughout a number of weeks.

Many have made the claim that a "die-off" effect is observed, similar in nature to the Herxheimer Effect[5].

Further information on the oral use of H_2O_2 may be acquired from a site dedicated to Walter O. Grotz, http://www.foodgrade-hydrogenperoxide.com/id79.html

There are many other uses for hydrogen peroxide for health purposes than simply topical use on sores, or intravenous therapy. With permission from ECHO[4], [now found at http://echoh2o2.squarespace.com/] the following is presented:

Other Uses for H2O2

Use 3% solution, except where 35% is highlighted.

Vegetable soak: Add 1/4 cup to a full sink of cold water. Soak light-skinned (like lettuce) 20 minutes, thicker skinned (like cucumbers) 30 minutes. Drain, dry and refrigerate. Prolongs freshness. If time is a problem, spray vegetables (and fruits) with a solution of 3%. Let stand for a few minutes, rinse and dry.

Leftover tossed salad: Spray with a solution of 1/2 cup water and 1 Tbsp. 3%. Drain, cover and refrigerate.

To freshen kitchen: Keep a spray bottle in the kitchen. Use it to wipe off counter tops and appliances. It will disinfect and give the kitchen a fresh smell. Works great in the refrigerator and kid's school lunch boxes.

Marinade: Place meat, fish, or poultry in a casserole (avoid using aluminum pans). Cover with hydrogen peroxide. Place loosely covered in refrigerator for 1/2 hour. Rinse and cook.

In the dishwasher: Add 2 ozs to your regular washing formula.

Sprouting seeds: Add 1 oz. to a pint of water and soak the seeds overnight. Add the same amount of hydrogen peroxide each time you rinse the seeds.

House and garden plants: Put 1 oz. in 1 quart of water. Water or mist plants with this solution.

Insecticide spray: Mix 8 ozs. white sugar, 4-8 ozs. hydrogen peroxide in 1 gallon of water.

Humidifiers and steamers: Mix 1 pint to 1 gallon of water.

Laundry: Add 8 ozs. to your wash in place of bleaches.

Shower: Keep a spray bottle of hydrogen peroxide in the shower. Spray your body after washing to replace the acid mantle of your skin that soap removes.

Facial: Use on a cotton ball as a facial freshner after washing. (Remember: **do not use 35% grade!**)

Rejuvenating detoxifying bath: Add 6 ozs. to 1/2 tub of water. May increase hydrogen peroxide up to 2 cups per bath. Soak at least 1/2 hour.

Alternate bath: Add 1/2 cup 35% H_2O_2 , 1/2 cup sea salt, and 1/2 cup baking soda or epsom salts to bath water and soak.

Foot soak: Add 1-1/2 ozs. 35% H_2O_2 to 1 gallon water and soak.

Athlete's foot: Soak feet nightly until condition is improved.

Mouthwash: Add a dash of liquid chlorophyll for flavoring if desired.

Toothpaste: Use baking soda and add enough to make a paste. Or just dip your brush in it and brush.

Douche or enema: Add 6 Tbls. to a quart of distilled water. 6 Tbls. is the maximum amount to use.

Pets: For small animals (dogs & cats) use 1 oz. to 1 qt. of water.

Agriculture: Use 8 ozs. 35% H_2O_2 per 1000 gallons of water. If you do not have an injector, start out by using 1 tsp. 35% H_2O_2 in the drinking cup at the stanchion.

Drinking water of ailing cows: Use 1 pt. to 5 gallons of water. To drench sick calves put 1/3 pt. bottle and fill remainder with water. Do this twice a day. For an adult cow use the same procedure but use a quart.

Foliage feed crops: put 5 to 16 ozs. of 35% H_2O_2 into 20 gallons of water. This is sufficient for 1 acre. Spray on plants early in the morning when the dew is still on them and the birds are singing.

Hydrogen peroxide has been a recognized medicinal source since at least the 1800's, has gone into disrepute, and now seems to lie in a sort of limbo so far as established medicine is concerned.

However, research has progressed forward on its use throughout the world and American doctors of a more open-minded view are persisting in learning its good effects.

Again I caution the reader that there is controversy between the use of oral hydrogen peroxide and use of IV (intravenous) treatment. You must study the issues and come to your own judgement. But please make an educated decision, and whichever you decide find a physician who knows what s/he is doing.

Stimulation of Oxidative Enzymes

Charles H. Farr, M.D., Ph.D. had used hydrogen peroxide clinically, and had reported on research that he performed that sheds a great deal of light on how H_2O_2 functions. Contrary to popular belief the use of H_2O_2 by either infusion or orally cannot supply as much oxygen as a good, deep breath. Instead, it is the stimulation of oxidative enzymes that does the useful trick. Dr. Farr's conclusions are appropriate and follow:

Dr. Farr says[6], "There are a number of commercial products [that] claim to contain more oxygen on a volumes percent basis than Hydrogen Peroxide and consequently this has been interpeted as meaning they would somehow have more biological activity. There is a great deal of confusion about the difference between the terms `Oxygenation' and `Oxidation' when applied to biochemical reactions. A product which contains more oxygen per molecule may or may not have biological activity.

"We reported[1] Intravenous Hydrogen Peroxide has an oxidative stimulatory effect when administered to man which appears to be independant of the amount of oxygen produced.

"Hydrogen Peroxide is a very simple molecule produced by almost every cell in the body. This amazing molecule, essential for life in both plant and animal, has been generally overlooked for it's role in oxidative metabolism. Every chemist knows any reaction must have an opposite reaction to balance the equation. This applies equally to reactions in the test tube and in living cells. The world seems to have been caught up in the idea that all biological oxidation is harmful because free-radicals may be produced. Free-radicals can cause lipid peroxidation and membrane damage. Consequently many products, containing anti-oxidants, are being promoted to prevent peroxidation. Some researchers[7], including this author, feel peroxidation serves a useful purpose in the biochemical balance and may need stimulating at times instead of prevention.

"Hydrogen Peroxide as an oxidizer, under certain catalytic conditions, can degrade into water and oxygen.

"The fact that Hydrogen Peroxide may increase oxygen tension in the tissue is of secondary importance. Any student of biochemistry knows the principal reaction of an oxidizer, such as Hydrogen Peroxide, is to accept electrons in the RedOx [reduction/oxidation] reactions of the body and has nothing to do with "Oxygen" or "Oxygenation." It is true Hydrogen Peroxide increases the *rate of oxidation* in the body[8], but this is not because it produces oxygen but rather it *stimulates oxidative enzymes.*

"Hydrogen Peroxide is a naturally produced purposeful molecule in the body. It functions to aid membrane transport, acts as a hormonal messenger, regulates thermogenesis (heat production), stimulates and regulates immune functions, regulates energy production and many other important metabolic functions. These effects can occur without increasing the amount of oxygen. It is purposely used by the body to produce Hydroxyl Radicals to kill bacteria, virus, fungi, yeast and a number of parasites. This natural killing or protective system has nothing to do with increasing the amount of available oxygen.

"The amount of oxygen produced by a therapeutic infusion of Hydrogen Peroxide is very small. A single breath of fresh air contains many times more oxygen than found in either a therapeutic infusion or in a few drops of 35% Food Grade Hydrogen Peroxide taken orally.

"Claims are being made that molecules containing Oxygen and Chlorine, or Chlorite ions will sterilize water, milk and almost anything to which they have been added. Chlorine is added to almost all public water supplies for the same purpose. The small amount of oxygen in these molecules has very little to do with this sterilization process. There are many more aerobic (requires oxygen) than anerobic (does not use oxygen) bacteria and increasing the oxygen supply may actually stimulate the growth of the aerobic bacteria. `Oxygen supply' or `Oxygenation' is not a credible basis for the promotion of these products. *Oxidation* is the key word and not *Oxygenation.*

"Oxidation is the removal of an electron from a molecule which changes electrical energy of the molecule into an oxidized state. The oxidizing agent which accepts the electron through this reaction becomes reduced. This reaction takes place in many biochemical reactions in which OXYGEN is *not* involved. In oxidative reactions in which Hydrogen Perxoide is involved, oxygen is released when the Hydrogen Peroxide, acting as an oxidizer, is reduced but it is the transfer of the electrons which is important and not the production of Oxygen.

"Manufacturers of products which claim to have the same effect as Hydrogen Peroxide may not have a good understanding of the biochemical role of Hydrogen Peroxide in the body. Some of these products claim to provide more oxygen molecules than Hydrogen Peroxide and that may be true but I know of no scientific evidence to show this enhances oxidative metabolism. Cancer and many other degenerative diseases are thought to be the results of poor cellular oxidative processes. They are not the results of a reduced supply of oxygen. Persons with anemias or severe lung disease may have an oxygen deficit but do not necessarily have a greater incidence of Cancer or chronic diseases. The problem is not the delivery of oxygen to the cells but utilization by the cells. Hydrogen Peroxide affects utilization or oxidation dramatically whereas hyper-oxygenated or chlorinated molecules have not been shown to be necessary in the body to improve oxidative metabolism[9]."

Many physicians and clinics are effectively using Hydrogen Peroxide intravenously with their patients.

There is a ton of literature favoring Hydrogen Peroxide treatment for various medical conditions[10].

We suggest that your study of H2O2 may be an important step in your search for good health. It's worth looking into!

References

1. International Bio-Oxidative Medicine Foundation, PO Box 13205, Oklahoma City, OK 73113-1205.

2. William Campbell Douglass, *The Cutting Edge*, PO Box 1568, Clayton, GA 30525. According to Douglass' paper, see: Docknell, *Inf./Immunity*, January 1983, pp. 456; Mallams, Finney & Balla, S.M.J., March 1962; Jay et. al., Tex *Rep. Biol. & Med.*, 22:106, 1964; Urschel, *Diseases of the Chest*, 51:180, 1967; Finney, et. al., *Angiology*, 17:223, 1966; *Hydrogen Peroxide — The Forgotten Miracle*.

3. Anthony di Fabio, *Chelation Therapy*, The Arthritis Trust of America/The Rheumatoid Disease Foundation, http://www.arthritistrust.org.

4. Walter O. Grotz, ECHO, 300 South 4th Street, Delano, MN 55328. ECHO for a small fee can provide you with a listing of abstracts dating back to 1920; also see their *Progress Report*, 2nd Edition.

5. Dr. Paul K. Pybus, Anthony di Fabio, *The Herxheimer Effect*, http://www.arthritistrust.org.

6. Charles H. Farr, M.D., Ph.D., *The Therapeutic Use of Intravenous Hydrogen Peroxide* (Monograph). Genesis Medical Center, Oklahoma City, OK 73139, Jan. 1987.

7. T.L. Dormandy, "In Praise of Peroxidation," *Lancet*, II (Nov. 12):1126, 1988.

8. Charles H. Farr, M.D., Ph.D., "Physiological and Biochemical Responses to Intravenous Hydrogen Peroxide in Man," *J ACAM*, 1:113-129, 1988.

9. "Why Hydrogen Peroxide?" *International Bio-Oxidative Medical Foundation Newsletter*, Vol. II, No. 1, Op.Cit., 1989.

10. Ed McCabe, *O2xygen Therapies*, Energy Publications, 99-RD1, Morrisville, NY 13408, 1988.

11. Leon Chaitow, "Bland Attacks 'Fad' for Hydrogen Peroxide," *Townsend Letter for Doctors*," May 1988, p. 204; from *Journal of Alternative & Complementary Medicine* (UK).

12. Jonathan Collin, M.D., "The H2O2 Crusades," *Townsend Letter for Doctors*, Op.Cit., June 1989, p. 322.

A Closer Look at Intravenous
Hydrogen Peroxide H202 ©
by Gordon Josephs, D.O., MD(H) Homeopathic Physician,
7315 Evans Road, Scottsdale, AZ 85260, (480) 998-0232
Intravenous Hydrogen Peroxide

PORTIONS OF THIS BOOKLET MAY BE REPRODUCED PROVDED THIS PAGE IS DISTRIBUTED WITH THE REPRODUCED PORTIONS.

In 1988, satisfied (EDTA) chelation patients began sending me lots of referrals. My patients particularly began sending me a lot of people with *emphysema, asthma, and chronic lung disease*. Well chelation therapy does have a benefit for these people, but chelation is best known for heart and circulation problems. I needed something that particularly worked well for *lung* problems.

I heard about intravenous hydrogen peroxide, and I heard that it was *terrific* for lung disease. I also heard that you had to be *very careful*, that the therapy could be *dangerous*. I heard *conflicting* stories from doctors, but *none of these doctors actually used intravenous hydrogen peroxide*. My search for the truth led me to a meeting of IBOM, the International Bio-Oxidative Medical Foundation, presided by Dr. Charles Farr, an MD in Oklahoma City.

I went to Dallas to an IBOM meeting for several days. There I was taught *exactly* how to *safely* administer hydrogen peroxide intravenously. I was taught a *specific protocol*. At the meeting, IBOM doctors were speaking *from experience* about the various things for which they found peroxide useful. To my very great amazement, I learned that peroxide was good for a *great many things* beside lung problems.

GENERAL INFORMATION ABOUT PEROXIDE

There are lots of studies which demonstrate that peroxide does the following:

1. Peroxide *stimulated the immune system*.

2. Peroxide *killed* a dozen different *pathogenic bacteria*, and killed many *viruses*, and *yeast and fungus* too!

3. Peroxide even *improved circulation* and *unblocked arteries*, like chelation did!

4. It caused debris deep down in the lungs to be *expelled*!

5. It got rid of all kinds of *chronic pains*, but nobody was certain why.

6. It *oxygenated the body*, better than if you got into a $100,000 hyperbaric oxygen chamber!

7. Peroxide even destroyed some cancerous tumors!

And the list of things went on and on. I'd bore you to tears if I read off the list. It turns out that there are over 6000 articles in the medical literature about peroxide.

So **if peroxide does so much good, why isn't it being used more by**

doctors? The answer has to do with money and stupidity.

For example, drug companies would like doctors to prescribe a $60 antibiotic, not a dollars worth of peroxide! You have to understand that the drug companies fill the medical journals with expensive and really slick advertising. Because of these ads, doctors perceive that drugs are the state of the art. Nobody advertises hydrogen peroxide. Peroxide is not patentable. Who's going to promote peroxide when *anyone* and *any drug company* can make it?

Then, some doctors are just plain stupid. They don't even wash hands between examining patients, which was proven to reduce hospital infections by Dr. Semmelweis a hundred years ago. It took doctors 40 years to accept the electrocardiogram as useful!

Well, it's been over 60 years since peroxide was found to be miraculous. In 1929 there was a worldwide flu epidemic. There was no drug to kill the flu virus (and there still isn't), so some people with poor immune systems died from it. 84% of those who developed *influenza pneumonia* died.

Well in 1929, doctors took patients dying from influenza pneumonia, and for the first time in history gave them intravenous hydrogen peroxide. 48% of them lived! Yes, I'm telling you that there's been an antiviral remedy for over *60 years* and doctors seem ignorant of it all.

Dr. Charlie Farr, who I consider my *guru*, did a great **study on flu** victims just a few years ago. He gave 44 patients with the flu a peroxide treatment and told them to return the next day if they were not better. Seven returned (note: *all seven* that returned had a prior history of lung problems). He gave them a second peroxide treatment and told them to return if they were not better. Two returned and they required a third dose. How's that for anti-viral action? You see, if you come early to the doctor with a virus it can be knocked out.

ASTHMA, EMPHYSEMA, AND CHRONIC LUNG DISEASE

Well, what about *emphysema, asthma, and chronic lung disease*? It turns out that IV peroxide can do something special, something that no other substance I know of can do. It can *clean* the lungs!

Ask a pathologist what color a baby's lungs are. He'll tell you they're *pink*. At autopsy, 50 or more years later, those lungs are gray-black . . . . filled with *soot and grime*, from the air we breathe, that could not be eliminated by the body. It's harder to transfer oxygen from the air you breathe through soot-covered air sacks. Well here's great news. . . . Intravenous peroxide *burns* the soot and debris, and *lifts it off the surface* of the air sacks. Then you cough this *gunk* up, get it out of your body, and you can breathe easier after that. **Nothing else in medicine has this action.**

This miracle isn't always met with joy. All the patient knows is that they took a peroxide treatment and began coughing more than ever. They've got to understand that *this coughing is good*. The coughing can begin right as the peroxide IV is dripping, or after the IV has been completed. This reaction to peroxide may occur for three to six treatments, after which it ceases. The job is done! The air sacs of the lungs have been cleaned.

The coughing doesn't always occur. Instead of coughing, the loose debris is often brought up in the sputum (the mucus and phlegm in the throat), and then swallowed, without the patient even being aware of it.

HOW MANY TREATMENTS ARE NEEDED FOR LUNG PROBLEMS?

For *asthma, emphysema, or chronic lung disease*, peroxide treatments should be taken once per week for at least ten treatments. **It takes some time for the changes to occur in chronic disease.** You must not say to yourself, "Well, I'll just try two or three treatments and see if it's any good for me." That's not how peroxide works. And frankly, *I don't really want you to start peroxide unless you intend to finish a reasonable series.* That's because I don't want anyone condemning peroxide unless they've given it a proper try. Peroxide is good therapy, used correctly. For asthma, emphysema, and chronic lung disease, this means taking at least ten treatments over ten weeks.

HOW MANY TREATMENTS ARE NEEDED FOR MOST PROBLEMS?

Now maybe you've heard that peroxide could fix you up *in just one or two treatments*. Well that *can* be the truth . . . . it just depends upon what disease we're talking about. For example, I had a man come to me who was suffering with **temporal arteritis**. Temporal arteritis causes terrible, one-sided head pain around the eye and the temple. I had a man come to me who had been to dozens of doctors and top notch pain centers. He was loaded up on every manner of drug. A smile came over this man's face as the *first IV* was dripping. He could feel his pain going away. He took a second treatment, and it was gone! That was six months ago, and he hasn't been back! So you see, for some things it *can* be a matter of a couple treatments. I hope that you will meet personally with me or with your "peroxide" doctor, and discuss how many treatments are likely to be needed for your condition.

WHAT DIAGNOSES RESPOND TO PEROXIDE?

Let me tell you about some other random cases, and how peroxide worked. First, let's talk about **shingles** (also called **herpes zoster**). Just one or two treatments taken for a couple days in a row, and one more a week later generally does the trick! I had a patient with AIDS and shingles. It took about six treatments over the course of two weeks, not bad considering a battered immune system. Sometimes the pains that may linger after shingles (**post herpetic neuralgia**) responds to a peroxide series. I think it's because there's still live virus deep in the nerve root.

I believe that **Bell's Palsy** (of the face) is also from a virus similar to shingles, because my peroxide treatments have relieved the condition over a week or two.

For **colds**, or **the flu**, I've already told you that one or two treatments are generally sufficient.

I had a woman with **malignant melanoma with metastasis to her lymph nodes**. She was in awful pain. She wanted one treatment every day. When she got it, she felt no pain, was active and busy. Without a daily treatment, she was miserable and could not function.

A lot of **chronic painful conditions** respond to peroxide. I believe that all chronic pain comes *ultimately* from insufficient oxygen getting into the effected area of the body. (Activation of oxidative enzymes.) Peroxide gets the oxygen into the tissue and the pain leaves. Nevertheless, the official line is that we *don't understand why peroxide helps chronic pain*. There's no telling the best way to give the peroxide for chronic pain. One might need it once a week or once a day. I've recently learned that slowly infusing the peroxide all day long, using an infusion pump, can get rid of constant pain much better than just a short IV (my thanks to Dr. Jesse Stoff for that finding).

For disorders of **blocked arteries**, such as **angina pectoris**, or **peripheral artery blockage in the legs**, Dr. Charlie Farr says that one peroxide each week, *plus two chelation treatments each week, works the best*. I think that's a perfectly fine schedule, and about ten weeks of treatment should be considered minimal. 15-20 weeks would be really good.

If your **immune system** is down, and you get sick a lot, take one treatment a week for ten weeks or twenty, (you'll need a variety of nutritional supplements too). Here the peroxide stimulates the production of T-helper cells and causes white cells to make interferon, and lots more.

Let's talk about **chronic fatigue syndrome**. Chronic fatigue is *not* one disease. It more than likely is a name given to hundreds of *not-yet-diagnosed* problems in a person. What I mean is that there may be someone with undiagnosed parasites, dragging their body around, exhausted. Well that's chronic fatigue. And so is undiagnosed Epstein-Bar virus infection, and so is malabsorption with mineral deficiency. My point is that there obviously is no *magic bullet remedy* for what is called chronic fatigue, because the causes of chronic fatigue are varied. The underlying cause of each individual's chronic fatigue needs to be determined and treated with the most suitable remedy or remedies. Peroxide is likely to help many chronic fatigue patients, because peroxide has so many actions.

For IBOM's list of diagnoses for which peroxide has been found useful, please see INDEX A at the end of this [article].

IS PEROXIDE THE MAGIC BULLET?

Well *if there were a magic bullet*, it might well be IV peroxide, because peroxide has so many different actions. It can kill considerable numbers of viruses, bacteria, fungi, yeast, parasites, and even some tumor cells! It can boost the immune system by improving the number and quality of various blood cells. It can improve circulation, improve heart function, and provide oxygen to the brain. It can relieve pain. It can destroy toxic environmental chemicals inside your body and quiet allergies. **Can you think of anything more likely to help an unknown, undiagnosed, hidden illness?**

MIXING OTHER SUBSTANCES IN THE PEROXIDE IV

It was once believed that the doctor could not add any other substance into the peroxide IV bottle. It was believed that either the peroxide would be destroyed, or that the added substance might be destroyed. Recently, however, studies have determined that certain vitamins and minerals can be added into a peroxide infusion. Sadly, vitamin C cannot be added. Fortunately, *magnesium* can be added.

Magnesium is my personal favorite mineral (if there is such a thing). That's because magnesium *lowers blood pressure, relaxes artery walls and thus promotes increased circulation, reduces anginal chest pains, reduces irregular heart rhythms, relaxes muscles, alleviates muscle cramps, reduces anxiety levels, and increases energy production in every cell in your body*! Also, for reasons that we don't yet fully understand, magnesium reduces the likelihood of infusion site discomfort, arm pain. As far as I'm concerned, I'm going to add magnesium to just about every peroxide IV I can.

Other *trace minerals* can be added to a peroxide IV also. And *B-Complex Vitamins* and *B-12* can be added. So now it is possible to give the patient more for his money. With one treatment infusion, the doctor may be able to accomplish more by providing the body with needed nutrients as well as peroxide.

ISN'T PEROXIDE HARMFUL?

Peroxide is extremely well tolerated by the human body. This may come as a surprise to you. After all, if peroxide kills so many things, then why doesn't it kill us? The answer is the enzyme CATALASE. Catalase, found throughout the human body causes hydrogen peroxide to change into *harmless* oxygen and water. Viruses don't have catalase, so the peroxide destroys them. Humans have catalase in their cells, and are not destroyed by peroxide.

When you get an infection, your white blood cells surround the germs and kill them. Well exactly HOW does the white blood cell kill germs? Let me tell you something that 9,999 out of 10,000 MDs don't know. Your white blood cells produce a little *hydrogen peroxide*, and they bathe the germs in the peroxide, and this kills the germs! It has always been peroxide that *naturally* cured infection in your body!

Did you know that hydrogen peroxide is made in the atmosphere, and that it comes down in our rainwater, and it kills off a certain amount of living organisms in the soil? If it were not for this peroxide, the earth's surface would be putrid from bacterial overgrowth. What I'm trying to convey to you, is that peroxide is a wonderfully natural, beneficial molecule.

This is not to say that peroxide cannot be harmful. Humans can tolerate just so much of the stuff, and that's why **you should have peroxide treatments only from a well trained physician**. As far as I'm concerned, if the doctor hasn't studied the IBOM protocols, he's not prepared to do a good job with peroxide.

POSSIBLE SIDE EFFECTS

There are some POTENTIAL side effects to IV peroxide. I say *potential* because, in truth, I hardly ever see undesirable side effects. But I want you to know about them. Here in Arizona, where my office is located, intravenous hydrogen peroxide is considered *experimental*. I may give you peroxide treatments, but I must follow all the rules and regulations for doing *experimental medicine*. Foremost is that you be fully informed about what I am about to do, and that includes understanding potential side effects. So here goes.

1. The most common side effect is **vein inflammation**, right where the IV is going in your arm. There can be pain, and if it occurs, there's little to do except change the location of the needle. If you have a big vein, such as in the elbow crease, that's a great place to place the IV. The bigger the vein, the less likely any discomfort. Magnesium is added to the IV and this reduces the likelihood of any pain also.

2. You can get a **red streak** up your arm, starting right where the needle is inserted. There are *two kinds* of red streaks. One kind of streak is *completely harmless* and goes away within 20 minutes of finishing the IV. The other red streak *means that the vein is getting inflamed,* and we've got to change the needle insertion.

3. A few people get a **chest sensation, with a shortness of breath feeling** after the infusion has been running for a while. It was thought that this was oxygen bubbling off in the lungs . . . . but that's not so. We don't know what causes this sensation, but we know that it's okay to continue the infusion. I prefer to slow the infusion down anyway,or discontinue it, if you've had most of the treatment.

4. Another side effect is **chills**. You can feel a little chilly because peroxide can throw off temperature regulation for a short while.

5. The next side effect is called a **Herxheimer Reaction**, also called **a die-off reaction**. Actually, it's a good sign, but you don't think so when it's happening. If you've got a lot of candida (or yeast) or a lot of infection, when the peroxide kills the yeast, your body will react to the dead, disintegrating yeast until it is eliminated from the body. You can have **chills, nausea, body aches, weakness and headaches** during this time. It can happen following one, two, or three treatments, and then it ceases. You can't predict in whom it will happen. If you get a Herxheimer reaction, why not look on the bright side? Your candida is on the way out! You are about to feel better.

6. Finally, because **peroxide intensifies the anticoagulant action of the drug Coumadin**, the doctor has to reduce the Coumadin dose *if you're taking it*.

That's pretty much the downside of peroxide therapy.

Question: If there was nothing wrong with you, and you took peroxide therapy for no reason at all, would it be harmful? Absolutely not! It would act like a *tune-up* to your body.

PEROXIDE IN AUSTRALIA, ENGLAND, AND FOREIGN COUNTRIES

Here in the USA we use a concentration of peroxide which has been shown to be very safe. But higher concentrations (as much as *four times* higher) have been used both in the USA and in foreign countries. The results using higher concentrations seem to be better, and I'm often tempted to use them. The problem is that higher concentrations *can irritate and cause sclerosing of veins*. **Sclerosing means that the inflamed walls of the veins develop a scar tissue within them, which makes them tender to the touch,**

and hard or ropy. The condition could go away in a few weeks or may *never* go away.

Now a patient with cancer may say, "Look, I want the strongest dose that you think may help me. My life is on the line, and I don't give a damn about some tender, hard veins." On the other hand, a person with shingles or the flu, may not care to risk permanent change in a vein, just to improve the likely outcome of their *temporary* dilemma. Here in Arizona, I'm sworn to go with the safer protocol . . . . *unless you sign a written waiver*, saying that you understand the risk, and you desire to take the risk.

SIGNING INFORMED CONSENTS

Regardless what concentration of peroxide is to be used, you are going to have to sign a permit before the doctor is going to perform IV peroxide on you. That's because the bulk of doctors in the USA consider peroxide *non-customary, experimental, unnecessary, weird, strange, or unusual* therapy. So the doctor who gives peroxide needs to protect his reputation by getting full-disclosure releases called *informed consents*. I've always been honest with my patients, and told them that my permits basically say, *"I can do anything I like to you, but you can't do anything to me!"* At my office you'll be asked to sign no less than two consents!

WILL INSURANCE OR MEDICARE PAY?

No! Most medical insurance companies, including Medicare, have been financially depleted by paying for large numbers of expensive surgeries and procedures. Segments of the health care industry profit from these surgeries and procedures, *and* they are politically powerful. Physicians who review claims for insurance companies often favor the extremely expensive or risky procedures while refusing payment for a more beneficial, far less expensive and often safer therapy. While insurance companies do not specifically exclude peroxide therapy in their policies, patients often have to resort to the courts in order to collect their insurance benefits.

HOW TO BEGIN PEROXIDE THERAPY

Each state is different, but in general, if you're going to start peroxide therapy, you're going to have to follow some rules established for receiving an *experimental* therapy because that's what peroxide is *usually* considered.

That means that you will likely need a *history and a physical exam* which goes somewhat beyond just your chief complaint. *Some lab work or other tests* might be needed also. You should obtain your past medical records which support your diagnosis, so that repeating tests becomes unnecessary and the diagnosis becomes clearer.

Now, if you've got the flu, for example, well then you've got the flu and there's no time nor reason to do a pile of tests. A short examination and history is all you'll need before sitting down for your treatment. But for any chronic illness the doctor will want to talk to you for a while and design a plan for treating the problem, using peroxide, and anything else which might be useful.

Now that you know the facts, I hope that you will schedule an appointment with your peroxide doctor real soon.....,

Index A

DIAGNOSES TREATED BY VARIOUS CLINICIANS USING I.V. PEROXIDE WITH VARYING DEGREES OF SUCCESS
(c/o L.B.O.M.)

1. Asthma
2. Emphysema
3. Chronic Obstructive Lung Disease (COPD)
4. Cardiovascular Disease
5. Cerbrovascular Disease
6. Alzheimer
7. Peripheral Vascular Disease
8. Arrhythmias (Irregular heart rhythms)
9. Influenza
10. Herpes Simplex (Cold Sores)
11. Herpes Zoster (Shingles)
12. Temporal Arteritis
13. Migraine headaches
14. Cluster headaches
15. Vascular headaches
16. Coronary artery spasm with angina
17. Chronic Epstein-Bar Virus infection, infectious mononucleosis
18. Diabetes Type H
19. HIV Infections
20. Hepatitis
21. Parasitic infections, various
22. Fungal infections, various
23. Bacterial infections, particularly chronic unresponsive infections
24. Candidiasis
25. Chronic pain syndromes, various
26. Pain of metastatic cancer
27. Environmental allergies
28. Early multiple sclerosis
29. Rheumatoid arthritis

In the original booklet, *A Closer Look at Intravenous Hydrogen Peroxide*, Dr. Gordon Josephs acknowledged Phyne Pharmaceuticals for absorbing the cost of the booklets for free distribution to physicians.

Lyme Arthritis Disease
by Anthony di Fabio

Lyme disease is far more widespread than our established medical profession and state health authorities are willing to admit. Virtually every state is a source of the spirocheate that causes this disability.

One reason for the unwillingness to admit the truth is the assumption that vacationing visitors will avoid the state, and so there is very often denial, or, at the least, a lack of funds for an objective study of the diseases's geography and health influence.

Current medical practices are generally inefficient and often a failure, leaving a percentage of the Lyme arthritis vicitms with the horrible prospects of a life that will continually go downhill.

One can understand that tourist money is involved in denial of Lyme arthritis' widespread existence. One cannot comprehend denial of good treatments or denial of alternative treatments enforced by the medical powers that exist. We've known more than one doctor who has had their license threatened or revoked because they'd step out of the cookbook approved by state authorities. The fact that their alternative treatment worked was not a factor in authority's decisions.

A cookbook approach to the practice of medicine, by the way, is one of the most inefficient and deadliest of approaches to the practice of medicine. Only incompetent, ill-educated or ignorant authorities would insist on such approches for patients.

Discovery of Lyme Disease

Rheumatoid Disease, consisting of perhaps a 100 differently named medical phenomena, but all related to collagen tissue damage, seems to be a response to many different factors: bacterial, viral, protozoal, yeast/fungal, poor nutrition, allergy, aging (free radicals), and so on.

While it is not unusual for a person to respond to a particular, single treatment, most often what seems to be an incorrigible health problem must be tackled from many different sources at once, say, nutritional, medical, Candidiasis treatment, allergy treatment, chelation therapy, and so on, depending upon the person and the problem.

The unlucky invasion of *Borrelia burgdorferi*, the spiral-shaped microbe injected by at least one species of tick, *Ixodes scapularis*, seems to present the unwitting victim with arthritic symptoms that also may require more than one approach for its solution. Thankfully, if diagnosed early enough, antibiotics can easily wipe out the invading population, and bring about swift remission. The antibiotics, of course, should be heavily accompanied with *Lactobaccilus acididophilus*[1], so that while treating the Lyme Disease, we do not also unwittingly bring about a fungal infection of Candidiasis. There are about 1,200 cases of Lyme Disease reported across the United States each year; there were 1,282 cases reported in 1934.

The disease remains concentrated along the coastal plain of the Northeast and mid-Atlantic region, in the upper Midwest, and along the Pacific coast, although the disease has been reported in every state.

66

In a *Science News* report, researchers at the University of Connecticut Health Center in Farmington and the Yale-New Haven Hospital examined 70 children diagnosed with Lyme Arthritis Disease and found that only 53% actually harbored the Lyme-causing bacterium *Borrelia burgdorferi*. The remaining 47% had been misdiagnosed.[4]

There is some hysteria regarding the incidence of this disease, possibly due to extensive adverse publicity. One thousand two hundred and eighty-two cases out of perhaps several hundred thousand with tick bites is not exactly a national emergency, although for a percentage of those afflicted, the disease can be rather significant and even catastrophic.

Lyme disease has the following symptoms: begins with reddened area that doesn't itch, resulting from tick bite, but expands over time, measuring several inches across; clearing of bite area begins in the center resembling a bull's-eye; flu-like symptoms: chills, fever, fatigue, joint and muscle pain; may develop a rash which disappears in a few days; may have tingling and numbness; non-symmetrical joint problems; other symptoms may also occur; sometimes sensitivity to light, stiff neck, headache, sleepiness, mood changes and memory loss; swelling and aching joints for months or years at a time; and vague, migrating musculature pains.

The characteristics of Lyme Disease were first laid out in 1975 when two mothers were told that their children had Juvenile Rheumatoid Arthritis. The name "Juvenile" does not distinguish it's clinical pattern from that of "Adult" Rheumatoid Arthritis, but merely tells the parent that this horrible, crippling disease occurred in their child, a fact that most parents already know. What is new is the diagnoses of "Rheumatoid Arthritis."

These two mothers soon learned that many other children and adults in their geographical region were afflicted with the same symptoms, and since Rheumatoid Arthritis does not seem to cluster in a regional geography (with some exceptions), Dr. Stephen E. Malawista of Yale University, among others, began to look for a source of this apparently new disease. Dr. Malawista discovered that many of his patients suffered from a range of symptoms among which might be those that resembled Rheumatoid Arthritis.

The cause of Lyme Disease was determined to be a microbe transmitted by a tick, in this first instance, from the species *Ixodes capularis*. Since this tick was common in the grasses and woods near Lyme, Connecticut, the cluster of symptoms obtained the name "Lyme Disease."

As Dr. Willy Burgdorfer, who worked for Rocky Mountain Laboratories in Hamilton, MT, identified the damaging microbe, the bacteria was named *Borrelia burgdorferi*, which is a spiral-shaped bacterium similar in shape to the spirochete, *Treponema pallidum*, which causes syphilis.

Since this initial set of discoveries, it's clear that similar diseases have existed in Australia, Africa, Europe and Asia. It also appears in every one of the states in the United States, but seems to be particularly common in northern California, Minnesota and the northeast.

Infection by *Borrelia burgdorferi* occurs chiefly in the spring, summer or early fall, because of the life cycle of the *Ixodes scapularis* tick.

Three Stages of *Borrelia burgdorferi*

There are three stages to the life cycle of the tick, and at each stage they have a favorite host, although they will attach themselves to a range of animals, including the human species.

The larva from *Ixodes scapularis* emerges in the summer from eggs deposited in the spring, and attaches itself to a small vertebrate such as a white-footed mouse, where it imbibes its first meal. If this mouse is infected with *Borrelia burgdorferi* spirochetes, the larva feeding on the mouse's blood, will also become infected.

Later, the larva molts into a nymph, and during the spring and summer (usually mid-May through July) this nymph takes a second meal. If the larva was infected, it may very well pass *Borrelia burgdorferi* onto its second host. This nymph is now about the size of a small seed, say, a poppy seed, and is responsible for most human infections.

The nymph molts again, and by October is the size of a larger seed, like an apple's. Again this tick feeds, at least by winter or spring, and they also mate to produce eggs that begin the cycle all over again. Usually ticks do their mating on white-tailed deer, which is why they are referred to as a "deer tick".

In some regions of the United States, between 15 and 30 percent of the *Ixodes scapularis* nymph and adult ticks are infected with *Borrelia burgdorferi* — some 50 percent of adult ticks are infected. The adult ticks are more likely to infect humans because they have had more opportunity, throughout their life-cycle, to do so.

About 1 to 3 percent of adults who are bitten by the infected tick contract Lyme disease, meaning that a high percentage of those infected are able to master the infection.

The tick attaches itself to the skin of its host, where it takes its meal of blood. At this time *Borrelia burgdorferi* begins to multiply in the gut of the tick, whence it crosses into the tick's circulation system, migrating to the salivary glands and passing with the tick's saliva through the host's skin.

A tick must be attached to its host for 36 to 48 hours before an infectious dose of *Borrelia burgdorferi* is transmitted. This is fortunate, because most folks who are bitten by a tick will find it prior to the infectious event.

Lyme Disease Symptoms

Those infected by the bacteria *Borrelia burgdorferi* usually have a set of characteristic symptoms:

Stage I Symptoms

1. About 60% will notice a round rash called an erythema chronicum migrans (ECM), as doctors like to have a nice, neat name for everything they observe.

2. Three days to a month later there will be a redness at or near the site of the tick bite.

3. The reddened area does not itch or hurt, but it will expand over time until it may measure several inches across.

4. There is a clearing that begins in the center, as the rash enlarges, resembling a bulls-eye. Some may acquire the rash, but fail to see these characteristics because of the bite's location.

5. The rash may disappear within weeks or even days.

6. Days or weeks later, a variety of other early symptoms affecting many areas of the body appears, and these symptoms are thought to be from the spread of the spirochete to many different tissues through the blood stream. The symptoms will include flulike symptoms, such as chills, fever, fatigue, joint and muscle pains, and loss of appetite.

Stage II Symptoms

Weeks to months later, about 10% of those afflicted will experience transient heart dysfunction. There will be varying degrees of heart blockage. Neurologic abnormalities include headaches, profound fatigue, meningitis, cranial nerve problems (neuropathies), including fascial palsies, and sensory and motor nerve problems.

Cardiac problems occur with 5 to 10 percent of those infected, if they have been untreated. Usually this condition is not noticed by the infected person, but can be detected by a physician. The heart irregularities persist for but a week to 10 days and probably will not require the use of a pacemaker.

Early symptoms may also include mild musculoskeletal disturbances, where patients complain of vague, migrating pain without swelling in muscles, tendons or joints. The jaw, the temporomandibular joint, may be affected. These symptoms, too, will decrease in weeks to months.

However, in about a half a year after the initial infection, 50% of those infected (without treatment) will suffer episodes of obvious arthritis, including the symptoms of swelling and discomfort in one or more joints, but often the knee.

Stage III Symptoms

Ten percent of those who reach the "arthritic" point will go on to suffer chronic Lyme Arthritis. These patients will find joints swelling for months at a time, or certain joints will become enlarged and achy for a year or more.

In these latter stages, joints, the central nervous system and the skin may be involved. Arthritis can develop from a few weeks to several years after Stage I. Sixty percent suffer at least one episode of arthritis if untreated. Usually the joint arthritis is but one-sided, and migration of the joint pain may prefer the larger joints, especially the knees.

Attacks may last for weeks or months, although they may also become less frequent over time and eventually disappear, leaving about 10% with damaged joints.

Sometimes neurological problems also appear, in about 20 percent of untreated patients, including Bell's palsy. Bell's palsy is one of our listed "Rheumatoid Diseases," a collagen tissue disease, and so there must be more than one causation for that affliction[2].

Other neurological afflictions include meningitis (sensititivty to light, stiff neck, headache), encephalitis (sleepiness, mood changes, memory loss), and radiculoneuropathy, where the roots of nerves that stem from the spinal cord to the periphery of some level of the body becomes irritated. These regions may be painful, tingle, or even go numb.

In traditional Rheumatoid Arthritis, a joint affected on one side of the body will also have a matching joint affected on the other side of the body. This is not true for Lyme Arthritis where only one joint may be affected on one side of the body.

Although the skin, heart, joints and nervous system are usually targeted, as the *Borrelia burgdorferi* bacteria can invade any system in the body, every organ or system in the body can also produce its own variation of symptoms. This ability to invade all human systems, too, is a similarity to the syphilis spirochete.

Traditional and Untraditional Treatments

Thankfully, if diagnosed early enough, antibiotics can easily wipe out the invading population, and bring about swift remission. (The antibiotics, of course, should be heavily accompanied with *Lactobaccilus acididophilus*1 so that while treating the Lyme Disease, we do not also unwittingly bring about a fungal infection of candidiasis.)

The key to solving Lyme Arthritis is early diagnoses and antibiotic treatment. Early diagnoses can be difficult, especially when the characteristic rash is not present. Since flulike symptoms can arise from many different sources, as described in Dr. Paul Pybus' *The Herxheimer Effect*[3], it becomes most difficult for a physician to make an early diagnoses. The patient's history, especially their recent exposure to woods, ticks, and bites, and especially noting the characteristic bulls-eye lesions on the skin, all are most important for early diagnosis.

Although a definitive test for *Borrelia burgodrferi* bacteria is possible, the test is presently a low-yield procedure. A direct examination of body fluids and tissues is not recommended because there will be so few organisms found. There are no good blood tests that can make an early diagnoses of Lyme Arthritis within the time length required for an early diagnosis, although surely someone, somewhere is working on or has developed such an early test, probably based on DNA of the microorganism. Blood testing for antibodies to Lyme bacteria is generally not necessary or helpful in early stage disease, but it can help in diagnosis in later stages. (Antibodies are produced by the body to attack the bacteria and can be evidence of exposure to the bacteria. These antibodies can be detected using a laboratory method called an enzyme-linked immunosorbent assay [ELISA].) Antibodies, however, can be false indicators of disease, since they can persist for years after the disease is cured. Moreover, false-positive tests in patients with nonspecific findings (those that are not specifically suggestive of Lyme disease) can lead to confusion. Currently, the confirmatory test that is most reliable is the Western Blot assay antibody test. More accurate tests are being developed. The study of body serums, serology, using indirect immunofluorescent assay or enzyme-linked immunoabsorbant assay has a slow antibody response and is positive in but 50% of Stage I infections, and should antibiotics be used, the test is often aborted.

Since Lyme Arthritis is potentially disabling, extreme vigilance must be taken by those who traverse woods and grasses, but overall, it may not cause serious problems for more than 10 percent of those who have received *Borrelia burgdorferi* through a tick bite.

Many who think they have Lyme Arthritis actually suffer from other forms of disease states, but among those who are found among the 10 percent seriously affected, there seems to be no good solution to the problem, because, after the early stage of the disease, antibiotics seem to be ineffective.

The primary problems with traditional treatments consists of the following: (1) Inability to diagnose the disease early without specific noting of the bulls-eye lesions, or having at hand an accurate, clear, case history. This delay affects treatment response by use of antibiotics, and often also causes over-extended usage of antibiotics; (2) Over-extended usage of antibiotics increases overgrowth of organisms-of-opportunity in the intestinal tract, such as *Candida albicans*, which condition also creates additional disease states, including some that mimic various arthritides forms, and also increases food allergies over time; (3) Many treated cases linger with pain, increasing systemic damage, and lessened vigor over many years, often ending up with damaged organs and joints.

There is hope, however.

Alternative Treatments

Anti-Amoebic (Anti-Microbial) Treatment

Gus J. Prosch, M.D., Jr. formerly of Birmingham, Alabama suggested a trial of the Rheumatoid Arthritis or Rheumatoid Disease treatment protocol as recommended by The Arthritis Trust of America/The Rheumatoid Disease Foundation: "I've seen Lyme Arthritis Disease clear up after using a course of anti-microorganism drugs as recommended by Professor Roger Wyburn-Mason for Rheumatoid Diseases.

"Although Lyme Arthritis Disease, and other diseases such as Gout, Carpal Tunnel Syndrome, and Tendinitis are not supposed to be the same kind of diseases as Rheumatoid Arthritis, I've seen them all respond one time or another to the same treatment we use for Rheumatoid Arthritis."[19]

In the case of Lyme Arthritis Disease, Dr. Prosch will give metronidazole (or one of the other 5-nitroimidazoles described) in heavier doses, for a longer period of time than recommended for Rheumatoid Disease.

Artificial Fever and Herbs

Agatha Thrash, M.D. and Calvin Thrash, M.D. write that "About one-third of patients with chronic infectious arthritis derive substantial benefits from fever treatments, one-third derive only moderate benefits, and one-third little or no help.

"In gonococcal arthritis, swelling and pain is often astonishingly helped. Patients suffering from [Osteoarthritis] receive temporary benefit, and the fever treatments may be used along with general arthritis treatment of diet and physical conditioning."[24]

The Case of John Woodworth

Agatha M. Thrash, M.D., Uchee Pines Institute, Seale, Alabama was visited by a 54 year old Caucasian with Lyme Arthritis Disease. John had typical symptoms of pain in the joints, neurologic symptoms and specific rash beginning with a small, raised, red area and spreading concentrically outward with fading in the mid-portion.

Dr. Thrash administered a series of 15 fever treatments in which the mouth temperature was brought up to 103 degrees Fahrenheit as many times as possible during the 15 treatments, each day. John took five treatments, then skipped 2 days and repeated this schedule 3 times.

Dr. Thrash writes: "Once in a great while a person with Lyme Disease does not clear completely with the first series of 15 treatments and must take a second series. This was the case with John Woodworth. We waited 3 weeks between series to give the body a good chance to reset the immune system. Fever enhances the effectiveness of the immune system, but the body adapts to the fever and the response begins to weaken after about 5 days. For this reason we skip 2 days each week and rest 1 to 3 weeks between series."

John also was given golden seal and echinacea, the first being anti-bacterial, and the second being a boost to the immune system. "The way to make it is by bringing a quart of water to a gentle simmer, adding 1 tablespoon of golden seal root powder and 1 heaping tablespoon of echinacea (chopped whole plant). It should be simmered for 20 to 25 minutes, cooled, strained, and drunk throughout the day. Make it up fresh every day.

"On the first day in chronic cases, and for 5 to 10 days during the acute phase, the patient should take 2 quarts of the tea daily. The patient should also take Nutri-biotic[TM] (grapefruit seed extract) obtainable from any health food store. Put 6 to 15 drops in a quart of water or tea and drink 2 quarts a day."

Dr. Thrash says that "We have had several typical cases of Lyme Disease, complete with the tick bite and rash, which have been treated with a series of artificial fever treatments. None of them, including John Woodworth, has had further illness, as long as 2 years follow-up later."[18]

Homeopathic Remedy
According to Stephen Tobin, D.V.M.

Stephen Tobin, D.V.M.,[31] is a veterinarian in a Lyme Arthritis Disease infested region. He's treated many cases of Lyme Disease in dogs, cats and horses.

After trying a number of homeopathic remedies, he settled on Ledum (Genus Epidemicus) in a 200 or 1M potency, three times a day for three days. Dr. Tobin says, "Every animal treated this way has shown immediate improvement, whether they were only recently infected or have had the disease for years, treated or not with antibiotics. A number of pet owners, on seeing how well it cured their companions, took it themselves, with equally good results.

"As a preventative, I use the *Borrelia burgdorferi* nosode 60X, giving one dose daily for one week, then one dose per week for one month, then one dose every six months, the same way I administer all the nosodes I give in place of vaccinations.

"I have had only one failure in almost two hundred animals so treated. This is more effective than the vaccine for Lyme Disease used in dogs, which often has the effect of producing symptoms of Lyme Disease, including lameness, swollen joints, lethargy, inappetance (lack of appetite), kidney failure, and cruciate degeneration (cross-shaped as in the cruciate ligaments of the knee)

"I have seen no side effects from the nosode itself."

According to Dr. Catherine Russell

Although rare in Mexico, Dr. Catherine Russell,[30] Guadalajara, Mexico, successfully treats Lyme Arthritis Disease just as she would any other arthritis. She uses proteolytic enzymes, niacinamide 500 mg 3 X daily, and homeopathic symptomatic medicine according to individual symptoms and modalities. Sometimes she also uses herbs, especially stinging nettle which she picks and prepares herself, especially when a lot of uric acid is involved.

Venus Fly Trap Carnivora Treatment

Carnivora is an extract of the Venus Fly Trap plant (*Dionaea muscipula*) that was developed by the German oncologist (cancer specialist) Helmut Keller, M.D.

According to medical reporter Morton Walker, D.P.M.,[22] "Since 1981, over 2,000 patients have been treated with Carnivora. Among them has been President Ronald Reagan who received the substance postoperatively following his operation for malignant polyps of the colon. The President took Carnivora drops for their healing and preventive powers against cancer recurrence."

"Actor Yul Brynner also received dosages of Carnivora in injections and/ or Carnivora drops." Yul Brynner's lung tumor's were rapidly diminishing in size until he foolishly followed the recommendation of a New York City oncologist and failed to keep up with the remedy."

"Carnivora has a proven 82 to 87% remission rate for most types of carcinoma when the patient's immune system has not been compromised by conventional, allopathic chemotherapy or radiation therapy."[22]

As Carnivora is a relatively new product, no one knows how many different organisms it can inhibit, or kill. In addition to its immune stimulating properties, the Carnivora extract "has been used successfully for the treatment of chronic diseases including most forms of cancer, neurodermitis, ulcerative colitis, Crohn's disease, multiple sclerosis, all types of herpes infections, primary chronic polyarthritis, and almost any immune deficiency state," and AIDS.

After it's use, Harvey Bigelsen, M.D. was so impressed with the reduction of pleomorphic organisms in a patient's blood that he ordered a supply of Carinvora for his own use.[22] Pleomorphic organisms are microorganisms that change form and function depending upon their surrounding environmental conditions.

Dorothea M. Linley, M.D.

Dorothea M. Linley, M.D. says, "In August 1986, I came down with a flu-like illness: pains in muscles, back, headache, fatigue and even my hair was painful. Fever and migrating arthritis followed by cardiac fibrillation which was controlled by oral magnesium. A blood test for Lyme disease was positive. . . .

"It settled in my knees, the left swelling so severely I needed crutches. I took 1 gram of tetracycline daily for 3 weeks and then 2 grams daily for three more weeks. Then my stomach rebelled and it was stopped.

"I was left with 50% reduced motion in both knees. Three months later I learned that the North (negative, south seeking) magnet would reduce swelling and pain. I applied a North pole magnet to both knees for 30 minutes twice a day[5]. In one week my knee flexion was doubled. In 6 months flexion was almost normal except for something that didn't feel right in the middle of the joint.

"Two months later I experimented with germanium sesquioxide[6]. On a dose of 900 mg daily the right knee returned to normal in 3 days and after reducing the dose to 300 mg daily, the left knee took about 2 months to become normal . . . .

"I was 5 years without any symptoms.

"In May 1992 my left knee started swelling and a blood test was positive for Lyme. Whether this was a new case or a return of the first attack I do not know. What I did know was that I had no desire to take antibiotics again. I had just finished treatment for Candidiasis[7].

"In mid-July I learned about Carnivora [*Dionaea muscipula*, Venus Fly Trap plant extract] from Morton Walker's article in the *Townsend Letter for Doctors*[8]. I learned that Carnivora would kill bacteria, yeast, parasites and viruses without harming beneficial intestinal bacteria.

"I believe the Carnivora has killed the Lyme bactria as well as Candida overgrowth. I lost 10 pounds, my skin is younger looking, my bowels are functioning normally for the first time in my life, my fingernails are hard and growing well, and my digestion is improved, needing fewer digestive aids.

"I hope my story will help those many patients suffering from chronic illness which may be due to Lyme. I was fortunate in that I did not take antibiotics until after a positive blood test. Those who treat symptoms clinically typical of Lyme before developing a positive blood test will never test positive and thus obscure the diagnosis. There are many people out there in this situation."

Neurokinesiological Testing and Herbal Remedies of Louis Marx, M.D.
Louis Marx, M.D. Recommended Treatment

Louis J. Marx, M.D.[11] combines neurokinesiology as a research and diagnostic tool with herbal programs.

A simple explanation of kinesiology given by Dr. Marx is that "if you touch a blocked acupuncture point while testing a muscle, that muscle will test weak. . . . Kinesiology is a technique for testing the integrity of the energy supply to an organ, as evidenced by a specific muscle. It uses the concept of organ-muscle linkage. . . . Any muscle can be used.

"Neurokinesiology differs from applied and other forms of kinesiology by not relying on the organ-muscle linkage . . . it tests directly through the nervous system . . . Dr. Calvin Alldredge has developed reflex points for the various known and unknown infections, hormonal system, nutritional status and toxic substance. By testing through the nervous system we are getting responses from the body's innate intelligence."

In Dr. Marx's *Neurokinesiological Testing and Herbal Remedies*, writing on herbal remedies (tinctures or capsules), he says, " Most programs last about three weeks. Usually, the patient experiences an improvement from a program within a day or two. However, during the third week after beginning a program, the patient may feel a decline in well-being and may develop new symptoms. It is very important to understand what is happening to avoid discouragement and loss of confidence in the treatment.

Here are more books by Louis J. Marx, M.D., *Healing Dimensions of Herbal Medicine, Neurokinesiological Testing and Herbal Remedies*; Ventura, CA 93003.

"What really happens is that the herbals have just about resolved those problems being treated, and the immune system no longer has to concern itself with those specific disorders. Therefore, the immune system starts attacking another group of infections, etc. This can happen a number of times with some patients. However, each group of new programs brings more energy and well-being than the prior programs. Expect this and explain it to the patient so they will not get discouraged.

"Sometimes a patient may present a specific complaint and testing identifies a specific factor as causing that complaint. However, after taking the program for that problem, the symptom remains. If you retest, you will identify another basis for the symptom which was not identified in your first examination. It is like the problem has layers to it, and as one layer is uncovered, a deeper one surfaces. Occasionally, you may need to treat two or three factors before there is a final resolution of the complaint. Usually the response is rapid enough and dramatic enough to leave little doubt about the benefit of the herbal programs."

Dr. Marx, using neurokinesiological testing and herbal remedies, has developed a combination of herbal recommendations for almost every disease condition. These include, but are not limited to, viruses (assorted, intestinal, liver, herpes, wart, immune, life force), parasites, bacteria, Mycoplasma, rickettsia, yeast/fungi, onco genes (involved in cancer), and even the will to live.

Dr. Marx says, "Once you learn the system, you can apply it to any remedy. You can test your foods, supplements, drugs, etc.

"The drops can be put in water or juice, or taken directly into the mouth. The amount of alcohol ingested is negligible, and many reformed alcoholics tolerate the tincture well without inducing a craving for alcohol.

"The capsules are best taken after meals. The capsules and tinctures do not need to be taken at the same times of day. All the tinctures or extracts can be taken together. If there are six bottles of liquids to be taken, they all can be put in a small amount of juice. Shake and drink followed by some extra juice to chase down the taste. It is actually better to squeeze the dropper top and squirt out one dropper full. It is more accurate than counting out the drops.

That's because some of the liquids are thicker, therefore, have larger drops.

"If the extracts or tinctures are too thick, just add a few drops of water to the bottles.

"Most herbal programs contain three bottles — one bottle of cut dried herbs in capsules. There are 70 caps to each bottle. The other two are one half ounce bottles of liquid extracts or tinctures. On each of these bottles are letters AO, RVO, VO, JRVO just before the program name. These letters stand for the extractants used in making the formula. A stands for alcohol, O stands for oil, R stands for rice water, V stands for vinegar, and J stands for fruit juice. T stands for tincture, and so (T)-(AO) stands for tincture of oil in an alcohol base. SPIRO- (L) would stand for the Lyme Spirochete.

Louis J. Marx, M.D. recommends that herbal remedies be ordered from Monastery of Herbs, PO Box 3123, Granada Hills, CA . There are other good sources, but best one check through a health professional, as many herbs are either not what they are supposed to represent, or have been degraded throughout its delivery and storage cycle.

In the case of Lyme Arthritis Disease, Dr. Marx recommends the use of:

(T)-(AO)   SPIRO-(L) @ 30 drops/day for 1/2 Fld. Oz
(T)-(RVO) SPIRO-(L) @ 30 drops/day for 1/2 Fld. Oz
Herbal Blend   SPIRO-(L) @ 4 Capsules/day for 50 Caps.

The Case of Pearl Bennette Atkin, R.N., M.A., C.S.

Where Carnivora extract helped one person, it seemed to become a burden for another. Pearl Atkin, RN, MA, CS, Briarcliff Manor, New York, fought against Lyme disease, to win. Healer Atkin[10] wrote to *Townsend Letter for Doctors* for advice in November 1992, saying:

"In June of 1984 I attended a professional conference in the wooded town of Armonk, New York. Within a couple of weeks I had flu-like symptoms — aches and pains all over my body, especially a headachy feeling each afternoon, and discomfort in my coccyx area. After the summer cold the aches and pains subsided, but I continued to experience a 'hypoglycemia-type' of late afternoon problem, which I took care of with a fruit and nut snack, and sometimes with an ounce or two of vodka.

"But even after that, I was still left with an aching coccyx, and at that point I decided my mattress had to be traded for a softer, more luxurious type — such as deep innerspring, or foamy and waterbed types. I had always thought that a waterbed was decadent — until that summer. When I first tried out a waterbed, I was able to get comfortable on it in a second — and my coccyx felt good in any position!

"Then, after about six weeks of these unpleasant symptoms, as I was finally sleeping a little more comfortably at night, . . . an official from the conference that I had attended 8 weeks before called to ask how I felt, and asked if I had [any of about 40 symptoms] — and I'd experienced many of them. I had recently turned 50, and felt that [age] was the reason — now I knew differently — I had Lyme [Arthritis] Disease.

"I was given the name of a Westchester Lyme [Arthritis Disease] specialist. I called him, then went for a consultation, and told him about my symptoms. Blood was drawn, and I was put on 7-10 days of tetracycline 240 mg 4 times a day. I was informed that, although I had not had the classic bull's-eye — I had had a rashy welt initially on my forehead that I thought was poison ivy — two weeks later it had spread down to my neck and chin areas — I would know it was 'Lyme' if, after taking each tetracycline capsule I would have an exacerbation of the headachy, flu-like symptoms. That's exactly what happened. I continued taking the capsules until the exacerbation experience stopped — and then for a few more days — which was a total treatment of about 10-12 days. Yet the blood work was negative.

"During and for some time after the treatment period, I continued to be troubled, frequently, by the peculiar headaches, though I had hardly ever had headaches before. And these felt different from any I had experienced before. As they were miraculously cured, almost instantaneously, by a shot of vodka, it was my treatment of choice whenever they returned.

"That was the summer of 1984. Very gradually, over many months, the headaches became less frequent and less intense. But two years later, in 1986, my headachy symptoms flared again, and I again went on tetracycline 500 mg 4 times a day for 7-10 days. It did the trick this second time also.

"Two years later, in 1988, there was a third episode. I had the headachy feeling again, and the doctor gave me a choice of 7 days in the hospital with an intravenous (IV) drip of penicillin (which was the treatment of choice at that moment in time) — or I could try 7-10 days of tetracycline 500 mg again.

"I opted for the oral treatment, and took more vodka every afternoon with my snack parties!

"The headache receded to a low level that was tolerable and I went on about my life. [During these episodes, the first two measurements for Lyme antibodies (titers) were negative — but I understand that false negatives are common; then a third sample was taken, but that one was lost.]

"But now I'm right in the middle of it again — my fourth serious episode. This past summer I went to Eastern Europe on a genealogical tour and when I returned home I had a protracted case of 'jet lag.' One day I noticed a rashy welt in my pubic/groin area, and the next day I had 103 degree F temperature. I called my gynecologist — but he was on vacation. His 'covering' doctor called back, and we ran through the 'could be's — and came up with my fourth recurrence of Lyme Disease.

"He prescribed 500 mg of tetracyline 4 times a day again for 7-10 days. The temperature and rash were gone immediately! When I called my gynecologist the next week, he said I should continue on the tetracycline for 1 month — that was the protocol for Lyme this year.

"By the second week, however, the tetracycline was giving me nausea, queasiness, stomach and abdominal discomfort, and I was having headaches around the clock. So I called a doctor friend (an internist), and he changed me to Amoxicillin (straight penicillin 500 mg 3 times a day), for another 2 weeks.

"That treatment gave me back my appetite, and took the worst of the headaches away. But what else is it doing to my poor system? I've been taking *Lactibaccilus acidophilus*[1] to counteract the killing of the good intestinal microrganisms.

". . . I've paid no attention to Lyme Disease therapies the last few years, because I've had other things to deal with personally and professionally that seemed more important than a 'hypoglycemic headache' but now my spotlight [is] on Lyme Disease, . . ."

On December 1993, Pearl Atkin[12] described the great help she'd gotten, particularly from Lous Marx, M.D. of California. She wrote:

"I want to let you know how well I've been since you published my last 'Letter [in *Townsend Letter for Doctors and Patients*] . . . regarding my plea for help with my fourth Lyme Disease attack. Each time I have had a Lyme infection I have been treated with massive doses of antibiotics, but have nevertheless been left with a pattern of recurrent headaches identical to those experienced during the initial acute Lyme episodes. This last time the headaches were so severe that they were disorienting as well as disabling. For several months I could not remember what it was like to have a clear-thinking and pain-free head.

"One of your subscribers, Dr. Dorothea Linley from Connecticut, contacted me with information about a treatment that had been successful for her own chronic Lyme infection. She had been working with a nutritionist who advised Carnivora[22] (Venus Fly Trap extract) as part of a program that also included many vitamin supplements and glandulars. After I began this program my headaches cleared up about 70%. But each time I opened [and began using] a new bottle of Carnivora I had a recurrence of devastating flu-like symptoms[3] — high fever, and head and full body aches for 3 days. After three rounds of this (approximately 3 months) I stopped those treatments, as I decided to accept the 70% remission and live with it!

"At this time a physician — Dr. Louis Marx[11] — sent a copy of his herbal book to me, having earmarked the page on 'Spirochetes; Lyme Disease.' Reading this book, I was impressed with his work of the last 10 years on 'designer herbals' (with Dr. Clifford Alldridge), and called him to discuss my situation. He encouraged me to order the Spirochete-Lyme program — but told me to expect that it might not give me 100% relief, and also that I might need to do several more herbal programs, as one layer of disorder after another required attending to. . . .

"Within three days my headachy feeling that I have lived with for years was gone — and my head was clear as a bell! It was unbelievable, and extremely pleasurable."

Nutritional and Immune Support

The Case of Sarah Statesmyer

Sarah Statesmyer, age 16, came to the office of Robin Ellen Leder, M.D.,[29] in New Jersey, complaining of severe fatigue and episodes of debilitating joint pain, especially in her knees. Low energy made it extremely difficult for Sarah to do her work at a law firm on her bad days. She felt like she could barely walk. Her symptoms, she reported, had been ongoing since childhood.

Sarah's parents thought her problem stemmed from a tick bite years earlier, but a blood test was only suggestive of Lyme Arthritis Disease, and was not conclusive, probably because of the time that had passed since Sarah's first exposure to the *Borrellia burdorfi* organism. However, because of the described symptoms and probable history of Lyme Arthritis disease, this condition was considered to be the most likely cause of Sarah's problem.

Dr. Leder discussed traditional, possibly long-term, antibiotic therapy with Sarah, and also the importance of supporting the immune system in chronically symptomatic Lyme Arthritis Disease patients.

Sarah and her family chose to begin treatment using the nutritional approach offered by Dr. Leder.

To help design a diet that would benefit Sarah, Dr. Leder began by having Sarah take a six hour glucose tolerance test and a special blood test for food allergies. She was found to be quite hypoglycemic (tendency to low blood sugar), and also to have sensitivities to a number of foods.

Sarah's diet was changed and she was required to eat a minimum of five to six times per day, and every meal or snack was to include some form of protein. All foods that Sarah was allergic or sensitive to, according to her blood test, were eliminated from her diet.

Dr. Leder, according to her custom, also asked Sarah to eliminate other common foods that have a history of being allergenic, even though they were not on Sarah's list, and, in addition, to cut out any other foods that had any remote history suggestive of allergy.

A broad spectrum of nutritional supplements and plenty of water completed Sarah's program.

"With the help of an exceptionally supportive family, Sarah's symptoms literally disappeared, her energy was restored to a level normal for a healthy young woman, and, during several months of follow-up, no further flare-ups of her joint pain occurred."

Universal Oral Vaccination

When former Iowa Congressman Berkley Bedell[13] testified before the U.S. Senate Health Appropriations Subcommittee Chaired by Senator Tom Harkin, also of Iowa, on June 24, 1993, he gave witness to a powerful and obviously safe method of solving Lyme Arthritis Disease.

He described a procedure whereby the killed bacteria, *Borrelia burgdorferi*, was injected above a cow's udder, above the base of the teat, (where the antigen or allergen is sure to reach the cistern) prior to the birth of her calf. Colostrum — the cow's first milk after the calf is born — is processed into whey — the liquid left after milk has been coagulated by the aid of a coagulating enzyme called rennet.

Congress Bedell also gave witness to the effects of an over-powerful, suppressive governmental organization that would prevent people from trying every 1-1/2 hours for a few weeks the whey of this milk to learn if their Lyme Arthritis Disease will disappear. He reports that the company that cured him "dares not sell such a medicine, because of FDA regulations."[21]

Later the same farmer that cured Congressman Bedell of his Lyme Arthritis Disease prepared a homeopathic remedy which, Bedell reports, had 80-90% success in treating patients for whom conventional treatments had not been effective.

When specific personalities in the U.S. Department of Agriculture were shown in court to have falsified data regarding this patent — apparently as part of governmental suppression (although according to one source there may have been personality conflicts also) — it became only the second patent in U.S. history to receive by vote of U.S. Congress an additional 16 year lifetime protection.

On April 2, 1968, a patent number 3,376,198,23 "Method of Producing Antibodies in Milk," was granted to William E. Petersen, St. Paul, MN and Berry Campbell, Monrovia, California, assigned to Collins Products, Inc., Waukon, Iowa. Other patents for additional discoveries have since been granted to Mary E. Collins and Robert A. Collins (Patent No. 4,402,938; September 6, 1983; Gregory B. Wilson and Gary V. Paddock (March 28, 1989); Robert A. Collins and Philip F. Weighner (Patent No. 4,843,065; June 27, 1989); Robert Collins K (Patent No. 5,102,669; April 7, 1992)

The original work on development of the cows'-milk vaccine was performed at the University of Minnesota, School of Biochemistry under the direction of the patent asignees. (Porter: *Biological Abstracts* 1953, p. 951, par. 10, 185). In August, 1951, Dr. Porter, then "working on his doctoral thesis, suggested the possibility of manufacturing antibodies in the cow's udder by infusion of antigen into the udder of a lactating cow." (Patent No. 3,376,198)

A spokesman for a group that prefers not to be identified, says that the protective element "seems to be a system of peptides that is produced by the cow. . . . Basic research beginning in the late sixties was directed to identify the active products (biological and chemical) in the whey product. This has proven very difficult and especially because the activity is not an antibody per se, but appears to be the action of a low molecular weight material. [Complement, the end product of killing microorganisms, was discovered; 5,000 or less Daltons in molecular weight. See "Immune System Protection from Foreign Invaders" and "Universal Oral Vaccine," http://www.arthritistrust.org.]

"Several important activities can be found in the product that is produced by infusion of specific antigens into the udder (above the udder into the cistern) of a cow after collecting the colostrum and milk for the final product production. These are being researched.

Many people have used the product, and it seems not to matter whether the cow's colostrum is used, made into whey, the cow's milk is used, or a homeopathic remedy is prepared, whether or not pasteurized, whether or not lypholized (freeze dried), or pasteurized and lypholized — all are effective, although transfer factor, an additional protective substance, as described in one patent seems to be of higher yield in the colostrum.

Reminiscent of what has become the routine human use of dimethylsulfoxide (DMSO) or antiobiotics restricted by law to veterinarians and those practicing husbandry, marked "Not For Human Use," some dairy farmers purchase colostrum products for their animals' disease protection, but use the products on themselves with success.

Those with access to a cow can purchase standardized antigens (killed) or allergens from biological supply sources which can be innoculated through the cow's udder or into the base of the udder (into the cistern) at the proper time before calving. A variety or blend of organisms or substances — pollen, cat, dog, or cow hair if one is allergic, or specific antigens against a given disease condition — will result in a milk product — colostrum — that will cure and protect from an equally large and varied number of pathogenic organisms or allergens, respectively.

In homeopathic remedies produced by Beaumont Bio-Med, Waukon, Iowa, conditions claim to be aided are Rheumatism, Rheumatoid Arthritis, coughing, respiratory, sore throat, skin conditions, acne blemishes, upset stomach, cold and flu, diarrhea and impetigo.

(See "Universal Oral Vaccine" and "Homeoapthy for for Arthritics," http://www.arthritistrust.org.)

A few homeopathic remedies based on the described principles can be obtained from Beaumont Bio-Med, Waukon, Iowa.

As a general principle, this method (cow's specially prepared whey) will vaccinate safely against any allergen or antigen — any substances which when introduced into the body create antibodies such as allergenic pollens, house dust, animal hairs, or micro-organism proteins.

According to Patent Number 3,376,198, antigenic protections can be developed against "bacteria, viruses, proteins, animal tissue, plant tissue, spermatozoa, rickettsia, metazoan parasites, mycotic molds, fungi, pollens, dust and similar substances. . . . exemplary antigens include: bacterial — *Salmonella pullorum, Salmonella typhi, Salmonella paratyphi, Staphylococcus aureus, a Streptoccus agalactiae, g Streptococcus agalactiae, Staphylococcus albus, Staphylococcus pyogenes*, *E. Coli* pneumococci, streptococci, and the like; viral — Influenza type A, fowl pox, turkey pox, herpes simplex and the like; protein — egg albumin and the like; tissue — blood and sperm."

Protected, according to this and a later patent, were mice, cows, goats, chickens and pigs.

For allergy prevention, one can use a mixture of hair (cats, dogs, cattle), making a vaccine. (Many milk-producing farmers become allergic to cow's hair.) Other allergens, such as pollens, can also be introduced, such that many other allergies can be beneficially affected.

It's also good for chickenpox, cold sores, genital herpes, *Cryptocides sporidium*, and for anti-inflammatory conditions, as it is heavy with complement and anti-complement (C3B), substances that assist in the destruction of invasive organisms.

According to a source,[23] "One North Dakota support group uses this substance for multiple sclerosis with beneficial results."

In a 1984 study reported in *Medical Microbiology and Immunology*[32] IgA-rich cow colostrum containing anti-measles lactoglobulin resistant proteases was orally administed to patients with MS. Measles-positive antibody colostrum was orally administered every morning to 15 patients with multiple sclerosis at a daily dosage of 100 ml for 30 days. Similarly, measles-negative antibody control colostrum (< 8) was orally administered to 5 patients. Of 7 anti-measles colostrum recipients, 5 patients improved and 2 remained unchanged. Of 5 negative (< 8) recipients, 2 patients remained unchanged and 3 worsened. These findings suggested the efficacy of orally administered anti-measles colostrum in improving the condition of MS patients ($P < 0.05$).

The Case of Dorthy Johnson

Dorothy Johnson[28], 49 years-of-age, was diagnosed at the Mayo Clinic with multiple sclerosis, a slowly progressive Central Nervous System disease characterized by patches of demyelinated nerve tissue of the brain and spinal cord. Demyelination is the loss of insulative protective tissues that surround nerve tissue.

Dorothy suffered from varied and multiple neurological symptoms and signs, such as shakiness, numbness in legs, difficulty in climbing stairs, tingling in hands and feet, cramping of legs, and other symptoms.

Although multiple sclerosis may go into remission and then recur, often with greater severity, over a period of four years Dorothy became progressively worse, until she met Herb Saunders, a farmer who had been treating people for various conditions by the use of specially prepared colostrum from a cow.

Dorothy took 4 tablespoons of colostrum a day for two years, and gradually improved, until all of her symptoms disappeared.

When some symptoms did reappear after a period of time without the colostrum, her husband obtained three more bottles of specially prepared colostrum, and again the symptoms disappeared. She has continued without symptoms for several years.

The Case of Judith Toliver

Dorothy's experience was repeated by that of Judith Toliver,[28] 26 years-of-age, who was wheel-chair bound. Her blood was injected into the cistern of a cow, and the prepared colostrum given to her in the same manner as that described for Dorothy. After one year of treatment, she was able to walk upstairs with a cane.

Other Diseases

Early work using the described principle for Rheumatoid Arthritis involved staphylococcus and streptococcus killed organisms injected as antigens into the cow's cistern, the successful results thus strongly supporting the infectious nature of Rheumatoid Arthritis. As many forms of Rheumatoid Diseases and related diseases seem to have an infectious and/or allergenic component, such as Ankylosing Spondilitis, Candidiasis, Crohn's disease,

Fibrositis, Fibromyalgia, food allergies, rhinitis, and so on, this form of protection may be all-inclusive, inexpensive, and all-important.

According to one spokesperson,[23] "The homeopathic remedy derived from this process has been found useful for various forms of arthritis."

One hundred gallons of milk is taken from an innoculated cow, casein and fat separated by ultra-centrifuge, and pasteurized. It is then lypholized — freeze dried — that is the water is taken out under cold temperature. The resulting powder can then be used sub-lingually, or made into homeopathic remedies, or any other reasonable means for introducing it into the human or animal body.

The suppression of safe, workable treatments continues: The Minnesota diary farmer, Herb Saunders, 66, who cured Congressman Bedell, was prosecuted in St. James, Minnesota by the state prosecuting attorney for practicing medicine without a license. Herb was selling bovine colostrum ("first milk") as a potential cure for cancer. "Saunders would sell each patient a cow for $2,500, but keep the cow on his farm. He would inject a sample of each patient's blood into the cow's udder [cistern], and then sell the colostrum to the cow's owner for $35 a bottle. Saunders told an undercover state agent who posed as a cancer patient that he would 'cough out' his cancer within months if he would take colostrum, [and] refrain from chemotherapy.

"After two weeks of [court] trial — the longest this small community had ever seen — the result was a hung jury. The 6-person jury voted 5-1 to convict, but the last holdout, a part-time social studies teacher, apparently couldn't decide whether Saunders was practicing medicine without a license or offering an alternative type of care that is not medical practice."[26]

Former Iowa CongressmaN Berkley Bedell provided $21,000 for Saunders' defense.

"The Watonwan County attorney's office stated that it planned to retry Saunders." Herb Saunders was indeed tried a second time, resulting in a hung jury more pronounced than the first time.[26]

To make these kinds of obviously safe treatments available to all, avoiding great costs and suffering under ineffective traditional treatments, each person is advised to write to his/her U.S. Senators and Representatives in support of freedom-of-choice-in-medicine legislation, and also to support similar bills at each state level.

Perhaps the reader would like to know why governmental agencies and other vested interests have not followed up the work of developing and distributing "antigen specific" colostrum.

Antigen specific colostrum can easily be manufactured through the wide-spread milk industry that would treat and cure virtually everyone of any disease based on microorganisms or allergens. If any country or company wre to follow this path the whole of the pharmaceutical vaccination industry would be wiped out! (See "Universal Oral Vaccine" at http://www.arthritistrust.org.)

There's no restriction on manufacturing and selling antigen specific colostrum to veternarians and dairy farmers, but never, never to humans!

Royal Raymond Rife Technology

Superb technology was developed by Royal Raymond Rife under

sponsorship of the Timken ball-bearing funding. According to 1930's reports by physicians associated with the University of Southern California, cancer and other diseases were being cured.

After the FDA persecuted and destroyed Rife's work, his technology languished until James E. Bare, D.C. retraced Rife's frequency generating path, using modern technology. Dr. Bare and others have now produced results that seem to match, and in some respects exceed, Rife's work. As they cannot build or sell these devices without incurring the ire of FDA, they have made circuit diagrams, video tapes and internet data available to those who would like to build the devices themself. (See https://drparviz.wordpress.com/2011/05/08/136/ and numerous other websites.)

According to internet information, using this newly developed Rife instrument, frequencies 432, 484, 610, 790, and 864 will kill off the bacteria that causes Lyme disease.

Information can be obtained from James E. Bare, D.C. (Also see http://www.electroherbalism.com/Bioelectronics/RifeBare/)

At least one researcher, John Myers, D.C., has learned that Rife's hard-won frequency information can easily be obtained via use of applied kinesiology, thus determining appropriate polarity, frequency and wave form for killing microorganisms, erasing internal scar tissue, reducing tumors, and clearing up arterial plaques. Although the editor knows of a number of patients — including those suffering from lyme arthritis disease — who have been treated and cured by Dr. Myers, no proper documentation exists to pass along to others at this time.

References

1. See Anthony di Fabio, "Friendly Bacteria — *Lactobacillus acidophilus & Bifido bacterium*," The Arthritis Trust of America/The Rheumatoid Disease Foundation, 7111 Sweetgum Road, Fairview, TN 37062, 1989.

2. Anthony di Fabio, *Rheumatoid Diseases Cured at Last*, The Arthritis Trust of America/The Rheumatoid Disease Foundation, Op.Cit., 1985.

3. Dr. Paul K. Pybs, "The Herxheimer Effect," The Arthritis Trust of America/The Rheumatoid Disease Foundation, Op.Cit., 1992.

4. "Picking Out the Lymes From the Lemons," *Townsend Letter for Doctors*, 911 Tyler St., Port Townsend, WA. 98368-6541, May 1993, p. 408; reprint from *Science News*.

5. See, William H. Philpott, M.D., *Magnetic Resonance Bio-Oxidative Therapy for Rheumatoid and Other Degenerative Diseases*, The Arthritis Trust of America/The Rheumatoid Disease Foundation, Op.Cit., 1994.

6. See Anthony di Fabio, "Germanium," The Arthritis Trust of America/The Rheumatoid Disease Foundation, Op.Cit., 1989.

7. See Gus J. Prosch, Jr., M.D., "Candidiasis: Scourge of Arthritics," The Arthritis Trust of America/The Rheumatoid Disease Foundation, Op.Cit., 1994.

8. See Morton Walker, D.P.M., "The Carnivora Cure for Cancer, AIDS & Other Pathologies — Part II, *Townsend Letter for Doctors*, May 1992, #106, p. 329.

9. See Fred S. Kantor, "Disarming Lyme Disease," *Scientific American*, 415 Madison Avenue, New York, NY 10017-1111, September 1994, p. 34.

10. Pearl Atkin, R.N., M.A., CS, "My Experience With Lyme Disease," *Townsend Letter for Doctors*, Op.Cit., November 1992, p. 997.

11. Louis J. Marx, M.D., *Healing Dimensions of Herbal Medicine*, 3418 Loma Vista Road, Suite 1-A, Ventura, CA 93003, date unknown.

12. Pearl Atkin, R.N., M.A., CS, "Treatment of Lyme Disease," *Townsend Letter for Doctors*, Op.Cit., December 1993, p. 1220.

13. Congressman Berkely Bedell, "Bedell Testifies Before U.S., Senate," *Townsend Letter for Doctors*, Op.Cit., December 1993, p. 1229.

14. "Malaria Therapy: A Cure for Cancer and Aids?" *Journal of Longevity Research*, Vol.1/No.2, December 1994, p. 8.

15. Anthony di Fabio, "Lyme Disease: Arthritis by Infection," *The Art of Getting Well*, The Arthritis Trust of America/The Rheumatoid Disease Foundation, 7111 Sweetgum Road, Fairview, TN 37062, 1994.

16. *Textbook of Internal Medicine*, J.B. Lippincott Company, East Washington Square, Philadelphia, PA 19105, 1989.

17. Burton Goldberg Group, *Alternative Medicine: The Definitive Guide*, 1st edition, Future Medicine Publishing Co., Inc., 10124 18th St., Court E, Puyallup, WA 98371.

18. Personal communication from Agatha M. Thrash, M.D., November 2, 1995.

19. Personal communication from Gus J. Prosch, Jr., M.D., November 20, 1995.

20. Jwing-Ming Yang, *Arthritis — The Chinese Way of Healing and Prevention*, YMAA Publication Center, Yang's Martial Arts Association (YMAA), 38 Hyde Park Avenue, Jamaica Plain, Massachusetts 02130, 1991.

21. Personal letter from Berkley Bedell July 18, 1994.

22. Morton Walker, D.P.M., "The Carnivora Cure for Cancer, AIDS & Other Pathologies — Part I & II, *Townsend Letter for Doctors*, 911 Tyler St., Port Townsend, WA, 98368-6541, #95, p. 412; #106, p. 324.

23. Personal interview with, and correspondence from a scientist who chooses not to be identfied.

24. Agatha Thrash, M.D., Calvin Thrash, M.D., *Home Remedies*, Thrash Publications, Rt. 1, Box 273, Seale, Alabama 36875.

25. United States Patent 3376198.

26. "Minnesota Milk-Cure Case Ends with Mistrial," *Townsend Letter for Doctors*, 911 Tyler St., Port Townsend, Washington, 98368-6541, August/September 1995, p. 81; from *Minneapolis Star Tribune*, 3/16/95.

27. Malcolm Ritter, "Whey Could Prevent HIV Infection," *Wisconsin State Journal*, January 31, 1996, quoting the February *Nature Medicine*.

28. Personal interview with Dorothy Johnson.

29. Personal communication from Robin Ellen Leder, M.D.

30. Personal interview with Dr. Catherine Russell.

31. Stephen Tobin, D.V.M., "Lyme Disease," *Townsend Letter for Doctors*, 911 Tyler St., Port Townsend, WA, 98368-6541, January 1993, p. 63.

32. T. Ebina, et. al., *Med Microbiol Immunol*, Springer-Verlag, 173:87-93, 1984.

The following excellent article came from http://www.mercola.com, a site that is highly recommended for the latest in alternative omplementarviews.

Suggestions for Treating Chronic Fatigue Syndrome (CFS)
Charles Weber

During the early development of medicine, one diagnosed a disease according to classification of the observed symptoms. If the joints ached, for example, the disease was called "arthritis." Never mind that there can be as many as one hundred or more causations involved in creating joint pain — just call them all "arthritis!" This methodology does very little, if anything, to assist in diagnosing causation and thus determining remedies that work.

We could site numerous medical conditions where the naming of a disease by observed symptoms only produces a confused, unworkable set of proposed remedies.

Overlooked and certainly unknown by these medical pioneers was a fact that still has not gotten through many medical heads, that the body can only respond in a limited number of ways; and, that there can be a large multitude of causations for a given set of observable symptoms.

So, therefore, the A plus medical student is the one with a vast ability to memorize and can quote off by rote the given name of any set of observed symptoms — it being assumed, therefore, that by naming the symptoms one has named the disease and that this brilliance will lead to remedies that cure the disease.

Not so!

Modern laboratory tests have begun to shred this mystical method of diagnosis. Not completely has it disappeared, however. I'm very much afraid that Chronic Fatigue Syndrome is one of those catch-all nomenclatures that sounds erudite but, in fact, covers up the fact that the body is responding in its particular manner because of one or more stresses, not all of them clearly known.

One of us (Charles Weber) discusses Chronic Fatigue Syndrome from a broader perspective.

INTRODUCTION

Chronic fatigue syndrome (CFS) is a disease characterized by symptoms of extreme, long lasting fatigue, loss of memory [Marcel], impaired sleep, sore throat, muscle and joint aches, headache, cough, photophobia, night sweats, [Evengard] depression that has much lower ACTH and cortisol secretion than typical depression [Demitrack], lymph node pain, eye pain and fibromyalgia (muscle pain) [Bell DS] as well as white spots on MRI brain scans [Buchwald 1992] and single-photon emission computed tomography (SPECT) scans [Schwartz], loss of fingerprints in a third of the patients [Johnson p345], and a chronic low level activation of the immune system [Cannon] which last may be accounting for many of the non neurological symptoms, but all very variable, perhaps because different parts of the brain are attacked.

Women are much more often affected than men.

No one has been able to assign a definitive cause to it with certainty, although it has been proposed to be a hypochondria from misdiagnosis [Johnson p 126] or mass hysteria from reading newspaper articles proposed by the Center for Disease Control in the USA [Johnson p 135-138, 339, 342] (both very unlikely), an Epstein-Barr virus [Holmes] (because that virus antigen is often found in it as an opportunistic infection, but refuted [Buchwald 1988]), poor nutrition compounded by lack of exercise [Johnson p 685], a poison [Racciatti], or a retrovirus (because fragments were detected in some of its victims similar to retrovirus) [DeFreitas]. (The retrovirus work has ended because DeFreitas has become very sick and no one else has been competent to continue her work.) That it is caused by a virus which damages the immune system is highly probable since it comes on suddenly with flu like symptoms and shows up in clusters associated with social groups [Buchwald 1992]. Fragments of mycoplasma pathogen species have been found in CFS and fibromyalgia but they are probably opportunistic infections because when multiple species are found in the same patient it correlates with the length of time CFS was present [Nasralla].

The hypothesis that CFS is a psychosomatic illness has resulted in thousands of ruined and destitute lives. There probably has not been so ruinous a result from a failed hypothesis since governor Phips ended the Salem witch craft trials. Even the blood letting of the 18th century was fairly minor. After all, how much harm can you do removing a few drops of blood? The hypothesis by medical doctors that it was not necessary to wash hands for child birth caused many deaths, but at least these mothers were given a fairly quick end. The CFS victims could not collect insurance support or disability and descended into poverty.

That hypothesis was probably an important part of the chief cause of death, suicide. It is not only in the USA that the physical nature of this disease was denied. A young girl was taken away from her mother until the age of 18 because the mother dared to disagree with a doctor that the girl was faking her symptoms.

A poison can not be ruled out as at least a contributing factor [Bell IR], and may have been involved in the gulf war syndrome. Anthrax vaccine has been proposed as triggering gulf war syndrome with some convincing statistical evidence produced at some government hearings.

However, I believe there may have been other medical procedures at the same time. These brave men were denied support at first also.

There have been other names for the syndrome proposed. Yuppie flu was proposed because at first only higher income people had enough money saved to hire doctors or lobby officials. Chronic fatigue immune deficiency syndrome (CFIDS) was proposed because the immune system was distorted and it was hoped that this name would gain the victims some support and research funds. After all the magic letters "ID" had gained massive support for AIDS. It would be too bad if the early cavalier attitude toward CFS resulted in adopting such a cumbersome name. Fibromyalgia, which is widespread muscular pain, was proposed as a variant of CFS and probably is. The name "myalgic encephalomyelitis" (ME) was assigned to a similar disease by medical researchers in the British Commonwealth. Post viral fatigue syndrome (PVFS) and post infectious neuromyasthenia were also used.

DISCUSSION

So the cause is unknown. This leaves us with the problem of what to do about the disease currently while we wait for researchers to figure out what direction research should take and what causes it.

It has been proposed that poor nutrition and lack of exercise are contributing factors [Johnson p 685]. It certainly is plausible that a poorly nourished body would be more at risk. A vegetarian diet using lots of raw vegetables has significantly improved the symptoms of fibromyalgia with 19 out of 30 subjects reporting considerable improvement of all symptoms after a few weeks [Donaldson]. It would be a good idea to find out what in raw vegetables was responsible. That diet gave five to six thousand milligrams of potassium per day and 460 milligrams of magnesium. It has been discovered that magnesium injections mute the symptoms significantly [Takahasha][Cox]. So magnesium supplements may be in order for CFS people who eat junk food and maybe for everyone with CFS. However, magnesium was found to be normal in the red cells in CFS patients [Hinds] and magnesium is normal in blood cells during a magnesium deficiency as well, so red cell content can not be used in diagnosis.

A whole body (cell content) analysis of potassium has found that potassium averaged a little lower in CFS than the general population [Burnet] which general population is low in potassium in our society to start with. The CFS average was about two thirds of the highest values of healthy people. This is ominous because the highest values is the normalcy which the body attempts to attain since there is no storage of potassium in the body other than the tolerable range of soluble potassium in the cell fluid. It could be that potassium supplements are in order as well. Magnesium should be part of the experiment since potassium requires adequate magnesium in order to be absorbed effectively [Petersen][MacIntyre] and it is possible that inositol [Charalampous] is necessary also. While excessive salt intakes are detrimental, it is necessary to receive moderate amounts of sodium salt because extremely low intakes also increase potassium excretion. (See a marvelous and extensive article by Mildred Seelig on the relation of magnesium to CFS and FM, in which she suggests that CFS is a magnesium deficiency [Seelig]). I suspect it is not quite that simplistic. (http://www.mgwater.com/seelig.shtml)

Experiments must be performed with caution, however, because when a patient thought to be exhibiting symptoms of fibromyalgia was brought to 5.0 mEq/l in her blood (which is close to normal) she contracted paralysis [Gotze]. This may be because experiments have shown that people who have

CFS with muscle pain have normal serum potassium and so fibromyalgia must be a different variation of CFS. In monkeys the electrocardiogram in magnesium deficiency resembles that of high serum potassium (hyperkalemia) in spite of low serum potassium (hypokalemia) [Manitius p39]. So it is possible that lower cell potassium requires lower serum potassium for adequate nerve transmission, but the serum potassium does not drop correspondingly [Manitius p38]. If a magnesium deficiency does develop, half a year of supplements can be required for complete normalization of the affect of magnesium content on potassium. [Anonymous] If you wish to try increasing potassium by diet you may see a table which gives the relative values of potassium at; [http://members.tripod.com/~charles_W/table3.html]. Considerable increases in potassium are possible without the necessity of eliminating cooking and there is less danger of imbalances with other nutrients.

It may be that meals should be more than three times per day in smaller increments since the adrenal glands in CFS patients average smaller than other people [Scott & Dinan] and their depression has much lower ACTH and cortisol secretion [Demitrack] which may be partly from the smaller glands. There is a good chance damage to the part of the brain which controls the pituitary is a more important part of that low ACTH than gland size, and therefore cortisol also, by disruption of the brain-pituitary axis [Scott & Svec & Dinan].

Also smaller meals would help prevent surges of potassium too high for those with weakened kidneys to handle efficiently as well as possibly increasing the useful cell retention.

If you would like to explore nutrition there are severl good internet sites which list many good links organized in categories at and a good site on general health information by Dr Mercola at [http://www.mercola.com].

Exercise has also been found to be helpful in CFS by numerous experiments [Hakkinen][Mengshoel]. Both moderate and intense exercise has shown to be helpful [Hadhazy]. However, over training can precipitate CFS [Shephard] and exercise brings on a severe fatigue which lasts for days [Johnson p329-330, 491-492] so it seems to me that exercise should be mild (such as walking [Coutts]. This is supported by an experiment which showed that exercise in a pool gave less pain, anxiety, depression, and more days of feeling good [Jentoft] than terrestrial exercise and short, mild treadmill exercise caused no obvious problem [Clapp]. I suspect that many short periods of mild exercise across the day would be the preferred routine. I suspect across the day partly because clearance of blood through the liver in order to remove electrolyte hormones such as aldosterone [Messerli] (which removal decreases potassium losses and sodium retention) is probably an important part of the value of exercise. Even robust exercise had beneficial results in some of the symptoms other than the symptoms mentioned above [Hadhazy] but it is conceivable that these patients had a different part of their brain affected by the disease. Until researchers get it figured out it would be a good idea to approach exercise cautiously and moderately.

There are many clever devices which have been invented for other degenerative diseases. There is no reason why these devices can not be made available if they can be financed by society. Societal support would be necessary for most because severe CFS is so debilitating that it is impossible for some of these people to support themselves.

The most debilitating other infirmity than fatigue is loss of memory. CFS patients should carry maps with them showing the way home and notebooks with important information like phone numbers and grocery lists and this should help considerably. For those who have lost fingerprints [Johnson p345] a good ID should always be on them and perhaps name and number imprinted on their arm by a dye.

Another procedure which should be effective would be to carry cell phones with a button which automatically dials a central office which has people on duty familiar with the important information in the patients life and which has people skilled at giving emotional support in order to deal with the depression often present.

There is evidence of opportunistic herpes infection since 77% of CFS patients contain antibodies to HHV-6 EA as IgM and IgG [Patnaik]. It may be prudent for these CFS people also to eat sparingly of foods high in arginine continuously after CFS or maybe until tests determine that the immune peptide hormones [Patarca] and natural killer cells [Caligiuri] are all normal again. This is because the amino acid arginine accentuates the symptoms of herpes [McCune] and maybe even trigger a resurgence of a dormant infection such as shingles (dormant chicken pox). Foods high in arginine are peanuts, cashews (peanuts are 50% higher than cashews but cashews are substantial), chocolate, and seeds other than the grass derived grain.

Lysine supplements may be in order also because lysine helps to mute the effects of the herpes virus significantly, reducing the occurrence (when taken routinely during the disease), severity, and healing time of herpes simplex virus [Griffith]. It probably does so by interfering with the absorption of arginine by the virus.

You may see an excellent table of nutrients including amino acids at; [http://ndb.nal.usda.gov/] (just divide the values by the Kcal figure to get valid comparisons) and a table which shows lysine and arginine values by weight of food and lysine\arginine ratios at; [http://www.healthy.net/asp/templates/article.asp?PageType=article&ID=1744]. Those who have CFS should not be afraid to experiment with nutrients. The human body is very resilient. As long as you do not use a poison or procedure known to be harmful, there is not much chance that irreversible harm will transpire.

Experimenting has some risk but doing nothing is even riskier. If you do come across a nutrient, combination of nutrients, or procedure or other circumstance which produces perceptible positive or negative effects, perhaps you could see yourself clear to email the information into a site which is attempting to archive such experiences at; [http://scienceblog.com/7385/case-health-health-success-stories-blog/#ya4KAu2wWIRGJCSF.97]

As to NOT eating something, the chances of irreversible harm are vanishingly small. Of course your single case history is almost useless epidemiologically (the study of health statistics). However, perhaps it could become useful if you became a member of a group which keeps records and is willing to make the records public anonymously. Millions of people eat things about which no records are kept, such as hydrogenated oils. If they are not to be studied by the people who sell them, the federal agencies, or the universities, then it would be a good idea if the people who eat food to do so.

Just do not engage in any procedures out of the ordinary which go on interminably, especially medication or pain deadeners (analgesics) as pain deadeners have been proposed as a risk factor for CFS [Johnson p574]. Also several pain deadeners have been found to damage the kidneys. Among the prescription and over the counter medications that predispose patients to such damage are acetaminophen (Tylenol, Anacin-3, Liquiprin, Panadol, and Tempra) but not aspirin [Schwarz]. Kidney damage is extremely serious. Also it is plausible that anything which can damage kidney cells could damage immune cells as well.

The chance that a pain deadener will have any direct curative affect is vanishingly small, so it usually is better to tolerate the pain if at all possible.

Depression often shows up in CFS. Therefore it is almost certainly desirable for those who love the sufferer to apply as much emotional support as possible. Good jokes, camaraderie, and tactile approval (like hugs) will not cure the disease, but there is a good chance they will mute some of the symptoms and make an eventual defeat of whatever infection is involved a little more likely. Just be sure to make kissing or eating and drinking out of the same plate not part of the procedure because there is a suspicion that the last of the two is a risk factor. Guarding the sufferer from fear and staying warm will also probably prove to be advantageous since it has been shown that staying warm enhances immunity [Hanson] and fear is well known to affect the immune hormones.

When surgery is necessary for CFS patients it is imperative that doctors become familiar with contraindications for medication because CFS patients are very susceptible to adverse reactions from some anesthetics and other medications

CFS is potentially extremely dangerous to society because of its severity and length of recovery time. If a mosquito ever learns how to transmit it, the situation will be desperate for society. Therefore enormous research effort should be mobilized to not just ameliorate it, but like smallpox, to eradicate it.

REFERENCES

Also see <u>Soft Tissue Arthritis</u> by Anthony di Fabio and Paul Jaconello, M.D. on Amazon.com and on Kindle, book stores and at Arthritis Trust.org.

Anonymous 1994 Potassium and sodium and potassium in the skeletal muscle. Laeger Ugeskr 156; 4007-4010

Bell DS Bell KM Cheney PR 1994 Primary juvenile fibromyalgia syndrome and chronic fatigue syndrome in adolescents. Clin. Infect. Dis. Suppl. 1; S21-3.

Bell IR Baldwin CM Schwartz GE 1998 Illness from low levels of environmental chemicals: relevance to chronic fatigue syndrome and fibromyalgia. Am. J. Med. 105; 74S-82S.

Buchwald D Sullivan JL Leddy S Komaroff AL 1988 "Chronic Epstein-Barr virus infection" syndrome and polymyalgia rheumatica. J. Rheumatol. 15; 479-82.

Buchwald D Chenet PR Peterson DL Henry B Wormsley SB Geiger A Ablashi DV Salahuddin SZ Saysinger C

Biddle R et al 1992 A chronic illness characterized by fatigue, neurologic and immunologic disorders, and active human herpesvirus type 6 infection. Annals of Internal Medicine 116; 103-13.

Burnet RB Yeap BB Chatterton BE Gaffney RD 1996 Chronic fatigue syndrome: is total body potassium important? Med. J. Aust. 164; 384.

Caligiuri M, Murray C, Buchwald D, Levine H, Cheney P, Peterson D, Komaroff AL, Ritz J 1987. Phenotypic and functional deficiency of natural killer cells in patients with chronic fatigue syndrome. J. Immunol. 139(10):3306-13.

Cannon JG Angel JB Abad LW Vannier E Mileno MD Fagioli L Wolff SM Komaroff AL 1997 Interleukin-1 beta, interleukin-1 receptor antagonist, and soluble interleukin-1 receptor type II secretion in chronic fatigue syndrome. J. Clin. Immunol 17; 253-261.

Charalampous FC 1971 Metabolic functions of myoinositol: VIIII - Role of inositol in Na+-K+ transport and in Na+ and K+ activated adenosine triphosphate of KB cells. Journal of Biol. Chem> 246; 455 & 461.

Clapp LL, Richardson MT, Smith JF, et al. Acute effects of thirty minutes of light-intensity, intermittent exercise on patients with chronic fatigue syndrome. Phys. Ther. 1999;79:749-56.

Coutts R Weatherby R Davie A 2001 The use of a symptom "self report" inventory ro evaluate the acceptability and efficiency of a walking program for patients suffering with chronic fatigue syndrome. .J. Psychosom. Res. 51; 425-29.

Cox IM, Campbell MJ, Dowson D. 1991 Red blood cell magnesium and chronic fatigue syndrome. Lancet Mar 30;337(8744):757-60.

Demitrack MA, Dale JK, Straus SE, Laue L, Listwak SJ, Kruesi MJ, Chrousos GP, Gold PW 1991 Evidence for impaired activation of the hypothalamic-pituitary-adrenal axis in patients with chronic fatigue syndrome. J. Clin Endocrinol. Metab. 73(6): 1224-34.

DeFreitas E Hilliard B Cheney PR Bell DS Kiggunde E Sankey D Wroblewska Z Palladino M Woodward JP Koprowski H 1991 Retroviral sequences related to human T-lymphotropic virus type II in patients with chronic fatigue immune dysfunction syndrome. Proc. Natl. Acad. Sci. 88; 2922-2926.

Donaldson M Speight N Loomis S 2001 Fibromyalgia syndrome improved using mostly raw vegetarian diet: an observational study. BMC Complimentary and Alternative Medicine 1;7.

Evengard B Schacterle RS Komaroff 1999 Chronic fatigue syndrome: new insights and old ignorance. Journal Intern. Med. 246; 455-469.

Gotze FR Thid SK Kyllerman M 1998 Fibromyalgia in hyperkalemic periodic paralysis. Scand. Journal of Rheumatol. 27; 383-384.

Hadhazy VA Ezzo J Creamer P Berman BM 2000 Mind-body therapies for the treatment of fibromyalgia; a systematic review. J. Rheumatol. 27; 2911-8.

Hinds G, Bell NP, McMaster D, McCluskey DR. 1994 Normal red cell magnesium concentrations and magnesium loading tests in patients with chronic fatigue syndrome. Ann. Clin. Biochem. Sep;31(Pt 5):459-61.

Hanson, D.E.; Murphy, P.A.; Silicano, R.; Shin, H.S. 1983 The effect of temperature on the activation of thymocytes by interleukin I & II. Journal of Immunol. 130: 216, 1983.

Holmes GP et al 1987 A cluster of patients with a Chronic Mononucleosis-like Syndrome: Is Epstein-Barr virus the cause? Journal of the American Medical Association 257; 2297-302.

Jenthoft ES Kvalik AG Mengshoel AM 2001 Effects of pool based and land-based aerobic exercise on women with fibromyalgia / chronic widespread pain. Arthitis Rheum. 45; 42-7.

Johnson H 1997 Osler's Web. Penguin's Books, Ontario Canada.

MacIntyre I & Davidson D 1958 The production of secondary potassium depletion, sodium retention, nephrocalcinosis and hypercalcemia by magnesium deficit. Biochem. Journal 70; 456-462.

Scott LV Svec F Dinan T 2000 A preliminary study of dehydroepiandrosterone response to low-dose ACTH in chronic fatigue syndrome and in healthy subjects. Psychiatry Research 97; 21-28

Manitius A 1965 Some physiological effects of magnesium deficiency p28. in: Electrolytes and Cardiovascular Diseases, Bajusz E, editor. S. Karger, New York

Marcel B, Komaroff AL, Fagioli LR, Kornish RJ 2nd, Albert MS. 1996 Cognitive deficits in patients with chronic fatigue syndrome. Biol Psychiatry 1996 Sep 15;40(6):535-41.

Mengshoel AM Haugen M 2001 Health status in fibromyalgia - a follow up study. J. Rheumatol. 28; 2085-9.

Messerli FH, et al 1977 Effects of angiotensin II on steroid metabolism and hepatic blood flow in man.. Circ.Res 40; 204-207.<p>

Nasralla M, Haier J, Nicolson GL.1999 Multiple mycoplasmal infections detected in blood of patients with chronic fatigue syndrome and/or fibromyalgia syndrome. Eur. J. Clin. Microbiol. Infect. Dis. Dec;18(12):859-65

Patarca R Klimas NG Lugtendorf S Antoni M Fletcher MA 1994 1994 Dysregulated expression of tumor necrosis factor in chronic fatigue syndrome interelations with cellular sources and patterns of soluble immune mediator expression. Clin Infect. Dis. Jan 18 Suppl. 1; s147-s153.

Patnaik M Komaroff AL Conley E Ojo-Amaize EA Peter JB 1995 Prevalence of IgM antibodies to human herpesvirus 6 early antigen (p41/38) in patients with chronic fatigue syndrome. J. Infect. Dis. 172; 1364-67.

Petersen VP 1963 Potassium and magnesium turnover in magnesium deficiency. Acta Med. Scand. 174; 595-604

Racciatti D Vecchiet J Ciccomancini A Ricci F Pizzigallo E 2001 Chronic fatigue syndrome following toxic exposure.. Sci. Total Environ. 270; 27-31.

Schwartz A, Perez-Canto A. 1998 Nephrotoxicity of antiinfective drugs. Int. J. Clin. Pharmacol. 36(3):164-7.

Scott LV Dinan TG 1999 Small adrenal glands in chronic fatigue syndrome: a preliminary computer tomograph study psychoneuroendocrinology 24; 759-768.

Scott LV Svec F Dinan T 2000 A preliminary study of dehydroepiandrosterone response to low dose ACTH in chronic fatigue syndrome and in healthy subjects. Psychiatry Research.97; 21-8.

Schwartz RB, Garada BM, Komaroff AL, Tice HM, Gleit M, Jolesz FA, Holman BL. 1994 Detection of intracranial abnormalities in patients with chronic fatigue syndrome:comparison of MR imaging and SPECT. Am. J. Roentgenol. 1994 Apr;162(4):935-41

Schwarz A, Perez-Canto A. 1998 Nephrotoxicity of antiinfective drugs Int. J. Clin. Pharmacol. Ther. 36(3):164-7.

Seelig M 1998 Review and hypothesis: Might patients with chronic fatigue syndrome have latent tetany of magnesium deficiency? Journal of Chronic Fatigue Syndrome 4 (2).

Mycoplasmic Theory of Rheumatoid Disease According to Thomas McPherson Brown, M.D.

by

Harold W. Clark, Ph.D. (Mycoplasma Research Institute) as reported by Joseph Mercola, D.O. © **2000;**

Introduction by Anthony di Fabio

Introduction

When I (Anthony di Fabio) first suffered from "galloping" rheumatoid arthritis my family doctor knew only to provide me with pain relievers while the damage to my joints "galloped" on, and the pain intensified daily. I eventually learned of the Roger Wyburn-Mason, Ph.D., M.D. treatment based on the theory that an amoeba was the culprit of the disease. We were never able to prove Wyburn-Mason's theory, but we did know that he'd been treating folks on a worldwide basis since the 1960s, and getting them well. I got well in six weeks.

Then, later, after a number of medical doctors and I had founded the Rheumatoid Disease Foundation/The Arthritis Trust of America, we all learned of the Thomas McPherson Brown, MD. treatment based on his theory that a mycoplasma was the chief culprit in those who suffered from rheumatoid arthritis.

Since the Roger Wyburn-Mason treatment took only six weeks — at best twelve weeks — to test out, and the McPherson Brown treatment took as long as a year or even two years, it always seemed foolish that most medical doctors leaned toward the Brown treatment first.

It mattered not to our new foundation which theory was correct. I believe I speak for all rheumatoid disease victims everwhere when I say that we don't care which theory is correct. We only want the joint damage to stop and the pain to quit, which also means that we're only barely interested in symptomatic treatment as offered by the majority of medical practitioners.

The following, therefore, is considered by us to be another method of getting well. There can never be too many such methods in our opinion.

Roger Wyburn-Mason, Ph.D., M.D. treatment protocol for rheumatoid disease is rather well defined in his *The Causation of Rheumatoid Disease and Many Human Cancers* and numerous books published by this foundation written by or with Anthony di Fabio.

Nature of the Disease

The progressive immunologic rheumatoid diseases are characterized by periodic and chronic symptoms. The discovery of more effective forms of sustained therapy are handicapped by one significant fact: in nearly all forms of chronic arthritis, the causative factors although suspected remain unknown. An infectious agent has long been thought to initiate rheumatoid arthritis and related diseases previously designated "chronic infectious disorders" and "collagen vascular disorders." As recommended for many years high priority should be given to an intensive search for latent, slow acting microbes such as the ubiquitous and unique mycoplasmas that as a viable irritant could cause persistent inflammation.

In the immunologic disorders, such as the rheumatoid diseases that may incubate for years, the immune system becomes over-reactive. In their efforts to destroy the irritating agents the influx of digestive enzymes from the activated white blood cells (Wbc) start to destroy the surrounding tissues causing the inflammatory symptoms. The Wbcs are also activated to produce neutralizing antibodies against the invading germs. The antibodies combine with the germs in their effort to help contain the infection. When the antibodies combine with the germs or antigens they form "immune complexes" that activate the Complement enzyme system which in turn can also destroy both irritating germs and surrounding tissues. Both Lupus and rheumatoid arthritis are characterized by the deposition of immune complex in kidneys and other tissues along with the erosion of blood vessels.

Mechanistic Treatment

By eliminating the cause(s) the mechanistic approach can be more effective and less costly in controlling and preventing chronic disease activity. This is unlike the symptomatic treatment approach that temporarily relieves symptoms. Basically there are three therapeutic targets: 1) to search for and eliminate the microbial cause(s) and metabolic defects. 2) to identify and block immune complex formation, and 3) to control and eliminate inflammation, pain, and fatigue. The elimination of the microbial root cause should be the primary target. The less pathogenic or nonvirulent microbes would be less reactive requiring less antibiotic treatment.

Three Prong Prescription

1. *Antibiotics;* such as minocyclines, in low pulsed doses should be directed at inhibiting the microbial cause and preventing the disease. The multi prong tetracyclines can also act as antioxidants, immunosuppressants, and protein synthesis inhibitors.

2. *Immunosuppressants;* that come in many different forms of alternatives including low dose prednisone that blocks the immune complex formation and the activation of Complement which promotes tissue destructive inflammation.

3. *Antiinflammatory antioxidants;* such as dietary supplements and the nonsteroidal antiinflammatory drugs (NSAIDs) to eliminate and prevent the tissue destructive inflammation.

Several other major contributing factors affecting the occurrence and severity of the rheumatoid disorders must also be considered in selecting the most effective treatment. These include variable factors such as: Health, Diet, Exposure, physical & mental Stress. The most effective treatment is Good Health that is individually controlled by ones' Diet, and exposures to physical and mental Stress. The goal of many alternative therapies is helping to achieve maximum good health with natural dietary supplements and both physical and mental stimulants. In addition fixed factors that include: Age, Gender, and Genetic succeptability, all of which can help, hinder or predispose the therapeutic success. The treatment, for optimum benefits, should be individually adjusted for ones' age, body size, and gender. Even though the symptoms on the surface are similar the underlying mechanisms can be different.

(From the book: *"Why Arthritis? Searching for the Cause and the Cure of Rheumatoid Diseases"* Copyright by Harold W. Clark, Ph.D., used by permission.)

Dr. Brown's Antibiotic Treatment Plans

In his medical practice the late Thomas McPherson Brown, M.D. seemed to have a treatment protocol, a plan, for each rheumatoid patient that included some form of anti-mycoplasma antibiotics. Using different medications and dosages made it difficult to statistically compare and evaluate any single therapy. Medications were often changed trying to find both a tolerable and effective therapy. As new drugs became available they were continuously evaluated. For example tetracycline dosages varied from 10 mg. to 1000 mg. or from daily to weekly with oral and intravenous administration including several days of hospitalization. A significant study of 98 hospitalized rheumatoid arthritis patients treated over a five year period found that over 70 were substantially improved using the variable antibiotic treatment plan which was anything but the standard infection plan of 1 gm./day for 10 days.

The protocols weren't just drugs and antibiotics as Dr. Brown was also interested in the psychosocial aspects of illness and patient care. With extensive interviews the treatment also focused on both the patient and their family and not simply the disease. He worked extensively with a team of rehabilitation experts in helping to alleviate and solve the underlying patient problems. A good example of comprehensive medicine was the support by John L. Lewis, president of the Miners Union, that provided total care of the West Virginia miners' medical problems. Although not discussed in his book *The Road Back* Dr. Brown was also the director of a multi discipline medical Rehabilitation Center that also pursued the causes and the solutions to the related physical and mental health problems associated with rheumatoid diseases. The Allied Health staff proved essential for the therapeutic effectiveness.

Like their diverse rheumatoid patients, doctors after leaving school and with experience developed their own theories and philosophy of patient care that are a little different from their professor's and others. A consensus of what is the right medicine, a protocol for all patients, is not the question or the issue as medicine is more of an art than a science. There are many skilled artists and also 171 different wide ranging forms of arthritis. Most symptoms have suspected or unknown causes and become chronic or are short lived with periods of spontaneous remission. Because of the many different kinds and severity of symptoms many will require more than antimicrobials for control and eradication. Eventually with control comes prevention of the various forms of arthritis with regulated living and application of improved and alternative therapies. In his treatment plans Dr. Brown promoted a

Mechanistic approach in searching for the cause and cure of rheumatoid diseases. Because of the many targets Symptomatic treatment requires multiple medications that further complicate the protocol and the evaluation of safe and effective results. Prescribing a treatment for the primary causes provides a direction for the evaluation of effectiveness. For nearly forty years Dr. Brown was considered a maverick who's antibiotic treatment plan was criticized as unproven quackery and who's strong personality convinced patients they were better. Now today after the antibiotic approach has been extensively tested and proven to be safe and effective in rheumatoid diseases both doctors and patients are finding the treatment beneficial.

Dr. Thomas McPherson Brown [was] the chairman of the Arthritis Clinic of Northern Virginia. A world renowned leader in arthritis research and treatment, Dr. Brown has served as a consultant to the White House and has been a member of the National Research Council and the Food and Drug Administration's Arthritis Advisory Committee.

He is a graduate of Swarthmore College and Johns Hopkins Medical School. Dr Brown has served as Chief Resident in Medicine at Johns Hopkins and as a Resident at the Rockefeller Institute Hospital. He has held several prestigious positions, including Director of Arthritis Research at the Veterans Hospital in Washington, D.C., and Chairman of the Department of Medicine at George Washington University School of Medicine for a twenty year period. He founded the Arthritis Institute of the National Hospital for Orthopaedics and Rehabilitation in 1970.

His work on rheumatoid arthritis dates back to the late 1930's during his tenure at the Rockefeller Institute when a colleague, Dr. Albert Sabin, found a strain of mycoplasma in a mouse while studying the disease, Toxoplasmosis. Dr. Sabin injected another mouse with this mycoplasma strain and the second mouse contracted arthritis. During this same period, Dr. Brown had been researching for an unknown virus in rheumatic tissues. No virus was found but one culture of joint fluid revealed mycoplasma. Subsequently, he found the same agents in the cultures from the genital tracts of men and women.

Dr. Sabin had found that the mouse strain of mycoplasma was susceptible to gold salts and Dr. Brown and his coworkers found this to be true of human strains as well. This prompted the search for a non toxic antimycoplasma substance to substitute for gold. Such a substance was found with tetracycline antibiotics.

These findings suggested the initial use of antibiotic therapy in rheumatoid arthritis. A clinical finding which encouraged the pursuit of this approach was the Herxheimer reaction common to both gold and tetracycline with the initiation of treatment.

The concept of an infectious agent as a trigger of autoimmune diseases is not new. Indeed cross reactions between group A streptococcal antigens and human myocardium elicit autoantibodies that have been associated with acute rheumatic fever. Several microorganisms (bacteria, mycoplasmas and viruses) [protozoans: ed.] have been proposed as likely etiologic agents for rheumatoid arthritis and animal arthritis. In particular the swine arthritis that mimics the disease in humans is known to be caused by a mycoplasma.

The recent report that Lyme arthritis, (which is known to result from a bacterial infection), can demonstrate rheumatoid arthritis like symptoms, and can be treated with antibiotics, has once again stimulated interest in the infectious theory.

Dr. Brown and his staff continued to conduct research to confirm his working hypothesis.

His clinical observations throughout the years regarding which classes and combinations of antibiotics, and routes and intervals of administration were more tolerable, while at the same time providing the most effective means of sustained control in patients is summarized below. It is significant that the only antibiotics effective in the long term management of rheumatoid disease are also the only antibiotics effective against mycoplasmas.

Arthritis affected tissues are very reactive, and early cases of arthritis respond to treatment much better than the most severe long standing cases.

Dosage and administration of drugs

Tetracycline: (250 mg. dosages in capsule form) are administered once a day, three times a week at the onset of treatment.

Non-steroidal Anti-inflammatory Drugs (NSAIDs): The concomitant use of NSAIDs varies. Aspirin is often given initially, followed by a variety of substitutes for cortisone.

Cortisone: To reduce the inflammatory barrier and allow penetration of the antibiotics, 7 to 5 mg. of prednisone may be administered to the patient simultaneously with the antibiotic. Preferably, no more than 10 mg. should be administered for flares. Larger doses when required should be given in short interrupted courses. It is of interest that the concomitant use of antibiotics with the steroids makes steroid withdrawal easier. The dosage of the drug must be kept low to avoid interfering with the immune system but high enough to reduce the hypersensitivity or allergic inflammatory reactions of the disease.

The therapeutic outline can be modified by the physician at any time using the following major guideline:

1. Titration of the antibiotic dosage
2. Treatment complex to be given in interrupted fashion
3. Aim to phase out steroids in time

Ampicillin: in the presence of streptococcal infection as determined by the presence of an ASO titer, and/or a strong history of streptococcal infection, 250 mg. of ampicillin to be taken once daily (preferably in the evenings) twice or three times a week is administered.

As treatment progresses, a gradual increase in the tetracycline dose, up to 500 mg. one to three times a day, three times a week, (Monday, Wednesday and Friday) is administered. Care should be taken not to administer the drug at too high a dosage too fast, to avoid an allergic reaction by the patient.

When remission becomes established, the antibiotics may be gradually phased out. When flare ups occur, short courses of antibiotics, should be given until no longer needed.

Intravenous Therapy

For patients who usually do not tolerate oral antibiotics, or those patients with a history of drug resistance from earlier treatment with a variety of drugs (e.g. gold, penicillamine, etc.), an intravenous regimen is followed.

Cleocin (the least irritating effective antibiotic for intravenous use) is given daily in the course of 5 to 7 days in the following manner: 300 mgm. cleocin in 250 cc. 5% dextrose solution given by intravenous drip for a period of 40 minutes for the first two days. The dose is increased to 600 mgm. and finally 900 mgm. on subsequent days.

Following the courses of intravenous therapy, the oral medication is usually more effective and acceptable. Thus the intravenous therapy serves as a booster.

Some patients are likely to develop a Jarisch Herxheimer (J H) reaction. The most likely candidates are those who present at the onset of the disease with high levels of gamma globulin, C reactive protein, BFT titer, anemia and low white cell count. When this J H reaction occurs, it is best to discontinue treatment, and to administer cortisone (not to exceed a maximum of 10 mg. to relieve flares) as well as symptomatic remedies.

The Jarisch Herxheimer reaction is rather brief, and when the symptoms subside, treatment should proceed by using a carefully titrated course of tetracyclines; e.g. starting with doxycycline, 50 mg. three times a day, and gradually increasing the dosage to 100 mg.

When it is determined that the patient's symptoms have stabilized as may be observed by improvement in laboratory tests, (i.e. ESR, CBC, gamma-globulin, BFT titer (bentonite flocculation test; Rheumatoid Factor determination, etc.) the higher dose of antibiotics, i.e. tetracycline, 250 mg. to 500 mg. three times a week, etc. can be administered.

Anemia may be induced either by a spontaneous or drug related flare. Thus, the hemoglobin or hematocrit serves as a good therapeutic guide. Concurrently with the treatment, the patient's blood chemistry is monitored. This includes CBC, the platelet count: ESR, BFT, and C reactive protein. Urinalysis screening is also performed.

Tests for MCF (mycoplasma complement fixing antibodies), BFT and Kunkel Globulin (gamma globulin) determination are available for these analysis.

In his four decades of experience with antibiotics. Dr. Brown notes that significant benefits from this type of treatment require on the average one to two years. Some patients do experience a worsening of the condition during the first few months prior to. improvement; however; some patients were able to notice a dramatic improvement in their situation: as early as six weeks. The length of therapy varies widely depending on the extensiveness of the disease. In severe cases, it may take up to thirty months for the patient to gain sustained improvement, and the achievement of remission may take 3 to 5 years.

100

The primary importance of the antibiotic approach is that once remission is established it is generally permanent unlike the experience with other treatment approaches. It appears that the absence of drug toxicity allows suppression of antigen long enough for the body's immune system to take over. [The shorter Wyburn-Mason treatment results in permanent remission also. Ed:]

Persistence is usually required in seeking the right combination of antibiotic dosage and method of administration in the difficult cases that require reduction of sensitization to the antigen.

Although the antibiotic treatment approach is still considered experimental, Dr. Brown treated hundreds of patients successfully over a 40 year period, bringing many of them back from hopelessness to living healthy and productive lives.

Dr. Brown's Modified Protocol For Using Antibiotics In The Treatment Of Rheumatic Diseases Presented at the 32nd International Congress of the Great Lakes College of Clinical Medicine Baltimore, Maryland, September 25, 1999 by Joseph Mercola, D.O.

Introduction

Rheumatoid arthritis affects about 1 percent of our population and at least two million Americans have definite or classical rheumatoid arthritis. It is a much more devastating illness than previously appreciated. Most patients with rheumatoid arthritis have a progressive disability. More than 50% of patients who were working at the start of their disease are disabled after five years of rheumatoid arthritis. The annual cost of this disease in the U.S. is estimated to be over $1 billion.

There is also an increased mortality rate. The five-year survival rate of patients with more than thirty joints involved is approximately 50%. This is similar to severe coronary artery disease or stage IV Hodgkin's disease.

Thirty years ago, one researcher concluded that there was an average loss of eighteen years of life in patients who developed rheumatoid arthritis before the age of 50.

Most authorities believe that remissions rarely occur. Some experts feel that the term "remission-inducing" should not be used to describe ANY current rheumatoid arthritis treatment. A review of contemporary treatment methods shows that medical science has not been able to significantly improve the long-term outcome of this disease.

My Experience with the Dr. Brown's Protocol

I [Joseph Mercola, D.O.] first became aware of Doctor Brown's protocol in 1989 when I saw him on 20/20 on ABC. This was shortly after the introduction of his first edition of *The Road Back*.The newest version is *The New Arthritis Breakthrough* that is written by Henry Scammel. Unfortunately, Dr. Brown died from prostate cancer shortly after the 20/20 program so I never had a chance to meet him. By the year 2000, I will have treated over 1,500 patients with rheumatic illnesses, including SLE, scleroderma, polymyositis and dermatomyositis.

My application of Dr. Brown's protocol has changed significantly since I first started implementing it. Initially, I followed Dr. Brown's work rigidly with very little modification other than shifting the tetracycline choice to Minocin. I believe I was one of the first people who recommended the shift to Minocin, which seems to have been widely adopted at this time.

In the early 90s, I started to integrate the nutritional model into the program and noticed a significant improvement in the treatment response. I cannot emphasize strongly enough the importance of this aspect of the program. It is absolutely an essential component of the revised Dr. Brown protocol. One may achieve remission without it, but the chances are much improved with its implementation. The additional benefit of the dietary changes is that they severely reduce the risk of the two to six month worsening of symptoms that Dr. Brown described in his book.

In the late 80s, the common retort from other physicians was that there was "no scientific proof" that this treatment works. Well, that is certainly not true today. If one peeks ahead at the bibliography, one will find over 200 references in the peer-reviewed medical literature that supports the application of Minocin in the use of rheumatic illnesses. The definitive scientific support for minocycline in the treatment of rheumatoid arthritis came with the MIRA trial in the United States. This was a double blind randomized placebo controlled trial done at six university centers involving 200 patients for nearly one year. The dosage they used (100 mg twice daily) was much higher and likely less effective than what most clinicians currently use. They also did not employ any additional antibiotics or nutritional regimens, yet 55% of the patients improved. This study finally provided the "proof" that many traditional clinicians demanded before seriously considering this treatment as an alternative regimen for rheumatoid arthritis.

Dr. Thomas Brown's effort to treat the chronic mycoplasma infections believed to cause rheumatoid arthritis is the basis for this therapy. Dr. Brown believed that most rheumatic illnesses respond to this treatment. He and others used this therapy for SLE, ankylosing spondylitis, scleroderma, dermatomyositis and polymyositis.

Dr. Osler was also a preeminent figure of his time (1849-1919). Many regard him as the consummate physician of modern times. An excerpt from a commentary on Dr. William Osler provides a useful perspective on application of alternative medical paradigms:

Osler would be receptive to the cautious exploration of nontraditional methods of treatment, particularly in situations in which our present science has little to offer. From his reading of medical history, he would know that many pharmacologic agents were originally derived from folk medicine. He would also remember that in the 19th century physicians no less intelligent than those in our own day initially ridiculed the unconventional practices of Semmelweis and Lister.

Osler would caution us against the arrogance of believing that only our current medical practices can benefit the patient. He would realize that new scientific insights might emerge from as yet unproved beliefs. Although he would fight vigorously to protect the public against frauds and charlatans, he would encourage critical study of whatever therapeutic approaches were reliably reported to be beneficial to patients.

Nutritional Considerations

Limiting sugar is a critical element of the treatment program. Sugar has multiple significant negative influences on a person's biochemistry. Its major mode of action is through elevation of insulin levels. However, it has a similarly severe impairment of intestinal microflora. Patients who are unable to decrease their sugar intake are far less likely to improve.

One of the major benefits of implementing the dietary changes is that one does not seem to develop worsening of symptoms the first three to six months that is described in Dr. Brown's book. Most of my patients tend to not worsen once they start the antibiotics. I believe this is due to the beneficial effects that the diet has on the immune response. I ask all new patients to read my 6-page handout on the dietary changes. Rather than repeat it here, one could obtain the current version on my web site at www.mercola.com under the tab heading on the left side of the page entitled Read This First.

Antibiotic Therapy With Minocin

There are three different tetracyclines available: simple tetracycline, doxycycline, or Minocin (minocycline).

Minocin has a distinct and clear advantage over tetracycline and doxycycline in three important areas.

1. Extended spectrum of activity
2. Greater tissue penetrability
3. Higher and more sustained serum levels

Bacterial cell membranes contain a lipid layer. One mechanism of building up a resistance to an antibiotic is to produce a thicker lipid layer. This layer makes it difficult for an antibiotic to penetrate. Minocin's chemical structure makes it the most lipid soluble of all the tetracyclines.

This difference can clearly be demonstrated when one compares the drugs in the treatment of two common clinical conditions. Minocin gives consistently superior clinical results in the treatment of chronic prostatitis. In other studies, Minocin was used to improve between 75-85% of patients whose acne had become resistant to tetracycline. Strep is also believed to be a contributing cause to many patients with rheumatoid arthritis. Minocin has shown significant activity against treatment of this organism.

There are several important factors to consider when using Minocin. Unlike the other tetracyclines, it tends not to cause yeast infections. Some infectious disease experts even believe that it even has a mild anti-yeast activity.

Women can be on this medication for several years and not have any vaginal yeast infections. Nevertheless, it would be prudent to have patients on prophylactic oral *Lactobacillus acidophilus* and bifidus preparations. This will help to replace the normal intestinal flora that is killed with the Minocin.

Another advantage of Minocin is that it tends not to sensitize patients to the sun. This minimizes the risk of sunburn and increased risk of skin cancer. However, one must incorporate several precautions with the use of Minocin. Like other tetracyclines, food impairs its absorption. However, the absorption is much less impaired than with other tetracyclines. This is fortunate because some patients cannot tolerate Minocin on an empty stomach.

They must take it with a meal to avoid GI side effects. If they need to take it with a meal, they will still absorb 85% of the medication, whereas tetracycline is only 50% absorbed. In June of 1990, a pelletized version of Minocin became available. This improved absorption when taken with meals. This form is only available in the non-generic Lederele brand and is a more than reasonable justification to not substitute for the generic version. Clinical experience has shown that many patients will relapse when they switch from the brand name to the generic. It is strongly advised that only the non-generic brand name Minocin by Lederle be used.

However, many patients are on NSAID's which contribute to micro-ulcerations of the stomach which cause chronic blood loss. It is certainly possible they can develop a peptic ulceration contributing to their blood loss. In either event, patients frequently receive iron supplements to correct their blood counts. IT IS IMPERATIVE THAT MINOCIN NOT BE GIVEN WITH IRON. Over 85% of the dose will bind to the iron and pass through the colon unabsorbed. If iron is taken, it should be at least one hour before the minocin or two hours after. One recent uncommon complication of Minocin is a cell-mediated hypersensitivity pneumonitis.

Most patients can start on Minocin 100 mg. every Monday, Wednesday, and Friday evening. Doxycycline can be substituted for patients who cannot afford the more expensive Minocin. It is important to not give either medication daily, as this does not seem to provide as great a clinical benefit.

Tetracycline type drugs can cause a permanent yellow-grayish brown discoloration of the teeth. This can occur in the last half of pregnancy and in children up to eight years old. One should not routinely use tetracycline in children. If patients have severe disease, one can consider increasing the dose to as high as 200 mg three times a week. Aside from the cost of this approach, several problems may result from the higher doses. Minocin can cause quite severe nausea and vertigo. Taking the dose at night does tend to decrease this problem considerably.

However, if one takes the dose at bedtime, one must tell the patient to swallow the medication with TWO glasses of water. This is to insure that the capsule doesn't get stuck in the throat. If that occurs, a severe chemical esophagitis can result which can send the patient to the emergency room.

For those physicians who elect to use tetracycline or doxycycline for cost or sensitivity reasons, several methods may help lessen the inevitable secondary yeast overgrowth. *Lactobacillus acidophilus* will help maintain normal bowel flora and decrease the risk of fungal overgrowth. Aggressive avoidance of all sugars, especially those found in non-diet sodas will also decrease the substrate for the yeast's growth. Macrolide antibiotics like Biaxin or Zithromax may be used if tetracyclines are contraindicated. They would also be used in the three pills a week regimen.

Clindamycin

The other drug used to treat rheumatoid arthritis is clindamycin. Dr. Brown's book discusses the uses of intravenous clindamycin. It is important to use the IV form of treatment if the disease is severe. Nearly all scleroderma patients should take an aggressive stance and use IV treatment. Scleroderma is a particularly dangerous form of rheumatic illness that should receive aggressive intervention.

A major problem with the IV form is the cost. The price ranges from $100 to $300 per dose if administered by a home health care agency. However, if purchased directly from Upjohn, significant savings will be appreciated. A case of two-dozen 900 mg prefilled IV bags can be purchased directly from Upjohn for about $200. (2000 prices)

For patients with milder illness, the oral form is preferable. If the patient has a mild rheumatic illness (the minority of cases), it is even possible to exclude this from their regimen. Initial starting doses for an adult would be a 1200 mg dose once a week. Patients do not seem to tolerate this medication as well as Minocin. The major complaint seems to be a bitter metallic type taste, which lasts about 24 hours after the dose. Taking the dose after dinner does seem to help modify this complaint somewhat. If this is a problem, one can lower the dose and gradually increase the dose over a few weeks.

Concern about the development of C. difficile pseudomembranous enterocolitis as a result of the clindamycin is appropriate. This complication is quite rare at this dosage regimen, but it certainly can occur. It is important to warn all patients about the possibility of developing a severe uncontrollable diarrhea. Administration of the acidophilus seems to limit this complication by promoting the growth of the healthy gut flora.

If one encounters a resistant form of rheumatic illness, intravenous administration should be considered. Generally, weekly doses of 900 mg are administered until clinical improvement is observed. This generally occurs within the first ten doses. At that time, the regimen can be decreased to every two weeks with the oral form substituted on the weeks where the IV is not taken.

What To Do If Severe Patients Fail To Respond

The most frequent reason for failure to respond to the protocol is lack of adherence to the dietary guidelines. Most patients will be eating too many grains and sugars, which disturb insulin physiology. It is important that patients adhere as strictly as possible to the guidelines.A small minority, generally under 15%, of patients will fail to respond to the protocol described above despite rigid adherence to the diet.These individuals should already be on the IV Clindamycin.

It appears that the hyaluronic acid, which is a potentiating agent commonly used in the treatment of cancer may be quite useful. It seems that hyaluronic acid has very little to no direct toxicity but works in a highly synergistic fashion when administered directly in the IV bag with the Clindamycin. Hyaluronic acid is also used in orthopedic procedures. The dose is generally from 2 to 10 cc into the IV bag. Hyaluronic acid is not inexpensive as the cost may range up to $10 per cc.One does need to exert some caution with its use as it may precipitate a significant Herxheimer flare reaction.

Patients will frequently have emotional traumas that worsen their illness. Severe emotional traumas can seriously impair the immune response to this treatment. A particularly useful and rapid technique called Neuro Emotional Technique (NET) can be used to resolve this problem. Practitioners using this technique can be found by calling the One Foundation The ONE Research Foundation, 144 West D Street, Suite 107, Encinitas, CA 92024, Telephone: 800-638-1411 or 760-944-7383.

Anti-Inflammatories

The first non-aspirin NSAID (non-steroidal anti-inflammatory drug), indomethacin was introduced in 1963. Now more than 30 are available. Relafen is one of the better alternatives as it seems to cause less of an intestinal dysbiosis. If cost is a concern, generic ibuprofen can be used. Unfortunately, recent studies suggest this drug is more damaging to the kidneys. One must be especially careful to monitor renal function studies periodically. It is important for the patient to understand and accept the risks associated with these more toxic drugs.

Unfortunately, these drugs are not benign. Every year, they do enough damage to the GI tract to kill 2,000 to 4,000 patients with rheumatoid arthritis alone. That is ten patients EVERY DAY. At any given time patients receiving NSAID therapy have gastric ulcers in the range of 10-20%. Duodenal ulcers are lower at 2-5%. Patients on NSAIDs are at approximately three times greater relative risk for developing serious gastrointestinal side effects than are non-users.

Approximately 1.2% of patients taking NSAIDs are hospitalized for upper GI problems per year of exposure. One study of patients taking NSAIDs showed that a life-threatening complication was the first sign of ulcer in more than half of the subjects.

Celebrex has received much recent press due to its decreased toxicity to the gut. That is certainly a step in the right direction. Celebrex inhibits a specific type of prostaglandin and is called a COX2 inhibitor. A similar new drug introduced in 1999 is Vioxx. There was a report in early 1999 in the *Proceedings of the National Academy of Science*, which showed that these drugs might increase the risk of heart attack, stroke and blood clotting disorders.

Researchers found that the drugs suppress production of prostacyclin, which is needed to dilate blood vessels and inhibit clotting. Earlier studies had found that mice genetically engineered to be unable to use prostacyclin properly were prone to clotting disorders. Anyone who is at increased risk of cardiovascular disease should steer clear of these two new medications. Ulcer complications are certainly potentially life-threatening, but, heart attacks are a much more common and likely risk, especially in older individuals.

Risk factor analysis helps to discriminate those that are at increased danger of developing these complications.

Those associated with a higher frequency of adverse events are:

1. Old age
2. Peptic ulcer history
3. Alcohol dependency
4. Cigarette smoking
5. Concurrent prednisone or corticosteroid use
6. Disability
7. High dose of the NSAID
8. NSAID known to be more toxic

Studies clearly show that the non-acetylated salicylates are the safest NSAIDs. Celebrex and Vioxx likely cause the least risk for peptic ulcer. But as mentioned, they pose an increased risk for heart disease. Factoring these newer medications out would leave the following less toxic NSAIDs: Relafen, Daypro, Voltaren, Motrin, and Naprosyn. Meclomen, Indocin, Orudis, and Tolectin are among the most toxic or likely to cause complications.

They are much more dangerous than the antibiotics or non-acetylated salicylates. One should run an SMA at least once a year on patients who are on these medications. One must monitor the serum potassium levels if the patient is on an ACE inhibitor as these medications can cause hyperkalemia. One should also monitor their kidney function. The SMA will also show any liver impairment that the drugs might cause.

These medications can also impair prostaglandin metabolism and cause papillary necrosis and chronic interstitial nephritis. The kidney needs vasodilatory prostaglandins (PGE2 and prostacycline) to counter balance the effects of potent vasoconstrictor hormones such as angiotensin II and catecholamines. NSAIDs decrease prostaglandin synthesis by inhibiting cyclooxygenase, leading to unopposed constriction of the renal arterioles supplying the kidney.

One might consider the use of non-acetylated salicylates such as salsalate, sodium salicylate and magnesium salicylate (i.e., Salflex, Disalcid, or Trilisate). They are the drugs of choice if there is renal insufficiency. They have minimal interference with anticyclooxygenase and other prostaglandins.

Additionally, they will not impair platelet inhibition of those patients who are on every other day aspirin to decrease their risk for stroke or heart disease. Unlike aspirin, they do not increase the formation of products of lipoxygenase-mediated metabolism of arachidonic acid. For this reason, they may be less likely to precipitate hypersensitivity reactions. These drugs have been safely used in patients with reversible obstructive airway disease and a history of aspirin sensitivity.

They also are much gentler on the stomach then the other NSAIDs and are the drug of choice if the patient has problems with peptic ulcer disease.

Unfortunately, all these benefits are balanced by the fact they may not be as effective as the other agents and are less convenient to take. One needs to push them to 1.5-2 grams bid and tinnitus is a frequent complication.

One should warn patients of this complication and explain that if tinnitus does develop they need to stop the drugs for a day and restart with a dose that is half a pill per day lower. They repeat this until they find a dose that relieves their pain and doesn't give them any ringing.

Prednisone

One can give patients with severe disease a prescription for prednisone 5 mg. They can take one of them a day if they develop a severe flare-up as a result of going on the antibiotics. They can use an additional tablet at night if they are in really severe flare. Explain to all patients that the prednisone is very dangerous and every dose they take decreases their bone density. However, it is a trade-off. Since they will only be on it for a matter of months, its use may be justifiable. This is the first medicine they should try to stop as soon as their symptoms permit.

Blood levels of cortisol peak between 3 and 9 am. It would, therefore, be safest to administer the prednisone in the morning. This will minimize the suppression on the hypothalamic-pituitary-adrenal axis. Patients often ask the dangers of these medications. The most significant one is osteoporosis. Other side effects that usually occur at higher doses include adrenal insufficiency, atherosclerosis acceleration, cataract formation, Cushing's syndrome, diabetes, ulcers, herpes simplex and tuberculosis reactivation, insomnia, hypertension, myopathy and renal stones.

One also needs to be concerned about the increased risk of peptic ulcer disease when using this medicine with conventional non-steroidal anti-inflammatories. Persons receiving both of these medicines may have a 15 times greater risk of developing an ulcer.

If a patient is already on prednisone, it is helpful to give them a prescription for 1 mg tablets so they can wean themselves off of the prednisone as soon as possible. Usually one lowers the dose by about 1 mg per week. If a relapse of the symptoms occurs, than further reduction of the prednisone is not indicated.

Remission

The following criteria can help establish remission:
 *A decrease in duration of morning stiffness to no more than 15 minutes
 * No pain at rest
 * Little or no pain or tenderness on motion
 * Absence of joint swelling
 * A normal energy level
 * A decrease in the ESR to no more than 30
 * A normalization of the patient's CBC. Generally the HGB, HCT, & MCV will increase to normal and their "pseudo"-iron deficiency will disappear

* ANA, RF, & ASO titers returning to normal

The natural course of rheumatoid arthritis is quite remarkable. Less than 1% of patients who are rheumatoid factor seropositive have a spontaneous remission. Some disability occurs in 50-70% of patients within five years after onset of the disease. Half of the patients will stop working within 10 years. This devastating natural prognosis is what makes the antibiotic therapy so exciting.

Approximately one third of patients have been lost to follow-up for whatever reason and have not continued with treatment. The remaining patients seem to have a 60-90% likelihood of improvement on this treatment regimen.

That is quite a stark contrast to the numbers quoted above.

There are many variables associated with an increased chance of remission or improvement. The younger the patient is the better they seem to do. The more closely they follow the diet, the less likely they are to have a severe flare-up and the more likely they are to improve. Smoking seems to be negatively associated with improvement.

The longer the patient has had the illness and the more severe the illness the more difficult it seems to treat.

If patients discontinue their medications before all of the above criteria are met, there is a greater risk that the disease will recur. If the patient meets the above criteria, one can have them to try to stop their anti-inflammatory medication once they start to experience these improvements. If the improvements are stable for six months, then discontinue the clindamycin. If the improvements are maintained for the next six months, one can then discontinue their Minocin and monitor for recurrences. If symptoms should recur, it would be wise to restart the previous antibiotic regimen.

Overall, nearly 80% of the patients do remarkably better with this program. Approximately 5% of the patients continued to worsen and required conventional agents, like methotrexate, to relieve their symptoms.

Approximately 15% of the patients who started the treatment dropped out of the program and were lost to follow-up. The longer and more severe the illness, the longer it takes to cure. Smokers tend not to do as well with this program. Age and competency of the person's immune system are also likely important factors.

Dr. Brown successfully treated over 10,000 patients with this protocol. He found that significant benefits from the treatment require on the average one to two years. I have treated nearly over 1,500 patients and find that the dietary modification I advocate accelerates the response rate to several months. The length of therapy can vary widely. In severe cases, it may take up to thirty months for the patients to gain sustained improvement. One requires patience because remissions may take up to 3 to 5 years. Dr. Brown's pioneering approach represents a safer less toxic alternative to many conventional regimens and results of the NIH trial have finally scientifically validated this treatment.

[Contrast these facts with Wyburn-Mason trials. Whether or not Wyburn-Mason's treatment will work can be learned in six to twelve weeks at considerably lower c ost. Ed.]

Preliminary Laboratory Evaluation For Non-Rheumatologists

It is important to evaluate patients to determine if indeed they have rheumatoid arthritis. Most patients will have received evaluations and treatment by one or more board certified rheumatologists. If this is the case, the diagnosis is rarely in question and one only needs to establish some baseline laboratory data.

However, patients will frequently come in without having any appropriate workup done by a physician. Arthritic pain can be an early manifestation of 20-30 different clinical problems. These include not only rheumatic disease, but also metabolic, infectious and malignant disorders. These patients will require a more extensive laboratory analysis.

Rheumatoid arthritis is a clinical diagnosis for which there is not a single test or group of laboratory tests which can be considered confirmatory. When a patient hasn't been properly diagnosed, then one needs to establish the diagnosis with the standard Rheumatism Association's criteria found in the table at the end of the article.

One must also make certain that the first four symptoms listed in the table are present for six or more weeks.

These criteria have a 91-94% sensitivity and 89% specificity for the diagnosis of rheumatoid arthritis. However, these criteria were designed for classification and not for diagnosis. One must make the diagnosis on clinical grounds. It is important to note that many patients with negative serologic tests can have a strong clinical picture for rheumatoid arthritis.

The metacarpophalangeal joints, proximal interphalangeal and wrists joints are the first joints to become symptomatic. In a way, the hands are the calling card of rheumatoid arthritis. If the patient completely lacks hand and wrist involvement, even by history, the diagnosis of rheumatoid arthritis is doubtful. Rheumatoid arthritis rarely affects the hips and ankles early in its course.

Fatigue may be present before the joint symptoms begin. Morning stiffness is a sensitive indicator of rheumatoid arthritis. An increase in fluid in and around the joint probably causes the stiffness. The joints are warm, but the skin is rarely red. When the joints develop effusions, the patients hold them flexed at 5 to 20 degrees as it is too painful to extend them fully.

The general initial laboratory evaluation should include a baseline ESR, CBC, SMA, U/A, and an ASO titer. One can also draw RF and ANA titers to further objectively document improvement with the therapy. However, they seldom add much to the assessment.

Follow-up visits can be every two months for patients who live within 50 miles, and every three to four months for those who live farther away. An ESR at every visit is an inexpensive and reliable objective parameter of the extent of the disease. However, one should run this test within several hours of the blood draw. Otherwise, one cannot obtain reliable and reproducible results. This is nearly impossible with most clinical labs that pick up your specimen at the office.

Inexpensive disposable ESR kits are a practical alternative to the commercial or hospital labs. One can then run them in the office, usually within one hour of the blood draw. One must be careful to not run the test on the same countertop as your centrifuge. This may cause a falsely elevated ESR due to the agitation of the ESR measuring tube.

Many patients with rheumatoid arthritis have a hypochromic, microcytic CBC. This is probably due to the inflammation in the rheumatoid arthritis impairing optimal bone marrow utilization of iron. This type of anemia does NOT respond to iron. Patients who take iron can actually worsen if they don't need it as the iron serves as a potent oxidant stress. Ferritin levels are generally the most reliable indicator of total iron body stores. Unfortunately it is also an acute phase reactant protein and will be elevated anytime the ESR is elevated. This makes ferritin an unreliable test in patients with rheumatoid arthritis.

Fibromyalgia

One needs to be very sensitive to this clinical problem when treating patients with rheumatoid arthritis. It is frequently a complicating condition. Many times, patients will confuse the pain from it with a flare-up of their arthritis. One needs to aggressively treat this problem. If this problem is ignored, the likelihood of successfully treating the arthritis is significantly diminished.

Fibromyalgia is a very common problem. Some experts believe that 5% of people are affected with it. Over 12% of the patients at the Mayo Clinic's Department of Physical Medicine and Rehabilitation have this problem. It is the third most common diagnosis by rheumatologists in the outpatient setting. Fibromyalgia affects women five times as frequently as men.

Signs And Symptoms of Fibromyalgia

One of the main features of fibromyalgia is the morning stiffness, fatigue, and multiple areas of tenderness in typical locations. Most patients with fibromyalgia complain of pain over many areas of the body, with an average of six to nine locations. Although the pain is frequently described as being all over, it is most prominent in the neck, shoulders, elbows, hips, knees, and back.

Tender points are generally symmetrical and on both sides of the body. The areas of tenderness are usually small (less than an inch in diameter) and deep within the muscle. They are often located in sites that are slightly tender in normal people. Patients with fibromyalgia, however, differ in having increased tenderness at these sites than normal persons. Firm palpation with the thumb (just past the point where the nail turns white) over the outside elbow will typically cause a vague sensation of discomfort. Patients with fibromyalgia will experience much more pain and will often withdraw the arm involuntarily.

More than 70% of patients describe their pain as profound aching and stiffness of the muscles. Often it is relatively constant from moment to moment, but certain positions or movements may momentarily worsen the pain.

Other terms used to describe the pain are dull and numb. Sharp or intermittent pain is relatively uncommon.

Patients with fibromyalgia often complain that sudden loud noises worsen their pain. The generalized stiffness of fibromyalgia does not diminish with activity, unlike the stiffness of rheumatoid arthritis, which lessens as the day progresses.

Despite the lack of abnormal lab tests, patients can suffer considerable discomfort. The fatigue is often severe enough to impair activities of work and recreation. Patients commonly experience fatigue on arising and complain of being more fatigued when they wake up then when they went to bed. Over 90% of patients believe the pain, stiffness, and fatigue are made worse by cold, damp weather. Overexertion, anxiety and stress are also factors.

Many people find that localized heat, such as hot baths, showers, or heating pads, give them some relief. There is also a tendency for pain to improve in the summer with mild activity or with rest.

Some patients will date the onset of their symptoms to some initiating event. This is often an injury, such as a fall, a motor vehicle accident, or a vocational or sports injury. Others find that their symptoms began with a stressful or emotional event, such as a death in the family, a divorce, a job loss, or similar occurrence.

Pain Location

Patients with fibromyalgia have pain in at least 11 of the following 18 tender point sites (one on each side of the body):

1. Base of the skull where the suboccipital muscle inserts.
2. Back of the low neck (anterior intertransverse spaces of C5-C7).
3. Midpoint of the upper shoulders (trapezius).
4. On the back in the middle of the scapula.
5. On the chest where the second rib attaches to the breastbone (sternum).
6. One inch below the outside of each elbow (lateral epicondyle).
7. Upper outer quadrant of buttocks.
8. Just behind the swelling on the upper leg bone below the hip (trochanteric prominence).
9. The inside of both knees (medial fat pads proximal to the joint line).

Treatment Of Fibromyalgia

There is a persuasive body of emerging evidence that indicates that patients with fibromyalgia are physically unfit in terms of sustained endurance. Some studies show that cardiovascular fitness training programs can decrease fibromyalgia pain by 75%. Sleep is critical to the improvement. Many times, improved fitness will correct the sleep disturbance.

Allergies, especially to mold, seem to be another common cause of fibromyalgia. [Also see *Soft Tissue Arthritis* on Amazon.com, at bookstores and at Arthritis Trust.org. Ed.]

Exercise For Rheumatoid Arthritis

It is very important to exercise or increase muscle tone of the non-weight bearing joints. Experts tell us that disuse results in muscle atrophy and weakness. Additionally, immobility may result in joint contractures and loss of range of motion (ROM). Active ROM exercises are preferred to passive. There is some evidence that passive ROM exercises increase the number of WBCs in the joint. If the joints are stiff, one should stretch and apply heat before exercising. If the joints are swollen, application of ten minutes of ice before exercise would be helpful.

The inflamed joint is very vulnerable to damage from improper exercise, so one must be cautious. People with arthritis must strike a delicate balance between rest and activity. They must avoid activities that aggravate joint pain. Patients should avoid any exercise that strains a significantly unstable joint.

A good rule of thumb is that if the pain lasts longer than one hour after stopping exercise, the patient should slow down or choose another form of exercise. Assistive devices are also helpful to decrease the pressure on affected joints. Many patients need to be urged to take advantage of these.

Of course, it is important to maintain good cardiovascular fitness. Walking with appropriate supportive shoes is also another important consideration.

The Infectious Cause Of Rheumatoid Arthritis

It is quite clear that autoimmunity plays a major role in the progression of rheumatoid arthritis. Most rheumatology investigators believe that an infectious agent causes rheumatoid arthritis. There is little agreement as to the involved organism. Investigators have proposed the following infectious agents: Human T-cell lymphotropic virus Type I, rubella virus, cytomegalovirus, herpesvirus, amoeba and mycoplasma. This review will focus on the evidence supporting the hypothesis that mycoplasma is a common etiologic agent of rheumatoid arthritis.

Mycoplasmas are the smallest self-replicating prokaryotes. They differ from classical bacteria by lacking rigid cell wall structures and are the smallest known organisms capable of extracellular existence. They are considered to be parasites of humans, animals, and plants.

In 1939, Dr. Sabin, the discoverer of the polio vaccine, first reported a chronic arthritis in mice caused by a mycoplasma. He suggested this agent might cause human rheumatoid arthritis.

Dr. Thomas Brown was a rheumatologist who worked with Dr. Sabin at the Rockefeller Institute. Dr. Brown trained at John Hopkins Hospital and then served as chief of medicine at George Washington Medical School before serving as chairman of the Arthritis Institute in Arlington, Virginia. He was a strong advocate of the mycoplasma infectious theory for over fifty years of his life.

Culturing Mycoplasmas From Joints

Mycoplasmas have limited biosynthetic capabilities and are very difficult to culture and grow from synovial tissues.

They require complex growth media or a close parasitic relation with animal cells. This contributed to many investigators failure to isolate them from arthritic tissue. In reactive arthritis immune complexes rather than viable organisms localize in the joints. The infectious agent is actually present at another site. Some investigators believe that the organism binding in the immune complex contributes to the difficulty in obtaining positive mycoplasma cultures.

Despite this difficulty some researchers have successfully isolated mycoplasma from synovial tissues of patients with rheumatoid arthritis. A British group used a leucocyte-migration inhibition test and found two-thirds of their rheumatoid arthritis patients to be infected with *Mycoplasma fermentens*. These results are impressive since they did not include more prevalent Mycoplasma strains like *M. salivarium*, *M. ovale*, *M. hominis*, and *M. pneumonia*.

One Finnish investigator reported a 100% incidence of isolation of mycoplasma from 27 rheumatoid synovia using a modified culture technique. None of the non-rheumatoid tissue yielded any mycoplasmas. The same investigator used an indirect hemagglutination technique and reported mycoplasma antibodies in 53% of patients with definite rheumatoid arthritis. Using similar techniques other investigators have cultured mycoplasma in 80-100% of their rheumatoid arthritis test population.

Rheumatoid arthritis follows some mycoplasma respiratory infections. One study of over 1000 patients was able to identify arthritis in nearly 1% of the patients. These infections can be associated with a positive rheumatoid factor.

This provides additional support for mycoplasma as an etiologic agent for rheumatoid arthritis. Human genital mycoplasma infections have also caused septic arthritis.

Harvard investigators were able to culture mycoplasma or a similar organism, ureaplasma urealyticum, from 63% of female patients with SLE and only 4% of patients with CFS. The researchers chose CFS as these patients shared similar symptoms as those with SLE, such as fatigue, arthralgias, and myalgias.

Animal Evidence for The Protocol

The full spectrum of human rheumatoid arthritis immune responses (lymphokine production, altered lymphocyte reactivity, immune complex deposition, cell-mediated immunity and development of autoimmune reactions) occurs in mycoplasma induced animal arthritis. Investigators have implicated at least 31 different mycoplasma species.

Mycoplasma can produce experimental arthritis in animals from three days to months later. The time seems to depend on the dose given and the virulence of the organism.

There is a close degree of similarity between these infections and those of human rheumatoid arthritis.

114

Mycoplasmas cause arthritis in animals by several mechanisms. They either directly multiply within the joint or initiate an intense local immune response. Mycoplasma produces a chronic arthritis in animals that is remarkably similar to rheumatoid arthritis in humans. Arthritogenic mycoplasmas cause joint inflammation in animals by many mechanisms. They induce nonspecific lymphocyte cytotoxicity and antilymphocyte antibodies as well as rheumatoid factor. Mycoplasma clearly causes chronic arthritis in mice, rats, fowl, swine, sheep, goats, cattle and rabbits. The arthritis appears to be the direct result of joint infection with culturable mycoplasma organisms.

Gorillas have tissue reactions closer to man than any other animal. Investigators have shown that mycoplasma can precipitate a rheumatic illness in gorillas. One study demonstrated mycoplasma antigens occur in immune complexes in great apes. The human and gorilla IgG are very similar and express nearly identical rheumatoid factors (IgM anti-IgG antibodies). The study showed that when mycoplasma binds to IgG it can cause a conformational change. This conformational change results in an anti-IgG antibody, which can then stimulate an autoimmune response.

The Science of Why Minocycline Is Used

If mycoplasma were a causative factor in rheumatoid arthritis, one would expect tetracycline type drugs to provide some sort of improvement in the disease. Collagenase activity increases in rheumatoid arthritis and probably has a role in its cause. Investigators demonstrated that tetracycline and minocycline inhibit leukocyte, macrophage, and synovial collagenase.

There are several other aspects of tetracyclines that may play a role in rheumatoid arthritis. Investigators have shown minocycline and tetracycline to retard excessive connective tissue breakdown and bone resorption while doxycycline inhibits digestion of human cartilage. It is also possible that tetracycline treatment improves rheumatic illness by reducing delayed-type hypersensitivity response. Minocycline and doxycycline both inhibit phosolipases which are considered proinflammatory and capable of inducing synovitis.

Minocycline is a more potent antibiotic than tetracycline and penetrates tissues better. These characteristics shifted the treatment of rheumatic illness away from tetracycline to minocycline. Minocycline may benefit rheumatoid arthritis patients through its immunomodulating and immunosuppressive properties. In vitro studies demonstrated a decreased neutrophil production of reactive oxygen intermediates along with diminished neutrophil chemotaxis and phagocytosis. Investigators showed that minocycline reduced the incidence of severity of synovitis in animal models of arthritis. The improvement was independent of minocycline's effect on collagenase.

Minocycline has also been shown to increase intracellular calcium concentrations that inhibit T-cells.

Individuals with the Class II major histocompatibility complex (MHC) DR4 allele seem to be predisposed to developing rheumatoid arthritis. The infectious agent probably interacts with this specific antigen in some way to precipitate rheumatoid arthritis. There is strong support for the role of T cells in this interaction. Minocycline may suppress rheumatoid arthritis by altering T cell calcium flux and the expression of T cell derived from collagen binding protein. Minocycline produced a suppression of the delayed hypersensitivity in patients with Reiter's syndrome. Investigators also successfully used minocycline to treat the arthritis and early morning stiffness of Reiter's syndrome.

Clinical Studies

In 1970 investigators at Boston University conducted a small, randomized placebo-controlled trial to determine if tetracycline would treat rheumatoid arthritis. They used 250 mg of tetracycline a day. Their study showed no improvement after one year of tetracycline treatment. Several factors could explain their inability to demonstrate any benefits. Their study used only 27 patients for a one-year trial, and only 12 received tetracycline.

Noncompliance could have been a factor. Additionally, none of the patients had severe arthritis. Patients were excluded from the trial if they were on any anti-remittive therapy.

Finnish investigators used lymecycline to treat the reactive arthritis in *Chlamydia trachomatous* infections. The study compared the effect of the medication in patients with two other reactive arthritis infections Yersinia and Campylobacter. Lymecyline produced a shorter course of illness in the Chlamydia induced arthritis patients, but did not affect the other enteric infections-associated reactive arthritis. The investigators later published findings that suggested lymecycline achieved its effect through non-antimicrobial actions. They speculated it worked by preventing the oxidative activation of collagenase.

Breedveld published the first trial of minocycline for the treatment of animal and human rheumatoid arthritis. In the first published human trial, Breedveld treated ten patients in an open study for 16 weeks. He used a very high dose of 400 mg per day. Most patients had vestibular side effects resulting from this dose. However, all patients showed benefit from the treatment. All variables of efficacy were significantly improved at the end of the trial. Breedveld concluded an expansion of his initial study and observed similar impressive results. This was a 26-week double-blind placebo-controlled randomized trial with minocycline for 80 patients. They were given 200 mg twice a day. The Ritchie articular index and the number of swollen joints significantly improved ($p < 0.05$) more in the minocyline group than in the placebo group.

Investigators in Israel studied 18 patients with severe rheumatoid arthritis for 48 weeks. These patients had failed two other DMARD (disease-modifying antirheumatic drugs). They were taken off all DMARD agents and given minocycline 100 mg twice a day. Six patients did not complete the study, three withdrew because of lack of improvement, and three had side effects of vertigo or leukopenia. All patients completing the study improved. Three had complete remission, three had substantial improvement of greater than 50% and six had moderate improvement of 25% in the number of active joints and morning stiffness.

Criteria For Classification Of Rheumatoid Arthritis

Morning stiffness in and around joints lasting at least one hour before maximal improvement is noted.

Arthritis of three or more joint areas At least three joint areas have simultaneously had soft-tissue swelling or fluid (not bony overgrowth) observed by a physician. There are 14 possible joints: right or left PIP, MCP, wrist, elbow, knee, ankle, and MTP joints.

Arthritis of hand joints

At least one joint area swollen as above in a wrist, MCP, or PIP joint
Symmetric arthritis

Simultaneous involvement of the same joint areas (as in criterion 2) on both sides of the body (bilateral involvement of PIPs, MCPs, or MTPs) is acceptable without absolute symmetry. Lack of symmetry is not sufficient to rule out the diagnosis of rheumatoid arthritis.

Rheumatoid Nodules

Subcutaneous nodules over bony prominences, or extensor surfaces, or in juxta-articular regions, observed by a physician. Only about 25% of patients with rheumatoid arthritis develop nodules, and usually as a later manifestation.

Serum rheumatoid factor

Demonstration of abnormal amounts of serum rheumatoid factor by any method that has been positive in less than 5% of normal control subjects. This test is positive only 30-40% of the time in the early months of rheumatoid arthritis.

Radiological Changes

Radiological changes typical of rheumatoid arthritis on PA hand and wrist X-rays, which must include erosions or unequivocal bony decalcification localized to or most marked adjacent to the involved joints (osteoarthritic changes alone do not count).

Note: Patients must satisfy at least four of the seven criteria listed. Any of criteria 1-4 must have been present for at least 6 weeks. Patients with two clinical diagnoses are not excluded. Designations as classic, definite, or probable rheumatoid arthritis is not to be made.

Harold W. Clark, Ph.D. adds, "I'm not sure whether the tests (MCF, BFT, and Kunkle) are still available but should be included."

Bibliography

1.Pincus T, Wolfe F: Treatment of Rheumatoid Arthritis: Challenges to Traditional Paradigms. AnnInternMed 115:825-6, Nov 15 1991.

2.Pincus T: Rheumatoid arthritis: disappointing long-term outcomes despite successful short-term clinical trials. J Clin Epidemiol 41:1037-41, 1988.

3.Brooks PM: Clinical management of rheumatoid arthritis. Lancet 341 :286-90, 1993.

4.Pincus T, Callahan LF: Remodeling the pyramid or remodeling the paradigms concerning rheumatoid arthritis - lessons learned from Hodgkin's Disease and coronary artery disease. JRheumatol 17:1582-5, 1990.

5.Reah TG: The prognosis of rheumatoid arthritis. Proc R Soc Med 56:813-17, 1963.

6.Wolfe F, Hawley DJ: Remission in rheumatoid arthritis. J Rheumatol 12:245-9, 1985.

7.Kushner I, Dawson NV: Changing perspectives in the treatment of rheumatoid arthritis. JRheumatol 19:1831-34, 1992.

8.Pinals RS: Drug therapy in rheumatoid arthritis a perspective. Br J Rheumatol 28:93-5, 1989.

9.Klippel JH: Winning the battle, losing the war? Another editorial about rheumatoid arthritis. JRheumatol 17:1118-22. 1990.

10.Healey LA, Wilske KR: Evaluating combination drug therapy in rheumatoid arthritis. J Rheumatol 18:641-2, 1991.

11.Wolfe F: 50 Years of antirheumatic therapy: the prognosis of rheumatoid arthritis. J Rheumatol 17:24-32, 1990.

12.Gabriel SE, Luthra HS: Rheumatoid arthritis: Can the long term be altered? Mayo Clin Proc 63:58-68, 1988.

13.Harris ED: Rheumatoid arthritis: Pathophysiology and implications for therapy. NEngl JMed 322:1277-1289, May 3, 1990.

14.Schwartz BD: Infectious agents, immunity and rheumatic diseases. Arthr Rheum 33 :457-465, April 1990.

15.Tan PLJ, Skinner MA: The microbial cause of rheumatoid arthritis: time to dump Koch's postulates. J Rheumatol 19:1170-71. 1992.

16.Ford DK: The microbiological causes of rheumatoid arthritis. JRheumatol 18:1441-2, 1991.

17.Burmester GR: Hit and run or permanent hit? Is there evidence for a microbiological cause of rheumatoid arthritis? J Rheumatol 18:1443-7, 1991.

18.Phillips PE: Evidence implications infectious agents in rheumatoid arthritis and juvenile rheumatoid arthritis. Clin EXD Rheumatol 1988 6:87-94.

19.Sabin AB: Experimental proliferative arthritis in mice produced by filtrable pleuropneumonia-like microorganisms. Science 89:228-29, 1939.

20.Swift HF, Brown TMcP: Pathogenic pleuropneumonia-like organisms from acute rheumatic exudates and tissues. Science 89:271-272. 1939.

21.Clark HW, Bailey JS, Brown TMcP: Determination of mycoplasma antibodies in humans. Bacteriol Proc 64:59, 1964.

22.Brown Tmcp, Wichelausen RH, Robinson LB, et al: The in vivo action of aureomycin on pleuropneumonia-like organisms associated with various rheumatic diseases. J Lab Clin Med 34: 1404-1410. 1949.

23.Brown TMcP, Wichelhausen RH: A study of the antigen-antibody mechanism in rheumatic diseases. Amer JMed Sci 221:618, 1951.

24.Brown TMcP: The rheumatic crossroads. Postgrad Med 19:399-402, 1956.

25.Brown TMcP, Clark HW, Bailey JS, et al: Relationship between mycoplasma antibodies and rheumatoid factors. ArthrRheum 13:309-310, 1970.

26.Clark HW, Brown TMcP: Another look at mycoplasma. Arthr Rheum 19:649-50, 1976.

27.Hakkarainen K, et al: Mycoplasmas and arthritis. Ann Rheumat Dis 51: S70-72; l992.

28.Rook, GAW, et al: A reppraisal of the evidence that rheumatoid arthritis and several other idiopathic diseases are slow bacterial infections. Ann Rheum Dis 52:S30-S38; 1993.

29.Clark HW, Coker-Vann MR, Bailey JS, et al: Detection of mycoplasma antigens in immune complexes from rheumatoid arthritis synovial fluids. Ann Allergy 60:394-98, May 1988.

30.Wilder RL: Etiologic considerations in rheumatoid arthritis. Ann Intern Med 101 :820-21, 1984.

31.Bartholomew LE: Isolations and characterization of mycoplasmas (PPLO) from patients with rheumatoid arthritis, systemic lupus erythematosus and Reiter's syndrome. Arthr Rheum 8:376-388. 1965.

32.Brown TMcP, et al: Mycoplasma antibodies in synovia. Arthritis Rheum 9:495, 1966.

33.Hernandez LA, Urquhart GED, Dick WC: Mycoplasma pneumonia infection and arthritis in man. Br Med J 2: 14- 16. 1977.

34.McDonald MI, Moore JO, Harrelson JM, et al: Septic arthritis due to Mycoplasma hominis. Arth Rheum 26: 1044-47, 1983.

35.Williams MH, Brostoff J, Roitt IM: Possible role of Mycoplasma fermenters in pathogenesis of rheumatoid arthritis. Lancet 2:277-280 1970

36.Jansson E, Makisara P, Vainio K, et al: An 8-year study on mycoplasma in rheumatoid arthritis. Ann Rheum Dis 30:506-508, 1971.

37.Jansson E, Makisara P, Tuuri S: Mycoplasma antibodies in rheumatoid arthritis. Scan J Rheumatol 4: 165-68, 1975.

38.Markham JG, Myers DB: Preliminary observations on an isolate from synovial fluid of patients with rheumatoid arthritis. Ann Rheum Dis, S 1-7 1976.

39.Tully JG, et al: Pathogenic mycoplasmas: cultivation and vertebrate pathogenicity of a new spiroplasma. Science 195:892-4, 1977.

40.Fahlberg WJ, et al: Isolation of mycoplasma from human synovial fluids and tissues. Bacteria Proceedings 66:48-9, 1966.

41.Ponka A: The occurrence and clinical picture of serologically verified Mycoplasma pneumonia infections with
    emphasis on central nervous system, cardiac and joint manifestations. Ann Clin Res II (suppl) 24, 1979.

42.Hernandez LA, Urquhart GED, Dick WC: Mycoplasma pneumonia infections and arthritis in man. Br Med J2:14-16, 1977.

43.Ponka A: Arthritis associated with Mycoplasma pneumonia infection. Scand J Rheumatol 8:27-32, 1979.

44.Stuckey M, Quinn PA, Gelfand EW: Identification of T-Strain mycoplasma in a patient with polyarthritis. Lancet 2:917-920. 1978.

45.Webster ADB, Taylor-Robinson D, Furr PM, et al: Mycoplasmal septic arthritis in hypogammaglobuinemia. Br Med J 1 :478-79, 1978.

46.Ginsburg KS, Kundsin RB, Walter CW, et al: Ureaplasma urealyticum and Mycoplasma hominis in women with systemic lupus erythematosus. Arthritis Rheumatism 35 429-33, 1992.

47.Cole BC, Cassel GH: Mycoplasma infections as models of chronic joint inflammation. Arthr Rheum 22:1375-1381, Dec 1979.

48.Cassell GH, Cole BC: Mycoplasmas as agents of human disease. N Engl J Med 304: 80-89, Jan 8, 1981.

49.Jansson E, et al: Mycoplasmas and arthritis. Rheumatol 42:315-9, 1983.

50.Camon GW, Cole BCC, Ward JR, et al: Arthritogenic effects of Mycoplasma arthritides T cell mitogen in rats. JRheumatol 15:735-41, 1988.

51.Cedillo L, Gil C, Mayagoita G, et al: Experimental arthritis induced by Mycoplasma pneumonia in rabbits. JRheumatol 19:344-7, 1992.

52.Baccala R, Smith LR, Vestberg M, et al: Mycoplasma arthritidis mitogen. Arthritis Rheumatism 35:43442, 1992.

53.Brown McP, Clark HW, Bailey JS: Rheumatoid arthritis in the gorilla: a study of mycoplasma-host interaction in pathogenesis and treatment. In Comparative Pathology of Zoo Animals, RJ Montali, Gigaki (ed), Smithsonian Institution Press. 1980. 259-266.

54.Clark HW: The potential role of mycoplasmas as autoantigens and immune complexes in chronic vascular pathogenesis. Am J Primatol 24:235-243, 1991.

55.Greenwald, rheumatoid arthritis, Goulb LM, Lavietes B, et al: Tetracyclines imibit human synovial collagenase in vivo and in vitro. RhPn fol 14:28-32. 1987.

56.Goulb LM, Lee HM, Lehrer G, et al: Minocycline reduces gingival collagenolytic activity during diabetes. JPeridontRes 18:516-26, 1983.

57.Goulb LM, et al: Tetracyclines imibit comective tissue breakdown: new therapeutic implications for an old family of drugs. Crit Rev Oral Med Pathol 2:297-322, 1991.

58.Ingman T, Sorsa T, Suomalainen K, et al: Tetracycline inhibition and the cellular source of collagenase in gingival revicular fluid in different periodontal diseases. A review article. J Periodontol 64(2):82-8, 1993.

59.Greenwald rheumatoid arthritis, Moak SA, et al: Tetracyclines suppress metalloproteinase activity in adjuvant arthritis and, in combination with flurbiprofen, ameliorate bone damage. J Rheumatol 19:927-38, 1992.

60.Gomes BC, Golub LM, Ramammurthy NS: Tetracyclines inhibit parathyroid hormone induced bone resorption in organ culture. Experientia 40:1273-5, 1985.

61.Yu LP Jr, SMith GN, Hasty KA, et al: Doxycycline inhibits Type XI collagenolytic activity of extracts from human osteoarthritic cartilage and of gelantinase. JRheumatol 18:1450-2, 1991.

62.Thong YH, Ferrante A: Effect of tetracycline treatment of immunological responses in mice. Clin Exp Immunol 39:728-32, 1980.

63.Pruzanski W, Vadas P: Should tetracyclines be used in arthritis? J Rheumatol 19: 1495-6, 1992.

64.Editorial: Antibiotics as biological response modifiers. Lancet 337:400-1, 1991.

65.Van Barr HMJ, et al: Tetracyclines are potent scavengers of the superoxide radical. Br J Dermatol 117:131-4, 1987.

66.Wasil M, Halliwell B, Moorhouse CP: Scavenging of hypochlorous acid by tetracycline, rifampicin and some other antibiotics: a possible antioxidant action of rifampicin and tetracycline? Biochem Pharmacol 37:775-8, 1988.

67.Breedveld FC, Trentham DE: Suppression of collagen and adjuvant arthritis by a tetracycline. Arthritis Rheum 31(1 Supplement)R3, 1988.

68.Trentham, DE; Dynesium-Trentham rheumatoid arthritis: Antibiotic Therapy for Rheumatoid Arthritis: Scientific and Anecdotal Appraisals. Rheum Clin NA 21: 817-834, 1995.

69.Panayi GS, et al: The importance of the T cell in initiating and maintaining the chronic synovitis of rheumatoid arthritis. Arthritis Rheum 35:729-35, 1992.

70.Sewell KL, Trentham DE: Pathogenesis of rheumatoid arthritis. Lancet 341 :283-86, 1993.

71.Sewell KE, Furrie E, Trentham DE: The therapeutic effect of minocycline in experimental arthritis. Mechanism of action. JRheumatol 33(suppl):S106, 1991.

72.Panayi GS, Clark B: Minocycline in the treatment of patients with Reiter's syndrome. Clin Erp Immunol 7: 100-1, 1989.

73.Pott H-G, Wittenborg A, Junge-Hulsing G: Long-term antibiotic treatment in reactive arthritis. Lancet i:245-6, Jan 30, 1988.

74.Skinner M, Cathcart ES, Mills JA, et al: Tetracycline in the Treatment of Rheumatoid Arthritis. Arthritis and Rheumatism 14:727-732, 1971.

75.Lauhio A, Leirisalo-Repo M, Lahdevirta J, et al: Double-blind placebo-controlled study of three-month treatment with Iymecycline in reactive arthritis, with special reference to Chlamydia arthritis. Arthritis Rheumatism 34:6-14, 1991.

76.Lauhio A, Sorsa T, Lindy O, et al: The anticollagenolytic potential of Iymecycline in the long-term treatment of reactive arthritis. Arthritis Rheumatism 35: 195-198, 1992.

77.Breedveld FC, Dijkmans BCA, Mattie H: Minocycline treatment for rheumatoid arthritis: an open dose finding study. JRheumatol 17:43-46, 1990.

78.Kloppenburg M, Breedveld FC, Miltenburg AMM, et al: Antibiotics as disease modifiers in arthritis. Clin Exper Rheumatol 1 1(suppl 8):S113-S115, 1993.

79.Langevitz P, et al: Treatment of resistant rheumatoid arthritis with minocycline: An open study. J Rheumatol 19: 1502-04, 1992.

80.Tilley, B, et al: Minocycline in Rheumatoid Arthritis: A 48 week double-blind placebo controlled trial. Ann Intern Med 122:81, 1995.

81.Mills, JA: Do Bacteria Cause Chronic Polyarthritis? N Enel J Med 320:245-246. January 26, 1989.

82.Rothschild BM, et al: Symmetrical Erosive Peripheral Polyarthritis in the Late Archaic Period of Alabama. Science 241:1498-1502, Sept 16, 1988.

83.Clark, HW, et al: Detection of Mycoplasma Antigens in Immune Complexes From Rheumatoid Arthritis Synovial Fluids. Ann Allergy 60:394-398, May 1988.

84.Res PCM, et al: Synovial Fluid T Cell Reactivity Against 65kD Heat Shock Protein of Mycobacteria in Early Chronic Arthritis. Lancet ii:478-480, Aug 27, 1988.

85.Cassell GH, et al: Mycoplasmas as Agents of Human Disease. N Engl J Med 304:80-89, Jan 8, 1981.

86.Breedveld FC, et al: Minocycline Treatment for Rheumatoid Arthritis: An Open Dose Finding Study. J Rheumatol 17:43-46, January 1990.

87.Phillips PE: Evidence implicating infectious agents in rheumatoid arthritis and juvenile rheumatoid arthritis Clin Exp Rheumatol 6:87-94. 1988.

88.Harris ED: Rheumatoid Arthritis, Pathophysiology and Implications for Therapy. N Engl J Med 322:1277-1289, May 3, 1990.

89.Brown, TMcP, Clark, HW Bailey, JS, Gray, CW, A Mechanistic approach to treatment of rheumatoid-type arthritis naturally occurring in a gorilla, Trans. Clin. Climatol. Assoc. 1970, 82:227247.

90.Brown, TMcP, Bailey, JS, Iden, KI, Clark, HW, Antimycoplasma approach to the mechanism and the control of rheumatoid disease, In, Inflammatory Diseases and Copper (Ed) Sorenson, JRJ, Humana Press, NJ, 1982.

91.Clark HW: The Potential Role of Mycoplasmas as Autoantigens and Immune Complexes in Chronic Vascular Pathogenesis. Am J Primatol 24:235-243, 1991.

92.Wheeler HB: Shattuck Lecture Healing and Heroism. NEngl JMed 322:1540-1548, May 24, 1990.

93.Arnett FC: Revised Criteria for the Classification of Rheumatoid Arthritis. Bun Rheum Dis 38:1-6, 1989.

94.Braanan W: Treatment of Chronic Prostatitis. Comparison of Minocycline and Doxycycline. Urology 5:631-636, 1975.

95.Becker FT: Treatment of Tetracycline-Resistant Acne Vulgaris. Cutis 14:610-613. 1974.

96.Cullen, SI: Low-Dose Minocycline Therapy in Tetracycline-Recalcitrant Acne Vulgaris. Cutis 21:101-105, 1978.

97.Mattuccik, et al: Acute Bacterial Sinusitis. Minocycline vs.Amoxicillin. Arch Otolaryngol Head Neck Surgery 112:73-76, 1986.

98.Guillon JM, et al: Minocylcine-induced Cell-mediated Hypersensitivity Pneumonitis. Ann Intern Med 117:476-481, 1992.

99.Gabriel SE, et al: Rifampin therapy in rheumatoid arthritis. J Rheumatol 17: 163-6, 1990.

100.Caperton EM, et al: Cefiriaxone therapy of chronic inflammatory arthritis. Arch Intern Med 150:1677-1682, 1990.

101.Ann Intern Med 117:273-280, 1992.

102.Clive DM, et al: Renal Syndromes Associated with Nonsteroidal Antiinflammatory drugs. NEngl JMed 310:563-572. March 1 1994.

103.Piper, et al: Corticosteroid Use and Peptic Ulcer Disease: Role of Non-Steroidal Anti-inflammatory Drugs. Ann Intern Med 114:735-740, May 1, 1991.

104.Allison MC, et al: Gastrointestinal Damage Associated with the Use of Nonsteroidal Antiinflammatory Drugs. N Engl J Med 327:749-54, 1992.

105.Fries JF:Postmarketing Drug Surveillance: Are Our Priorities Right? JRheumatol 15:389-390, 1988.

106.Brooks PM, et al: Nonsteroidal Antiinflammatory Drugs Differences and Similarities. NEngl JMed 324:1716-1724, June 13, 1991.

107.Agrawal N: Risk Factors for Gastrointestinal Ulcers Caused by Nonsteroidal Anti-inflammatory Drugs (NSAIDs). J Fam Prac 32:619-624, June 1991.

108.Silverstein, F: Nonsteroidal Anti-Inflammatory Drugs and Peptic Ulcer Disease. Postgrad Med 89:33-30, May 15, 1991.

109.Gabriel SE, et al: Risk for Serious Gastrointestinal Complications Related to Use of NSAIDs. Ann Intern Med 115:787-796 1991.

110.Fries JF, et al: Toward an Epidemiology of Gastropathy Associated With NSAID Use. Gastroent 96:647-55, 1989.

111.Armstrong CP, et al: NSAIDs and Life Threatening Complications of Peptic Ulceration. Gut 28:527-32, 1987.

112.Murray MD, et al: Adverse Effects of Nonsteroidal Anti-Inflammatory Drugs on Renal Function. AnnInternMed 112:559, April 15, 1990.

113.Cook DM: Safe Use of Glucocorticoids: How to Monitor Patients Taking These Potent Agents. Postgrad Med 91:145-154, Feb. 1992.

114.Piper JM, et al: Corticosteroid Use and Peptic Ulcer Disease: Role of Nonsteroidal Anti-inflammatory Drugs. Ann Intern Med 114:735-740, May 1, 1991.

115.Thompson JM: Tension Myalgia as a Diagnosis at the Mayo Clinic and Its Relationship to Fibrositis, Fibromyalgia, and Myofascial Pain Syndrome. Mayo Clin Proc 65:1237-1248, September 1990.

116.Semble EL, et al: Therapeutic Exercise for Rheumatoid Arthritis and Osteoarthritis. Seminars in Arthritis and Rheumatism 20:32-40, August 1990.

117.O'Dell, J, Haire, C, Palmer, W, Drymalski, W, Wees, S, Blakely, K, Churchill, M, Eckhoff, J, Weaver, A, Doud, D, Erickson, N, Dietz, F, Olson,

R, Maloney, P, Klassen, L, Moore, G, Treatment of Early Rheumatoid Arthritis with Minocycline or Placebo: Results of a Randomized, Double-Blind, Placebo-Controlled Trial, Arthritis & Rheumatism, 1997, 40:5, 842-848.

118.Tilley, BC, Alarcón, GS, Heyse, SP, Trentham, DE, Neuner, R, Kaplan, DA, Clegg, DO, Leisen, JCC, Buckley, L, Cooper, SM, Duncan, H, Pillemer, SR, Tuttleman, M, Fowler, SE, Minocycline in Rheumatoid Arthritis: A 48-Week, Double-Blind, Placebo-Controlled Trial, Annals of Internal Medicine, 1995, 122:2, 81-89.

119.Bluhm, GB, Sharp, JT, Tilley, BC, Alarcon, GS, Cooper, SM, Pillemer, SR, Clegg, DO, Heyse, SP, Trentham, DE, Neuner, R, Kaplan, DA, Leisen, JC, Buckley, L, Duncan, H, Tuttleman, M, Shuhui, L, Fowler, SE, Radiographic Results from the Minocycline in Rheumatoid Arthritis (MIRA) Trial, Journal of Rheumatology, 1997, 24:7, 1295-1302.

120.Breedveld, FC, Editorial: Minocycline in Rheumatoid Arthritis, Arthritis & Rheumatism, 1997, 40:5, 794-796.

121.Breedveld, FC, Letters: Reply to Minocycline-Induced Autoimmune Disease, Arthritis & Rheumatism, 1998, 41:3, 563-564.

122.Fox, R, Sharp, D, Editorial: Antibiotics as Biological Response Modifiers, The Lancet, 1991, 337:8738, 400-401.

123.Greenwald, rheumatoid arthritis, Golub, LM, Lavietes, B, Ramamurthy, NS, Gruber, B, Laskin, RS, McNamara, TF, Tetracyclines Inhibit Human Synovial Collagenase In Vivo and In Vitro, Journal of Rheumatology, 1987, 14:1, 28-32.

124.Griffiths, B, Gough, A, Emery, P, Letters: Minocycline-Induced Autoimmune Disease: Comment on the Editorial by Breedveld, Arthritis & Rheumatism, 1998, 41:3, 563.

125.Kloppenburg, M, Breedveld, FC, Miltenburg, AMM, Dijkmans, BAC, Antibiotics as Disease Modifiers in Arthritis, Clinical and Experimental Rheumatology, 1993, 11: Suppl. 8, S113-S115.

126.Kloppenburg, M, Breedveld, FC, Terwiel, JPh, Mallee, C, Dijkmans, BAC, Minocycline in Active Rheumatoid Arthritis: A Double-Blind, Placebo-Controlled Trial, Arthritis & Rheumatism, 1994, 37:5, 629-636.

127.Kloppenburg, M, Mattie, H, Douwes, N, Dijkmans, BAC, Breedveld, FC, Minocycline in the Treatment of Rheumatoid Arthritis: Relationship of Serum Concentrations to Efficacy, Journal of Rheumatology, 1995, 22:4, 611-616.

128.Lauhio, A, Leirisalo-Repo, M, Lähdevirta, J, Saikku, P, Repo, H, Double-Blind, Placebo-Controlled Study of Three-Month Treatment with Lymecycline in Reactive Arthritis, with Special Reference to Chlamydia Arthritis, Arthritis & Rheumatism, 1991, 34:1, 6-14.

129.Lauhio, A, Sorsa, T, Lindy, O, Suomalainen, K, Saari, H, Golub, LM, Konttinen, YT, The Anticollagenolytic Potential of Lymecycline in the Long-Term Treatment of Reactive Arthritis, Arthritis & Rheumatism, 1992, 35:2, 195-198.

130.Paulus, HE, Editorial: Minocycline Treatment of Rheumatoid

Arthritis, Annals of Internal Medicine, 1995, 122:2, 147-148.

131.Pruzanski, W, Vadas, P, Editorial: Should Tetracyclines be Used in Arthritis?, Journal of Rheumatology, 1992, 19:10, 1495-1497.

132.Sieper, J, Braun, J, Editorial: Treatment of Reactive Arthritis with Antibiotics, British Journal of Rheumatology, July 1998.

133.Baseman, JB, Tully, JG, Mycoplasmas: Sophisticated, Reemerging, and Burdened by Their Notoriety, CDC's Emerging Infectious Diseases, 1997, 3:1, 21-32.

134.Franz, A, Webster, ADB, Furr, PM, Taylor-Robinson, D, Mycoplasmal Arthritis in Patients with Primary Immunoglobulin Deficiency: Clinical Features and Outcome in 18 Patients, British Journal of Rheumatology, 1997, 36:6, 661-668.

135.Hakkarainen K, Turunen, H, Miettinen, A, Karppelin, M, Kaitila, K, Jansson, E, Mycoplasmas and Arthritis, Annals of Rheumatic Diseases, 1992, 51, 1170-1172.

136.Hoffman, RH, Wise, KS, Letters: Reply to Mycoplasmas in the Joints of Patients with Rheumatoid Arthritis and Other Inflammatory Rheumatic Disorders, Arthritis & Rheumatism, 1998, 41:4, 756-757.

137.Schaeverbeke, T, Bébéar, C, Lequen, L, Dehais, J, Bébéar, C, Letters: Mycoplasmas in the Joints of Patients with Rheumatoid Arthritis and Other Inflammatory Rheumatic Disorders: Comment on the Article by Hoffman et al., Arthritis & Rheumatism, 1998, 41:4, 754-756.

138.Schaeverbeke, T, Gilroy, CB, Bébéar, C, Dehais, J, Taylor-Robinson, D, Mycoplasma fermentans, But Not M penetrans, Detected by PCR Assays in Synovium from Patients with Rheumatoid Arthritis and Other Rheumatic Disorders, Journal of Clinical Pathology, 1996, 49, 824-828.

139.Aoki, S, Yoshikawa, K, Yokoyama, T, Nonogaki, T, Iwasaki, S, Mitsui, T, Niwa, S, Role of Enteric Bacteria in the Pathogenesis of Rheumatoid Arthritis: Evidence for Antibodies to Enterobacterial Common Antigens in Rheumatoid Sera and Synovial Fluids, Annals of Rheumatic Diseases, 1996, 55:6, 363-369.

140.Blankenberg-Sprenkels, SHD, Fielder, M, Feltkamp, TEW, Tiwana, H, Wilson, C, Ebringer, A, Antibodies to Klebsiella pneumoniae in Dutch Patients with Ankylosing Spondylitis and Acute Anterior Uveitis and to Proteus mirabilis in Rheumatoid Arthritis, Journal of Rheumatology, 1998, 25:4, 743-747.

141.Ebringer, A, Ankylosing Spondylitis is Caused by Klebsiella: Evidence from Immunogenetic, Microbiologic,
     and Serologic Studies, Rheumatic Disease Clinics of North America, 1992, 18:1, 105-121.

142.Erlacher, L, Wintersberger, W, Menschik, M, Benke-Studnicka, A, Machold, K, Stanek, G, Söltz-Szöts, J, Smolen, J, Graninger, W, Reactive Arthritis: Urogenital Swab Culture is the Only Useful Diagnostic Method for the Detection of the Arthritogenic Infection in Extra-Articularly Asymptomatic Patients with Undifferentiated Oligoarthritis, British Journal of Rheumatology, 1995, 34:9, 838-842.

143.Gaston, JSH, Deane, KHO, Jecock, RM, Pearce, JH, Identification of 2 Chlamydia trachomatis Antigen, Recognized by Synovial Fluid T Cells from Patients with Chlamydia Induced Reactive Arthritis, Journal of Rheumatology, 1996, 23:1, 130-136.

144.Gerard, HC, Branigan, PJ, Schumacher Jr, HR, Hudson, AP, Synovial Chlamydia trachomatis in Patients with Reactive Arthritis/ Reiter's Syndrome Are Viable But Show Aberrant Gene Expression, Journal of Rheumatology, 1998, 25:4, 734-742.

145.Granfors, K, Do Bacterial Antigens Cause Reactive Arthritis?, Rheumatic Disease Clinics of North America, 1992, 18:1, 37-48.

146.Granfors, K, Merilahti-Palo, R, Luukkainen, R, Möttönen, T, Lahesmaa, R, Probst, P, Märker-Hermann, E, Toivanen, P, Persistence of Yersinia Antigens in Peripheral Blood Cells from Patients with Yersinia Enterocolitica 0:3 Infection with or without Reactive Arthritis, Arthritis & Rheumatism, 1998, 41:5, 855-862.

147.Inman, RD, The Role of Infection in Chronic Arthritis, Journal of Rheumatology, 1992, 19, Supplement 33, 98-104.

148.Layton, MA, Dziedzic, K, Dawes, PT, Letters to the Editor: Sacroiliitis in an HLA B27-negative Patient Following Giardiasis, British Journal of Rheumatology, 1998, 37:5, 581-583.

149.Mäki-Ikola, O, Lehtinen, K, Granfors, K, Similarly Increased Serum IgA1 and IgA2 Subclass Antibody Levels against Klebsiella pneumoniæ Bacteria in Ankylosing Spondylitis Patients With/Without Extra-Articular Features, British Journal of Rheumatology, 1996, 35:2, 125-128.

150.Morrison, RP, Editorial: Persistent Chlamydia trachomatis Infection: In Vitro Phenomenon or in Vivo Trigger of Reactive Arthritis?, Journal of Rheumatology, 1998, 25:4, 610-612.

151.Mousavi-Jazi, M, Boström, L, Lövmark, C, Linde, A, Brytting, M, Sundqvist, V-A, Infrequent Detection of Cytomegalovirus and Epstein-Barr Virus DNA in Synovial Membrane of Patients with Rheumatoid Arthritis, Journal of Rheumatology, 1998, 25:4, 623-628.

152.Nissilä, M, Lahesmaa, R, Leirisalo-Repo, M, Lehtinen, K, Toivanen, P, Granfors, K, Antibodies to Klebsiella pneumoniæ, Escherichia coli, and Proteus mirabilis in Ankylosing Spondylitis: Effect of Sulfasalazine Treatment, Journal of Rheumatology, 1994, 21:11, 2082-2087.

153.Svenungsson, B, Editorial Review: Reactive Arthritis, International Journal of STD & AIDS, 1995, 6:3, 156-160.

154.Tani, Y, Tiwana, H, Hukuda, S, Nishioka, J, Fielder, M, Wilson, C, Bansal, S, Ebringer, A, Antibodies to Klebsiella, Proteus, and HLA-B27 Peptides in Japanese Patients with Ankylosing Spondylitis and Rheumatoid Arthritis, Journal of Rheumatology, 1997, 24:1, 109-114.

155.Tiwana, H, Walmsley, RS, Wilson, C, Yiannakou, JY, Ciclitira, PJ, Wakefield, AJ, Ebringer, A, Characterization of the Humoral Immune Response to Klebsiella Species in Inflammatory Bowel Disease and

Ankylosing Spondylitis, British Journal of Rheumatology, 1998, 37:5, 525-531.

156. Wilkinson, NZ, Kingsley, GH, Sieper, J, Braun, J, Ward, ME, Lack of Correlation Between the Detection of Chlamydia trachomatis DNA in Synovial Fluid from Patients with a Range of Rheumatic Diseases and the Presence of an Antichlamydial Immune Response, Arthritis & Rheumatism, 1998, 41:5, 845-854.

157. Wollenhaupt, J, Kolbus, F, Weißbrodt, H, Schneider, C, Krech, T, Zeidler, H, Manifestations of Chlamydia Induced Arthritis in Patients with Silent Versus Symptomatic Urogenital Chlamydial Infection, Clinical and Experimental Rheumatology, 1995, 13:4, 453-458.

158. Alarcon, GS, Tilley, B, Cooper, S, Clegg, DO, Trentham, DE, Pillemer, SR, Neuner, R, Fowler, S, Letter: Another look at minocycline, Bulletin on the Rheumatic Diseases, 1996, 45(8), 6-7.

159. Amin, AR, Attur, MG, Thakker, GD, Patel, PD, Vyas, PR, Patel, RN, Patel, IR, Abramson, SB, A novel mechanism of action of tetracyclines: effects on nitric oxide synthases, Proceedings of the National Academy of Sciences of the United States of America, 1996, 93(24), 14014-14019.

160. Ayuzawa, S, Yano, H, Enomoto, T, Kobayashi, H, Nose, T, The Bi-Digital O-Ring Test used in the successful diagnosis & treatment (with antibiotic, anti-viral agents & oriental herbal medicine) of a patient suffering from pain & weakness of an upper extremity & Barre-Lieou syndrome appearing after whiplash injury: A case report, Acupuncture & Electro-Therapeutics Research, 1997, 22(3-4), 167-174.

161. Bitar, CN, Steele, RW, Use of prophylactic antibiotics in children, Advances in Pediatric Infectious Diseases, 1995, 10, 227-262.

162. Bluhm, GB, Sharp, JT, Tilley, BC, Alarcon, GS, Cooper, SM, Pillemer, SR, Clegg, DO, Heyse, SP, Trentham, DE, Neuner, R, Kaplan, DA, Leisen, JC, Buckley, L, Duncan, H, Tuttleman, M, Li, S, Fowler, SE, Radiographic Results from the Minocycline in Rheumatoid Arthritis (MIRA) Trial, Journal of Rheumatology, 1997, 24(7), 1295-1302.

163. Brandt, KD, Modification by oral doxycycline administration of articular cartilage breakdown in osteoarthritis, Journal of Rheumatology, 1995, Supplement 43, 149-151.

164. Breedveld, FC, Editorial: Minocycline in Rheumatoid Arthritis, Arthritis & Rheumatism, 1997, 40(5), 794-796.

165. Breedveld, FC, Letters: Reply to Minocycline- Induced Autoimmune Disease, Arthritis & Rheumatism, 1998, 41(3), 563-564.

166. Bullingham, R, Shah, J, Goldblum, R, Schiff, M, Effects of food and antacid on the pharmacokinetics of single doses of mycophenolate mofetil in rheumatoid arthritis patients, British Journal of Clinical Pharmacology, 1996, 41(6), 513-516.

167. Burton, IE, Moussa, KM, Sanders, PA, Agranulocytosis in rheumatoid arthritis associated with long-term flucloxacillin for staphylococcal osteomyelitis, Acta Haematologica, 1995, 94(4), 196-198.

168.Canvin, JM, Madhok, R, Letter: Minocycline in rheumatoid arthritis, Annals of Internal Medicine, 1995, 123(5), 392.

169.Caruso, I, Twenty years of experience with intra-articular rifamycin for chronic arthritides, Journal of International Medical Research, 1997, 25(6), 307-317.

170.Currie, BJ, Are the currently recommended doses of benzathine penicillin G adequate for secondary
    prophylaxis of rheumatic fever?, Pediatrics, 1996, 97(6, Part 2), 989-991.

171.Ebell, MH, Minocycline for rheumatoid arthritis, Journal of Family Practice, 1995, 40(5), 497-498.

172.Elkayam, O, Yaron, M, Zhukovsky, G, Segal, R, Caspi, D, Toxicity profile of dual methotrexate combinations with gold, hydroxychloroquine, sulphasalazine and minocycline in rheumatoid arthritis patients, Rheumatology International, 1997, 17(2), 49-53.

173.Evdoridou, J, Roilides, E, Bibashi, E, Kremenopoulos, G, Multifocal osteoarthritis due to Candida albicans in a neonate: serum level monitoring of liposomal amphotericin B and literature review, Infection, 1997, 25(2), 112-116.

174.Galland, L, Letter: Minocycline and rheumatoid arthritis revisited, Annals of Internal Medicine, 1995, 123(5), 392-393.

175.Griffiths, B, Gough, A, Emery, P, Letters: Minocycline- Induced Autoimmune Disease: Comment on the Editorial by Breedveld, Arthritis & Rheumatism, 1998, 41(3), 563.

176.Hanemaaijer, R, Sorsa, T, Konttinen, YT, Ding, Y, Sutinen, M, Visser, H, van Hinsbergh, VW, Helaakoski, T, Kainulainen, T, Ronka, H, Tschesche, H, Salo, T, Matrix metalloproteinase-8 is expressed in rheumatoid synovial fibroblasts and endothelial cells: Regulation by tumor necrosis factor-alpha and doxycycline, Journal of Biological Chemistry, 1997, 272(50), 31504-31509.

177.Herdy, GV, Editorial: The challenge of secondary prophylaxis in rheumatic fever [Portuguese, Original Title: Desafio da profilaxia secundaria na febre reumatica, Arquivos Brasileiros de Cardiologia, 1996, 67(5), 317.

178.Herdy, GV, Souza, DC, Barros, PB, Pinto, CA, Secondary prophylaxis in rheumatic fever: Oral antibiotic therapy versus benzathine penicillin [Portuguese, Original Title: Profilaxia secundaria na febre reumatica: Antibioticoterapia oral versus penicilina benzatina], Arquivos Brasileiros de Cardiologia, 1996, 67(5), 331-333.

179.Herrick, AL, Grennan, DM, Griffen, K, Aarons, L, Gifford, LA, Lack of interaction between flucloxacillin and methotrexate in patients with rheumatoid arthritis, British Journal of Clinical Pharmacology, 1996, 41(3), 223-227.

180.Houck, HE, Kauffman, CL, Casey, DL, Minocycline treatment for leukocytoclastic vasculitis associated with rheumatoid arthritis, Archives of Dermatology, 1997, 133(1), 15-16.

181.Iwata, M, Ida, M, Oda, S, Takeuchi, E, Nakamura, Y, Horiguchi, T, Sato, A, Bronchiolitis obliterans preceding rheumatoid arthritis: effect of clarithromycin [Japanese], Nippon Kyobu Shikkan Gakkai Zasshi ^Ö Japanese Journal of Thoracic Diseases, 1996, 34(11), 1271-1276.

182.Kassem, AS, Zaher, SR, Abou Shleib, H, el-Kholy, AG, Madkour, AA, Kaplan, EL, Rheumatic fever prophylaxis using benzathine penicillin G (BPG): two- week versus four-week regimens: comparison of two brands of BPG, Pediatrics, 1996, 97(6, Part 2), 992-995.

183.Kim, NM, Freeman, CD, Minocycline for rheumatoid arthritis, Annals of Pharmacotherapy, 1995, 29(2), 186-187.

184.Kloppenburg, M, Dijkmans, BA, Breedveld, FC, Antimicrobial therapy for rheumatoid arthritis, Baillieres Clinical Rheumatology, 1995, 9(4), 759-769.

185.Kloppenburg, M, Dijkmans, BA, Verweij, CL, Breedveld, FC, Inflammatory and immunological parameters of disease activity in rheumatoid arthritis patients treated with minocycline, Immunopharmacology, 1996, 31(2-3), 163-169.

186.Kloppenburg, M, Mattie, H, Douwes, N, Dijkmans, BA, Breedveld, FC, Minocycline in the treatment of rheumatoid arthritis: relationship of serum concentrations to efficacy, Journal of Rheumatology, 1995, 22(4), 611-616.

187.Kuznetsova, SM, Petrova, NK, Lecture: Antibiotics in the prevention of rheumatic fever [Russian, Original Title: Antibiotiki v profilaktike revmatizma (lektsiia)], Antibiotiki i Khimioterapiia, 1996, 41(2), 43-51.

188.Lai, NS, Lan, JL, Treatment of DMARDs-resistant rheumatoid arthritis with minocycline: a local experience among the Chinese, Rheumatology International, 1998, 17(6), 245-247.

189.Langevitz, P, Livneh, A, Bank, I, Pras, M, Minocycline in rheumatoid arthritis, Israel Journal of Medical Sciences, 1996, 32(5), 327-330.

190.Lauhio, A, Salo, T, Tjaderhane, L, Lahdevirta, J, Golub, LM, Sorsa, T, Letter: Tetracyclines in treatment of rheumatoid arthritis, The Lancet, 1995, 346(8975), 645-646.

191.McKendry, RJ, Is rheumatoid arthritis caused by an infection?, The Lancet, 1995, 345(8961), 1319-1320.

192.Meehan, R, Letter: Minocycline in rheumatoid arthritis, Annals of Internal Medicine, 1995, 123(5), 391-392.

193.Nordstrom, D, Lindy, O, Lauhio, A, Sorsa, T, Santavirta, S, Konttinen, YT, Anti-collagenolytic mechanism of action of doxycycline treatment in rheumatoid arthritis, Rheumatology International, 1998, 17(5), 175-180.

194.O'Dell, JR, Haire, CE, Palmer, W, Drymalski, W, Wees, S, Blakely, K, Churchill, M, Eckhoff, PJ, Weaver, A, Doud, D, Erikson, N, Dietz, F, Olson, R, Maloley, P, Klassen, LW, Moore, GF, Treatment of Early Rheumatoid Arthritis with Minocycline or Placebo: Results of a Randomized, Double- Blind, Placebo-Controlled Trial, Arthritis & Rheumatism, 1997, 40(5), 842-848.

195. Panush, RS, Thoburn, R, Should minocycline be used to treat rheumatoid arthritis?, Bulletin on the Rheumatic Diseases, 1996, 45(2), 2-5.

196. Patmas, MA, Letter: Minocycline in rheumatoid arthritis, Annals of Internal Medicine, 1995, 123(5), 391-392.

197. Paulus, HE, Editorial: Minocycline treatment of rheumatoid arthritis, Annals of Internal Medicine, 1995, 122(2), 147-148.

198. Pillemer, SR, Fowler, SE, Tilley, BC, Alarcon, GS, Heyse, SP, Trentham, DE, Neuner, R, Clegg, DO, Leisen, JC, Cooper, SM, Duncan, H, Tuttleman, M, Meaningful improvement criteria sets in a rheumatoid arthritis clinical trial: MIRA Trial Group, Minocycline in Rheumatoid Arthritis, Arthritis & Rheumatism, 1997, 40(3), 419-425.

199. Ryan, ME, Greenwald, rheumatoid arthritis, Golub, LM, Potential of tetracyclines to modify cartilage breakdown in osteoarthritis, Current Opinion in Rheumatology, 1996, 8(3), 238-247.

200. Sieper, J, Braun, J, Editorial: Treatment of Reactive Arthritis with Antibiotics, British Journal of Rheumatology, 1998, 37(7), 717-720.

201. Smith, GN Jr, Yu, LP Jr, Brandt, KD, Capello, WN, Oral administration of doxycycline reduces collagenase and gelatinase activities in extracts of human osteoarthritic cartilage, Journal of Rheumatology, 1998, 25(3), 532-535.

202. Tilley, BC, Alarcon, GS, Heyse, SP, Trentham, DE, Neuner, R, Kaplan, DA, Clegg, DO, Leisen, JC, Buckley, L, Cooper, SM, Duncan, H, Pillemer, SR, Tuttleman, M, Fowler, SE, Minocycline in rheumatoid arthritis: A 48-week, double-blind, placebo-controlled trial, MIRA Trial Group, Annals of Internal Medicine, 1995, 122(2), 81-89.

203. Trentham, DE, Dynesius-Trentham, rheumatoid arthritis, Antibiotic therapy for rheumatoid arthritis: Scientific and anecdotal appraisals, Rheumatic Diseases Clinics of North America, 1995, 21(3), 817-834.

204. Wilson, C, Senior, BW, Tiwana, H, Caparros-Wanderley, W, Ebringer, A, Antibiotic sensitivity and proticine typing of Proteus mirabilis strains associated with rheumatoid arthritis, Rheumatology International, 1998, 17(5), 203-205.

205. Yu, LP Jr, Burr, DB, Brandt, KD, O'Connor, BL, Rubinow, A, Albrecht, M, Effects of oral doxycycline administration on histomorphometry and dynamics of subchondral bone in a canine model of osteoarthritis, Journal of Rheumatology, 1996, 23(1), 137-142.

Biofeedback & Computerized Electrodermal Testing
by
Anthony di Fabio & Hector E. Solorzano, MD, D.Sc.

One of us, Anthony di Fabio, has visited Dr. Solorzano in Guadaljara, Mexico, several times. He's a remarkable doctor with a very open mind, choosing to work with inexpensive treatment modalities that show promise and effectiveness. I've constantly been amazed at the far-out processes he's been willing to explore, one or two of them so far out that I'd hesitate describing them because you'd not believe me!

In Mexico a student can go as far as they have the intelligence, peristence and grades to go. In Dr. Solorzano's case, as with many others like him, he was assigned to work with the indigent and poor folks in the far out hinterland by the government in return for his past education. Once he'd served his years with these folks, and having gained an appreciation for the ability of those in poverty to not pay, he accepted a position with the University of Guadalajara Medical School, but only if they would create for him, and assign him to a chair in Alternative Medicine. That's when I first met this good doctor.

At that time Dr. Solorzano was a surgeon, general practitioner and had even been to China to learn acupuncture.

Seldom does one doctor excell in so many disciplines!

The last time I visited Dr. Solorzano proudly demonstrated a variety of what I call computerized electrodermal testing machines. From time to time I've asked him for an article on one subject or another and this article relates to those machines which he describes as Biofeedback machines. In the United States and some European countries Biofeedback is viewed somewhat differently. The Association for Applied Psychophysiology and Biofeedback Certification, International Alliance and the International Society of Neurofeedback and Research arrived at a consensus definition in 2008. It's a discipline that continues to change and new versions are added constantly. It often uses electromyograph, electroencephalograph and electrocardiogram, among other devices. It's based on the concept that a wide variety of ongoing natural functions of the body occur at a level of awareness often termed as the "unconscious." The biofeedback process is designed to bring some of these processes under conscious control. However, the computerized electrodermal testing is designed chiefly to determine the state of one's organs or biological systems. One could make an argument that the two are related.

According to that definition computerized electrodermal testing does not yet reach the mark accepted by most biofeedback professionals. But, electrodermal testing can identify virtually anything wrong with a person — organ by organ, system by system — so that other remedies can be invoked. All of this is done by passing a small DC battery current through the body and comparing the results against stored signals inside the computer.

Some believe that computerized electrodermal testing is the future of medicine and will one day replace most costly testing devices and procedures now in use.

Biofeedback — and computerized electrodermal testing — are both practical approaches to diseases; Professor of Pharmacology and President of Biofeedback Society of Guadalajara, Dr. Hector Solorazano del Rio, M.D., D.Sc., says:

"Since the publication of the results of a study done by Dr. Eisenberg, in *The New England Journal of Medicine* on January 28th 1993, the interest in alternative medicine has increased enormously. He found that Americans spent $17 billion dollars in medical visits to alternative medicine practitioners. These patients preferred to spend their money than to receive the free medical orthodox consultation."

In 1992, the Office of Alternative Medicine (OAM) was opened as part of the National Institute of Health (NIH) with a starting budget of $2 million dollars. The increase of the demand to know more about these therapies has been so large that in October 21st, 1998 this OAM turned into the National Center for Complementary and Alternative Medicine (NCCAM) whose functions are to facilitate and drive biomedical research with a budget of $20 million dollars during that year.

When this article was written there were about 12 centers of the NCCAM that do research on alternative medicine in areas of specific diseases.

Then in 1994, the May issue of *Pediatrics* published for the first time in the history of the American conventional medicine a clinical study using homeopathy. Researchers of the University of Washington and Universidad de Guadalajara did it (Jacobs J., Jiménez LM, et al: "Treatment of acute childhood diarrhea with homeopathic medicine: A randomized clinical trial in Nicaragua," *Pediatrics* 93: 719-25, 1994).

The trends in alternative medicine use in the United States were reviewed and again Dr. Eisenberg found that the use of herbal remedies increased 380% and the use of high doses of vitamins rose 130% in a period of time of 7 years. At the time this article was written Americans spent around $27 billion dollars a year on this kind of therapy. Even some insurance companies pay for the alternative medicine treatments ("Trends in Alternative Medicine use in the United States,"1990-1997, *JAMA*, 1998;280:156-1575).

More attention was addressed to alternative medicine in 1998 when almost the whole issue of *JAMA* published on November 11th, was dedicated to the topic of alternative medicine.

A study done by the Office of Education Development, Harvard University, School of Medicine showed that 75 of the 125 schools of Medicine in the United States offered elective courses on alternative medicine. Thirty-eight courses of the 123 elective courses were offered by the Departments of Family Medicine and 14 courses were offered by the Departments of Internal Medicine ("Courses involving complementary and alternative medicine at US medical schools," *JAMA* 1998;(9)280:784-787, Wetzel MS, Eisenberg DM).

There is an advertisement that says: "Cancer Treatment Centers is the only group of hospitals in the country in which, the doctors of naturopathic medicine work side by side with the oncologists as an integral part of their treatment team against cancer". This statement would be incredible a few years ago.

Now I will attempt to present a clearer picture of biofeedback research.

The term feedback is defined as a method of controlling a system by reinserting into it the results of its past performance. We can learn to control our performance in sport by observing and acting upon the results of our previous results.

So biofeedback is simply a special kind of feedback. In this case, it can be the feedback of different parts of the body. It can be the brain, the heart, the muscles and so on. Then we got biofeedback training, which is the procedure that allows us to tune into our body functions and eventually to control them. It is really fascinating.

In a typical biofeedback training session an individual can on a device "see" his heartbeat and "hear" his brain waves. That means that he has the information he needs to start to control them.

Once a subject is able to recognize his brain waves, he soon learns how to control them at will. Nobody knows why this thing happens, but it does. And after a little practice, he will not need any aid, that is the biofeedback machine.

In holistic medicine, we are taught that the patient has the responsibility for and power over his own health. Biofeedback puts the emphasis on training rather than on certain medications or surgery.

Now that we realize that anybody has capacity to play an active role in combating his own medical conditions we must give the patient every available assistance in making that role as effective as possible. This is where we can say that biofeedback training comes in. Nowadays some doctors consider biofeedback training as the best tool we have to help the patients achieve control over the nervous system activities. Using this method, patients and physicians can cooperatively fight against disease. In this particular kind of fight, the patient becomes his own prescription to keep a good and lasting health (Karlins M. and Andrews L., *Biofeedback,* 1972, Warner Books Inc.)

One of the medical indications of biofeedback training is for the treatment of anxiety. When the patient learns to keep himself on the alpha level of brain-wave pattern he can bring down the level of anxiety at will.

The same way a patient who suffers migraine and tension headaches can regulate – through this biofeedback training – the blood flow to the head.

We know that 95 % of the people, who have been diagnosed as hypertensive, suffer the kind of hypertension known as "essential hypertension". This means that we cannot find a physical cause for this. biofeedback is an excellent and effective alternative treatment for all these patients.

In conventional medicine, we use hypnotic drugs for the treatment of insomnia. Some of them can suppress certain parts of the sleep cycle that may be important to psychological well-being (Pearlman, C., and Greenberg, R., "Medical-psycological implications of recent sleep research." *Psychiatry in Medicine,* 1970, 1, 261-276).

Electromyograph (EMG) biofeedback is also useful in the treatment of many neuromuscular disorders, including spasmodic tics and muscle cramps.

Dr. Weiss and Dr. Engel did an important study with 8 heart patients to see if they could learn how to control dangerous irregularities in their heartbeat by force of mental discipline only. The premature ventricular contractions increase the possibility of sudden death. What they found is that biofeedback really works.

At Universidad de Guadalajara, some years ago, Dr. Solorzano del Rio did clinical studies with patients who suffered of stuttering and others who suffered epilepsy. In both cases, biofeedback training helped all of the individuals.

In general, biofeedback may help drug addiction, neck injuries, hysterical deafness, stroke victims, opera singers, Raynaud´s disease patients, asthma and many more clinical conditions.

One unconventional use of biofeedback is to change our inner state, that is our consciousness. After the training, we do not need dangerous drugs to explore our inner self. We are able to change our minds without losing our heads.

We can easily learn how to slow down our brain-wave frequency, reaching alpha (8 to 13 cycles per second). Alpha is a mental state most often described as relaxed, passive and pleasant. Many people are able to get both an interhemispheric hyper synchronicity and an intrahemispheric hyper synchronicity. This helps people to develop their skills, including creativity. To us, it is a kind of modern electronic scientific raja yoga.

Some years ago, dreams were regarded as fluke occurrences. Now some investigators observe that these things correlate with bursts of eye movements that are today known as REM sleep. So suddenly dreams, instead of being wholly subjective experiences became real. So real that they can be measured and are valid objects for study.

Although features of biofeedback are common to computerized electrodermal testing, both practices and results may differ drastically.

There's a common principle that seems to run through applied kinesiology, electrodermal testing according to vol, and a few other subjects. We'll try to describe that essential commonality by stating as a first postulate, that the body knows how the body works.

Such a postulate may come as a great surprise to the reader as we are all of us are brought up to seek out academic, professional knowledge of those highly educated and trained to be physicians.

You can perform a search onlne for applied kinesiology and learn a great deal more than this brief introduction.

Here's a simple parlor experiment that anyone can try. A demonstration, in this case, is worth far more than a page full of words.

You'll need two people, yourself and another. Also you'll need a small amount of salt and a small amount of sugar. They do not have to be equal in volume or weight.

Have your partner stretch out one arm paralell to his/her chest. In the other hand the partner holds first the sugar. Ask your partner holding the sugar to resist the push you will use against his/her stretched out arm.

Now push the arm without the sugar quick and hard.

You will observe in every case that the person holding the sugar in the opposite hand will find that their arm muscles become week and the outstretched arm moves down easily.

Now do the same thing with your partner holding the salt.

Ah ha! The resistance is much stronger.

This is a description of a simple application of "applied kinesiology." The body holding the substances has just told both parties that salt is OK for the body but that sugar is not.

Medical doctors, chiropractors and others develop this kind of muscular difference into a very complex and accurate "yes" or "no" answer from the body.

You see, the body knows how the body works provided you ask a question that requires a simple "yes" or "no."

I urge you to search online for applied kinesiology to learn more.

Now let's look at computerized electrodermal screening. Here, again, the body answers faithfully on every question, but the results will depend upon how knowledgeable the operator is in asking the right questions.

A computer will contain a fantastic number of frequencies that will stand for the frequencies of specific microorganisms, cellular health, organ conditions, and system health conditions. Everything everywhere responds to specific frequencies.

A metallic probe is placed at specific acupuncture points that lie along one of the twelve meridians of the body. In the other hand the patient holds the other terminal. A tiny DC battery current is passed through the body whence the computer matches the patient's frequency responses back against the vast storage of frequency information in the computer.

Watching a skilled practitioner with a computer loaded with thousands of specifically identified frequencies is akin to watching miraculous diagnoses. Many of us declare that this approach to diagnosis and treatment is the future of medicine!

As it is recommended that you go online and read up on applied kinesiology, we also recommend that your go online and read up on computerized electrodermal testing.

We guarantee that you won't be disappointed!

Dr. Christ's Psoriasis Treatment!!!

by

Anthony di Fabio, Helmut Christ, M.D.

Permission to publish portions granted to *Townsend Letter for Doctors*, 911 Tyler St., Port Townsend, WA 98368-6541, June 1990, p. 351.

Also Rex Newnham, N.D., D.O. and Jonathan Wright, M.D., Gus J. Prosch, Jr., M.D.

Psoriasis is supposed to be incurable, but we've both seen patients cured.

This is a common, chronic, relapsing skin diesease. Itchy, scaly red patches and plaques may vary from severe to minor.

Mainstream medicine does not admit to any full understanding of the disease but does lump it, along with hundreds of other conditions, under an "immunological" title; i.e., a problem or defect of the immune system.

The Helmut Christ treatment protocol for Psoriasis is simple, and can be read without difficulty. We also present other treatment prossibilities.

Brief Background

In July of 1986 The ArthritisTrust of America/The Rheumatoid Disease Foundation brought to its Second National Medical Seminar, Dr. Helmut Christ, M.D. of Bisingen, West Germany, as a speaker.

One of Dr. Christ's subjects was "Psoriasis Under Control at Last".

Gus J. Prosch, M.D., referral physician (AL), was the first to try this new treatment on a patient with success. He obtained Psoriasis medicines from a pharmacy in Germany recommended by Dr. Helmut Christ.

Dr. Prosch's patient had tried everything possible, and he had reached a point of suicidal intent if this next treatment did not help, such was his despair.

Prosch proceeded with a successful trial.

On page 138 of *The Art of Getting Well*, (See Amazon.com at book stores and at Arthritis Trust.org) Helmut Christ, M.D. reported 100% successes[11].

Helmut, an Internist-physician who wished to be a general practitioner and did not choose to be a specialist on Psoriasis, as of this writing has treated 4.000 patients with Psoriasis, mostly by referral from successful patients and physicians. He did not invent the treatment, but rather received it from another physician who had had Psoriasis himself and who eventually developed the successful treatment protocol which has been tested in several universities and clinics.

It should be clear from the start that "Fumaric Acid" per se, is useless, but that "Fumaric Acid Monoethylester" and "Fumaric Acid di-Methylester" are the proper medicines.

There are those who sell "Fumaric Acid" alone for this treatment thereby misleading with a substance that will be of no effect whatsoever.

What is Psoriasis?

There are many forms of psoriasis, a skin disease characterized by the formation of scaly red patches on the extensor (following the muscles that perform extension) surfaces of the body.

Annularis Psoriasis in ring-shaped patches

Arthropathica   A form associated with chronic arthritis

Buccalis   Marked   by   white,   thickened patches in mucuous membrane of cheeks, gums, tongue

Circinata (See Annularis above)

Diffusa   Coalescence of large contiguous lesions   (Bakers, grocers', bricklayers itch, etc.)

Discoides Occurring in solid patches

Figurata Lesions in curved linear patterns

Follicularis   Small, scaly lesions located at openings of sebaceous and sweat glands

Guttata Occurs in small, distinct, irregular patches

Gyrata Having serpentine arrangement Inveterata with confluent lesions and thickening and hardening skin

Linguae (See **Buccalis** above)

Nummularis In circular patches that resembles coins

Osteacea In Old, thick, tough patches covered with scales resembling outside of oyster shells

Palmaris et plantaris Syphiloderm of palms or soles

Punctata Lesions consist of minute, red, pinhead shaped papules, often surmounted with pearly   scales

Pustular p. Lesions are covered with pustules

Rupioides Rupia-like crusts (skin   eruptions usually from syphilis)

Universalis Lesions over whole body

As one can easily see, these complex Latin terms are simply means for classifying various views of a skin condition and are not at all meaningful for the purpose of treating and controlling the disease except in certain few cases, such as Rupioides, which seems to be related to a known germ.

If you are one who suffers from Psoriasis, surely you know more about your symptoms than simply how to describe it. You know that it flares up worse then gets better from time to time, that it sometimes can create great embarrassment, pain, guilt — in short, it can indeed control your life.

According to Helmut Christ, M.D.: "It has now been established, that Psoriasis is not a SKIN DISORDER strictly speaking, but a T-cell-mediated autoimmune disease. The problem lies in the subcutaneous immune system. It is not a metabolic disorder as previously thought. It is an inherited disorder and is frequently brought on by factors like streptococcal infections, operations, antibiotics, depression, death of a family member and food-stuffs (spices, nuts, alcohol, chocolate, orange juice)."

We know that patients with Psoriasis have a higher incidence of Rheumatoid Disease than others.

What is Psoriasis?

Simply, it is a hyperproliferation (overgrowth) of the epidermis (outer skin covering), and the cell division is an enhanced 8-10 times normal.

Traditional Treatments

Many treatments are directed at interference with DNA synthesis and interruption of cell division as it is presumed by this treatment that this function is in error in our bodies.

Some patients move to warmer climates to increase sun exposure and humidity, although overexposure to sunlight can also aggravate the condition.

The traditional treatments for psoriasis include topical tars and ultraviolet light, keratolytics, anthralin and glucocorticosteroids. Current systemic therapies using psoralen-photochemotherapy or methotrexate are still largely investigational and may produce adverse effects. Besides blocking the abnormal rapid proliferation of psoriasis, methotrexate affects other normally rapidly growing tissues such as bone marrow, gastrointestinal tissues and hair roots.

Fluorinated steroids may be useful on a short-term basis for treatment of resistant, highly inflamed, or irritated plaques, but are not advisable for treatment of widespread psoriasis. Hydrocortisone creams are commonly used with mixed results for intetriginous (chafed) areas or on the face since they do not atrophy the skin. However, systemic steroids are generally contraindicated, as cessation is usually accompanied by rebound worsening of the disease.

PUVA (Psoralen and long-wave ultraviolet light) have been useful therapies but are still investigational. Side effects include phototoxicity with erythema and blistering, pruritis and nausea. Potential chronic side effects such as actinic damage and aging of the skin, carcinogenesis and cataract formation are of great concern. Moreover, patient compliance is generally poor. An average of 25 treatments given 2 or 3 times weekly are required for 80% clearing of Psoriasis. Patients who work outdoors do not like to wear goggles. Psoralen and long-wave ultraviolet light (PUVA) is only a palliative treatment and requires continued maintenance therapy. At Stanford University, experience with PUVA has shown that over 90% of patients develop recurrent psoriasis in the first year of therapy.

Crude coal tars, often combined with zinc and salicylic acid, has been a valuable adjunctive treatment for psoriasis. Coal tar products are able to suppress DNA synthesis in the epidermis within the first few hours after application. The Goeckerman regimen, combining coal tar with exposure to UV light, has induced remissions for several weeks and is a relatively safe method. Patient compliance is still a problem as these tars are messy and stain clothing. Some patients develop acanthomas (tumor or excessive development of skin). Coal tars also produce folliculitis (inflammation of hair folliculs). The absorbed mutagens may increase the risk of some forms of cancer. Crude coal tar is a mixture of 10,000 non-standarized components, which may create a potential problem of contact allergic sensitization.

The synthetic retinoids are a major advance in the treatment of both localized as well as generalized pusular Psoriasis. The dosage must be carefully monitored, as some patients experience a local recurrence of pustules with the lowered dosage. All of the important factors concerning toxicity and side effects of these drugs need to be considered carefully, especially the teratogenic effects. Some of the side effects are dose-dependent (e.g. dryness of the lips and oral mucosa) and are reversible after discontinuation of therapy. Other side effects include exfoliation (a falling off in scales or layers) of palms and soles, hair loss, conjunctivitis (inflammation of the layer that lines the eyelids), pruritis, paronchia, elevated serum lipids, muscle pain, neuralgia and hyperostosis (bone disorder). Considering the possible long-term effects of retinoid-induced lipid modulation on atherosclerosis and coronary artery disease, it is necessary to closely monitor the levels of serum lipids during therapy, particularly in patients with CHD risk factors. Some of the non-toxic therapies which may be used prophylactically in patients treated with retinoids include niacin (400 mg b.i.d) and L-Carnitine (250 mg b.i.d.).

Methotrexate is often used as a third-line therapy for patients with severe psoriasis (e.g. acute pustular Psoriasis, Psoriatic Arthritis, Psoriatic Erythroderma) unresponsive to other, less toxic therapies. Liver and renal functions must be carefully monitored prior to treatment. Severe liver disease, such as fibrosis and cirrhosis, may be present in patients with Psoriasis, especially in alcoholics. Unfortunately, no liver function tests are reliable indicators of severe liver toxicity. Other risk factors include obesity, diabetes and lowered renal function. One can minimize the risk by titrating the patient to the lowest possible dose to achieve and maintain adequate control, rather than 100% clearing of the

Recently ointments containing pimecrolimus and tacrolimus have been used which have an immunmodulating affect on the T-cells in the dermis.

Regardless of the treatment used, patient education remains a critical component in the present successful management of Psoriasis. Therefore patient education manuals and even support groups will enhance the prognosis of the disease and may even strengthen the base of patient referrals to a dermatologist's practice. Patients should be advised on those factors which make Psoriasis worse. Trauma and irritation of the skin, induced by rubbing, scratching or scrubbing off scales all can produce Psoriasis. Some throat and upper respiratory infections may flare Psoriasis and should be promptly treated by a physician. Some dermatologists are so absorbed in their subspecialty that they overlook the common patient complaints, normally encountered by a general practitioner (e.g. strep infections). Guttate Psoriasis (lesions that are drop shaped) particularly occurs in children and adolescents after strep infections.

Patients should be encouraged to discuss other illnesses besides their chief complaint. Most patients do not understand the fact that sun exposure should be used in moderation. While sunlight in moderation usually helps Psoriasis, sunburn may cause Psoriasis to flare up. A similar situation exists with topical steroids. Patients should be advised not to use these creams on areas in which the Psoriasis is cleared and to follow their dermatologist's directions carefully to preclude a rebound phenomenon. Stress and anxiety should be minimized.

Dietary recommendations are outlined in conjunction with our recommended treatment which is also **the new European fumaric acid protocol**.

Recent evidence points to abonormalities in the arachidonic acid metabolism in patients with Psoriasis. The cyclic AMP/cyclic GMP ratio is decreased in involved epidermis of Psoriasis compared with uninvolved epidermis from Psoriasis patients or epidermis from normal volunteers. The imbalance of the two cyclic nucleotides plays a central role in the pathogenesis of Psoriasis. Usually, tissue levels of free fatty acids are quite low. However, involved epidermis of Psoriasis contains high concentrations of free arachidonic acid. Elevated levels of the prostaglandin series leads to increased platelet aggregation. Fish oils, high in eicosapentaenoic acid and docosahexaenoic acids (EPA & DHA) are currently being used for normalizing aberations in the arachidonic acid cascade. It is interesting to note that the majority of patients with Psoriasis have elevated levels of cholesterol and triglycerides which may result from abnormal platelet behavior. Epidermal cells in Psoriatic lesions have a receptor for serum beta-lipoproteins. The rate of epidermal lipid synthesis may be regulated by serum lipoproteins. Dermatologists are encouraged to observe and control lipid abnormalities with Psoriasis.

One very promising treatment for Psoriasis is based on the use of fumaric acid ester. Clinical investigations with fumaric acid, an unsaturated dibasic acid, have been conducted in University Medical Centers in Switzerland, West Germany, Japan and the Netherlands and the results are promising. Fumaric acid is the transisomer of malic acid and an intermediate in the Krebs citric acid cycle. Fumaric acid ester has been used both topically and orally and a titration protocol has been suggested. (Cis and trans isomers often have different physical properties. Differences between isomers, in general, arise from the differences in the shape of the molecule or the overall dipole moment.)

Rationale for Use of Fumaric Acid Ester

Psoriasis is regarded as a disease having its origin in the immunsystem. A defect of fumaric acid metabolism is unlikely. Fumaric acid is the transisomer of malic acid. It is an important compound biochemically since it enters into the citric acid cycle. Fumarate is a by-product at certain stages in the arginine-urea cycle and in purine biosynthesis. Since the citric acid cycle is the center for energy production with the cell, fumaric acid must be present in every cell of the body as it is a by-product of the cycle. Although fumaric acid is not a foreign substance, it is metabolically very active.

In healthy individuals, fumaric acid is formed in the skin when it is exposed to sunlight (from the ultra-violet part of the spectrum). Apparently, patients suffering from Psoriasis have a biochemical defect in which they cannot produce enough fumaric acid and need prolonged exposure to the sun to produce it. This is one reason why patients frequently notice an improvement of their skin condition in the summer months and also explains, in part, the efficacy of PUVA treatment.

This protocol for the treatment of Psoriasis with fumaric acid capsules is based on several clinical studies conducted at the Beau Reveil Clinic in Leysin, Switzerland and the West End Hospital in den Haage, Netherlands. Studies were reported in the following journals: *Ned. Tijdschr. Geneeskd., Gann, Med. Msch., Biochem. Pharm., Arch. Derm. Res.* and *Arch. Derm. Forsch.*

Further references follow at the end of this article, but hereafter I shall follow the protocol as presented by Helmut Christ, M.D. and used by Gus Prosch, Jr., M.D. and other Arthritis Trust of America referral physicians.

Psoriasis Treatment Protocol

(From Helmut Christ, M.D.)

In healthy individuals, fumaric acid is formed in the skin when it is exposed to sunlight (from ultra-violet part of the spectrum). Apparently the patient suffering from Psoriasis cannot make fumaric acid that easily, so that he suffers a lack of the acid and needs a longer exposure to the sun to produce it. This is why these patients frequently notice an improvement of their skin condition in the summer months. The aim of our treatment is therefore not only the application of ointments and creams on the skin or its exposure to ultra-violet light, but the careful oral administration of the lacking fumaric acid ester. This is the basis of our treatment. **At no time is the patient treated with cortisone, either by mouth or on his skin.** (The patients frequently come from Dermatologists or University clinics, having been treated for years with Cortisone orally or as part of the ointment.)

What is fumaric acid?

Chemically it is an unsaturated dicarbonic acid and is part of the citric acid cycle.

CH - COOH

||

CH - COOH

As the citric acid cycle is the center for energy production within the cell, fumaric acid must be present in every cell of the body, being a by-product of the cycle. It is therefore not something that is foreign to the body. A lack of fumaric acid leads to the accumulation of half-products. These products, we believe, are responsible for the skin lesions in patients with Psoriasis. In administering the lacking fumaric acid slowly to the body, the Psoriasis can come to a halt. The administration of the acid should be slow, as it is a metabolically very active substance. However the administration of too little fumaric acid ester will result in a therapeutic failure, whereas too much can lead to heat waves and a drop in blood sugar. This is a very

141

rare occurrence.

The patient with Psoriasis may eat and drink everything that does not produce itching of the skin.

The rule is: If it itches today, then there was something in the food yesterday that his/her skin cannot tolerate. In this way every patient must eventually find out for themself what foods and spices their skin can tolerate and what foods should be avoided. I find it amazing that no Dermatologist or Skin clinic advises the patients in this way, but if one takes a careful history, the doctor will discover that many patients avoid certain food stuffs. A guideline for allowed foods is included. (See *Truth About Allergies & Addiction*, Anthony di Fabio, Warren Levin, M.D. www/ /arthritistrust.org.)

Other factors which can trigger off a relapse in the skin condition are acute illnesses accompanied by high temperatures, and conditions accompanied by accumulation of pus, like purulent tonsillitis, skin abscesses, root-abcesses of teeth, mycotic infections, cellulites, pyorderma, etc. These should be treated immediately and vigorously.

It is adviseable that the patient exercise frequently (jogging) and really sweat.

TREATMENT PROTOCOL
Fumaric Acid Ester Tablets (Strength I and II):

At the end of every evening the patient should take his tablet with a lot of fluid either tea, mineral water or preferably milk as this will reduce stomach acidity. If the patient gets an uneasy epigastric feeling after about an hour, he should take the capsule with a little sugar, as the blood sugar may drop a little at this time. (Of course diabetic patients will experience an improvement of their diabetic state — watch the fasting blood sugar a little more carefully. As Diabetes II has been shown to be caused by food allergies the patient should see *Magic Magnetic Medical Treatments* by William Philpott, M.D. at Amazon.com at bookstores and at Arthritis Trust.org)

The patient should not take the fumaric acid ester with coffee as this will increase gastric acidity, and cause more epigastric discomfort. If he wants to he can also take the tablet dissolved. After about 15 to 30 minutes he will notice a warm feeling and a tingling of the skin, the shoulder, and neck region up to the ear lobes. This reaction lasts approximately half an hour. This indicates that the metabolic process has started. Very rarely the reaction can also come on several hours after taking the tablet and occasionally it may be felt over the whole body. School children should be watched a little more carefully and should carry sweets with them, as they may experience a slight fainting after about 2 to 3 hours from a drop in blood sugar.

The fumaric acid ester tablets are the basis of the treatment, and they actually affect pH in the digestive tract, resulting in better digestion of foods. It is important for every patient to find out the right dose of fumaric

142

acid ester that he needs to keep his skin clear. The dosage may be very variable. If a certain dose does not lead to an improvement of the skin, he should increase the number of tablets every 2 to 3 weeks by ONE tablet (capsule) only. As long as he experiences a warm or tingling feeling in the neck and shoulders or as long as the lesions are slowly subsiding, he can stick to the same dose.

Fumaric Acid Ester Ointment

A compounding pharmacist will prepare this ointment for you. It should be used if the lesions are localized or confined only to the elbows and knees. Very small amounts should be rubbed into the skin lesions daily. An erythema (morbid skin redness) after the application is a good sign. DO NOT apply bandages together with the ointment — else the erythema will be very severe and the skin will burn. One may alternate the fumaric ointment with a salicylic acid ointment if the skin reaction is severe. Rub the ointment only on small areas and only on lesions which appear most active. If the skin tends to become very dry, apply a fattening ointment.

Fumaric Acid Ester Bath

Please notice that this solution should not be added to the bath, but also applied to the skin. The bottle should be mixed well before use. If the patient has very diffuse lesions over the whole body, he should use this solution and rub it very sparingly into the skin and wait for approximately 10 minutes (while the bath is being filled). **The water should not be too hot and the bath should not last longer than about 15 minutes.** When the lesions begin to subside, the ointment should be used for the remaining areas as described above.

Fumaric Acid Lotion

In West Germany Dr. Christ is using a lotion that is rubbed into the scalp immediately after washing the hair, so that it becomes diluted a little — else a slight burning sensation may occur. According to Christ, it is (translated from the German the best possible at this writing):

Fumaric Scalp Lotion Prescription

(*FS-Lotio*)

(RP!) Fumaric Acid	4.0
Monoethyl fumarate	4.0

Infiltrina   10.0 (Something to cause infiltration of scalp, like DMSO — dimethylsulfoxide, perhaps)

Solutio Cordes ad   100.0

MDS. (Place Where It is To Be Used): Scalp Lotion (*Kopfhaut-Lotio*)

General Measures

The natural course of the illness is one of remissions and relapses. If possible the patient should avoid stressful situations.

Dr. Christ suggests that any patient who is seriously interested in getting rid of Psoriasis, to drink absolutely no alcohol, at least until the skin is clear. If the patient's skin does not recover within a few weeks, he suggests to give the patient liver tablets, especially those metabolic products which are found in the fumaric acid cycle (L-Arginine, L-Citrulline, L-Aspartate and L-Ornithine). He would give these in the form of an injection intravenously every day for 2 to 3 weeks. Very frequently the patient will then experience a dramatic improvement of the skin.

It is most important to avoid wines of all kind, as these can produce a relapse. They should also not be used in cooking, gravies, etc.

Nuts of all kinds should be avoided, except almonds. Dissolved aromatic substances in the nuts are the cause of an exacerbation. Peanuts and products made of them (e.g. butter) must be strictly avoided, also mustard, pepper, curry, etc.

Most important for the treating physician to remember:

1. Always start the treatment with fumaric acid ester tablets of low concentration. Increase the number of tablets slowly, every 2 to 3 weeks. The maximum dose is 2 to 3 tablets of strength III. As long as the patient experiences the warm tingling feeling over the neck and shoulders, or as long as he notices that the skin lesions are slowly subsiding, he need not increase the dose.

2. Always remind the patient, that around the 10th to 14th day s/he might experience a slight worsening of itching, or may develop slight edema. This is only transient, if it does occur, and lasts only a few days. If really necessary, you might give a diuretic or antihistaminic preparation — usually it is not a problem.

3. The patient should **never get penicillin** vk. If an infection does have to be treated with an antibiotic, give any other drug except Pencillin VK and watch the patient a little more carefully regarding a relapse. Several other medications will also prevent skin improvement, namely the following ACE — inhibitors: (Angiotensin Converting Enzyme), Calcium-antagonists and beta-blockers, like propranolol.

4. Ointments should be applied very thin and should never be covered up (no bandages, no band-aids, etc.).

5. It is most important that the patient stick to the diet, at least for 2 to 3 months. Only when the skin has recovered completely, should s/he start adding spices to foods and try different foods to find out what his/her skin will tolerate.

6. I would not advise the patient to use ultra-violet light additionally. I doubt whether improvement of the skin is accelerated in this way — and besides, there are several reports from the United States of an increased rate of skin cancer.

7. When the skin is clear (no scars are left behind on healing) the patient may slowly try to reduce the number of fumaric acid tablets. If the skin does start to itch again, he must continue with the dose that kept the lesions away.

8. Reassure the patient that s/he is taking a harmless medication which is not foreign to his body and has no serious side-effects on the liver, kidney, etc. I reassure the patient by showing him the laboratory

144

data regarding hepatic and renal function.

9. *If the skin does not clear up, the patient is either not taking   his   medication correctly (that is   too   little medication), or s/he is not sticking to the diet, or the diagnosis   is incorrect.* Mycotic infections may mimic Psoriasis and antimycotic treatment should be tried if the fumaric acid ester treatment does not bring the expected improvement.

(Helmut Christ,M.D. says: "I am still waiting for the first patient who does not show an improvement — sometimes it just takes a couple of weeks longer!")

10. Additional recommendations (besides the diet) are that patients should also take Omega-3-fatty acids and Omega-6-fatty acids. This was a chance finding and was published in *The Lancet* Nr. 8582, p. 378-380.

Dietary Recommendations for Psoriasis

Foods to be Avoided

Meat: Pork

Spices: All types of aromatic seasoning, pepper, ginger, clove, nutmeg, caraway, anise (licorice), cinnamon, mustard, red pepper, seasoned foods, e.g. sausages, mixed seasoning, (seasoning salt), pre-spiced dishes (e.g. salami, luncheon meats, bouillon cubes), mayonnaise, orange syrup, candied lemon peel, lemon flavoring or extract.

Nuts: Filberts, Hazelnuts, peanuts, all products made of peanuts, e.g. butter, cakes, etc., peanut oil, walnuts, chocolate with nuts.

Alcohols: Wines of all sorts, wine-vinegar, cognac, champagne, sherry, vermouth, port, malaga, liqueur, all other alcohols or foods containing alcohols.

Foods Allowed

Meat: Fish, beef, venison, poultry.

Fruit: All types, tomatoes, fruit-vinegar.

Vegetables: All types, rice, potatoes, pasta, cabbages, saffron, legumes (without forbidden spices).

 Spices: garlic, onion, herbs, parsley, chives, peppercorn, etc.

Oils: olives, olive oil, saffron.

Nuts: coconuts, almonds, all products made of almonds. Pastries: Various kinds.

Highly Recommended

Hand-pressed fresh fruit juices, lots of beetroot-juice, carrot-juice, milk products (yoghurt, curd), sauerkraut, pickles without pepper, half-sour pickles.

This diet recommendation is that of both Helmut Christ, M.D. and Clinique Beau Reveil, CH 1854, Leysin Switzerland.

Remember Dr. Christ's statement:

If the skin does not clear up, the patient is either not taking   his/her   medication correctly (that is, too   little medication), or he/she is not sticking to the diet, or the diagnosis [of Psoriasis] is incorrect.

Psoriasis-Therapy of

Dr. med. Schafer and Dr. med. Christ
(Translated the best possible at this writing)
Salve:
1. Fumaric Acid Monoethylester   1.5
2. Skin Cream (DDD*)   15.0
3. DMSO (Dimethylsulfoxide)   8.0
4. Milk Acid Ethylester '   1.0
5. Glyoxylic Diureide   1.0
6. Eucerin anhydric to   50.0

* *Skin Cream (DDD) Composition: Salicylic Acid, Camphor, Chlorobutanol, Phenol, Methylsalicylate, Thymol.* This is a mixture of substances, in different strengths, available through pharmacies in Germany and England, and with these properties (according to German package insert): "DDD penetrates deep into the skin tissue and, because of its antiseptic and antibacterial force, it fights effectfully inflamation and pus instigators. DDD activates the metabolism process in the skin, promotes the blood circulation and provides better nutrition of the cells, better extraction of disease agitators and promotes the new formation of healthy, hardy tissue. Itching, tension in the skin, and pain sensations disappear most immediately after the application." (Produced in license of DDD Ltd., England by DDD Lab, 1000 Berlin, 30 Delta Clinic, 6078 New Isenburg.)

Psoriasis-Bath:
1. Fumaric acid Ester   100 g
2. Balneum Herb Bath   500 ml

Taken From the German From Helmut Christ

1. Fumaric Ester Powder Capsule I

Fumaric Acid Monoethylester — Metal Salts:

F. - Fe Salt	0.100g
F. - Ca Salt	0.400g
F. - Mg Salt	0.400g
F. - Li Salt	0.200g
F. - K Salt	0.200g
F. - Zn Salt	0.400g
F. - Cu Salt	0.020g
Fumaric Acid	0.600g
Fumaric Acid dimethyl Ester	0.600g

These constituents (to go into) 20 capsules. Generally, should be taken after meals, the   amount determined by the doctor.

NOTE: For the prescription it is sufficient to use / the name "Fumaric Powder Capsule I." For chronic therapy an amount of 120 capsules is recommended for the prescription.

2. Fumaric Powder Capsule II

Fumaric Acid Monoetheylester — Metal Salts:

F. - Ca Salt	1.0g

F. - Fe Salt	0.12g
F. - Cu Salt	0.02g
F. - Mg Salt	0.8g
Fumaric Acid dimethyl Ester	2.4g
Magnesium Carbonate	0.8g
Zincum Oxide	0.2g

These constituents (to go into) 20 capsules. Generally, should be taken after meals, the amount determined by the doctor.

NOTE: For the prescription it is sufficient to use the name "Fumaric Powder Capsule II." For chronic therapy an amount of 120 capsules is recommended for the prescription.

3. Fumaric Acid Bath

Fumaric Acid Ester	100.0
Balneum Herbal Oilbath	500.0

Usage: As soon as you have wet your body in the shower, you use this bath liquid, and after that use the powder on the skin lesions. After waiting 5 minutes for it to take effect, rinse off the whole body with water.

4. Fumaric Salve I

Fumaric Acid Monoethylester	3.0
Glyoxylic Diureide	3.0
Lactic Acid Ethyl Ester	3.0
DMSO	10.0
DDD — Soothing Skin Cream	40.0
Eucerin anlydricum to	100.0

Usage: According to instructions of doctor. Fumaric Salve I is for the patient with strong itching.

NOTE: For the prescription it is sufficient to use the name "Fumaric Salve I."

Helmut Christ, M.D. states that he has had no experience with items 5, 6, and 7 that follow, but they were so interesting, and they might be useful and so we include them .

5. Fumaric Salve II

Fumaric Acid Monoethylester	3.0
Glyoxylic Diureide	3.0
Decoderm Basis Cream	40.0
Eucerin With Water to	100.0

Usage: According to instructions of doctor. Fumaric Salve II is only for skin care.

NOTE: For the prescription it is sufficient to use the name "Fumaric Salve II."

6. (Scalp) Head Alcohol

Fumaric Acid	2.5
Fumaric Acid Monoethylester	2.5
DMSO	5.0
Spiritus Cordes to	100.0

Usage: According to instructions of doctor.

7. Fumaric Fingernail Polish

Griseofulvin	*0.01*
Fumaric Acid Monoethylester	*0.5*
Benzoic Acid Ethyl Ester	*0.3*
Mallebrin	*0.1*
Talcum	*0.05*
Cellulose Nitrate Lacquer to	*10.0*

Usage: According to instructions of doctor.

Over the past 6 years we were able to increase the success rate of the healing effect of the fumaric acid ester by the addition of thymus extract, the trace mineral selenium, zinc and vitamin B complex as intravenous infusion.

The following is an interesting letter from Helmut Christ, M.D. to Robert F. Cathcart, M.D., a copy forwarded to Anthony di Fabio at Christ's request, March 1, 1989:

"Thank you very much for your letter dated Dec. 1, 1988. Please excuse the long delay for answering, but as you guessed, I am being flooded with letters from physicians and patients in the U.S. wanting to know more about the treatment [Psoriasis, Ed:] and where they can get the medication.

"It appears that physicians in this country are slowly wakening up and becoming more and more alert to this very successful type of treatment and I just cannot cope any more. I am seriously considering having another physician to assist me.

"Other medications that interfere with the fumaric acid [ester] treatment — this is an interesting subject. I don't know why Beta-blockers, Calcium-antagonists and Angiotensin-converting-enzyme inhibitors prevent the psoriatic lesions from healing off. It could be a local effect at the site of the scales on the skin. However I believe that these drugs interfere in metabolic pathways, either in the citric acid cycle or the fumaric acid cycle, which is closely connected to the former. You are reading my thoughts by suggesting that fumaric acid [ester] may act as a type of antibiotic in the bowel killing . . . organism[s]. How else can you explain that Metronidazole gives some improvement in patients with psoriasis. Maybe one should try both substances in patients — 10% — who just don't want to get better. One should investigate this problem with bacteriological sensitivity tests.

"Another interesting aspect is that if you give these patients the metabolic products of the fumaric acid cycle, e.g, L-Citrulline, L-Argnine, L-Ornithine, L-Aspartate (The L-amino acids), intravenously you can watch the patient getting better week to week.

"As far as literature [scientific studies] goes, I have a large collection, but it is all in German! I would suggest that you order the capsules, ointment, bath and lotion for the scalp on a regular basis — BUT IN SMALL AMOUNTS — from our pharmacist[s] in Germany. I have heard from several patients in the U.S. that they are getting the fumaric acid [ester] from [name omitted] and some trace minerals and the whole thing doesn't help the patient at all. The secret is that it is important that the 'Ester' form of the fumaric acid has to be used and not fumaric acid as such, alone." [Ed. The compounding pharmacist was located in Canada and he did, indeed, sell Fumaric Acid rather than fumaric acid esther.]

On March 10, 1985, Christ transmitted to this author two addresses in West Germany that did supply the proper medicines. They were: Herr Horst Widmann, "Stadt — Apotheke", Friedrichstrabe 27, 7460 Balingen; and Herr Winfried Ertelt, "Hohenzollern — Apotheke", Steinhofenerstrabe 14, 7457 Bisingen. Also in the United States, **Cardiovascular Research Ltd. 1061-B Shary Circle, Concord, CA 94518 sold under the name of Psorex; phone 1-800-888-4585; (510)-827-2636.**

[I would like to apologize in advance for possible incomplete or mistaken translations of the materials forwarded to us by Helmut Christ, M.D.. Perry A. (Tony) Chapdelaine, M.D. is responsible for translations that are presented for which thanks are due.

Jonathan Wright, M.D. Recommendation

The October 2002 issue of *Nutrition & Healing*[12] provides a "Clinical Tip 108" which recommends adding a small amount (almost homeopathic) of nickel/bromide to the fumaric acid ester treatment. Such a pill is sold as Psorizide® Forte, available through Tahoma Clinic Dispensary, natural food stores, and compounding pharmacies. This substance was developed by Steven Smith, M.D. of Tulsa, Oklahoma, and apparently just one tablet a day, together with proper diet and fumaric acid ester treatment providesabout 90 percent relief.

Additional information (dated March 3, 1987): "We are finding that fumaric acid ester may dissolve too slowly if taken by capsules, even with two 10 ounce glasses of liquid. With some people it is important to empty capsule and dissolve the contents in juice, etc. to get high enough concentration in blood to initiate head and shoulders flush. It seems to vary widely from person to person."

We cannot leave this article without a reference to "Universal Oral Vaccine" found at the www.arthritistrust.org website, and also in several of our publications found on Amazon.com, at bookstores and at Arthritistrust.org, namely *Absolutely Phenomenal Medical Treatments.* In brief it is reported that psoriasis vanishes almost immediatly when covered with streptococcus antigen-specific colostrum. In the United States such substances are easily available for purchase by the dairy farmer and veterinarian but denied for humans, not because of safety or effectiv eness problems but mainly because the whole, sad, faulty structure of vaccinations would be endangered should this kind of knowledge become known to the masses. This immune milk is mentioned further on.

References

1. Chopra, D.P. & Flaxman, B.A. Comparative proliferative kinetics of cells from normal human epidermis and benign epidermal hyperplasia (psoriasis) *in vitro. Cell and Tissue Kinetics.* 7.69, 1974.

2. Weinstein, G.D. & Frost, P. Abnormal cell profliferation in psoriasis. *J. Invest. Derm.* 50:254, 1968.

3. Schweckendiek, W. Helilung von Psoriasis vlugaris. *Med. Msch.* 13:103-104, 1959.

4. Kuroda, Z. and Akao, M. Antitumor and anti-intoxication activities of fumaric acid in cultured cells. *Gann,* 72:777-782, 1981.

5. Hagedorn, K. et al. Fumarsauremonoathylester: Wirkung auf DNA-Synthese und erste tierexperimentelle Befunde. *Arch. Derm. Res.* 254:67-73, 1975.

6. Bruynzeel, D. Kan fumaarzuur worden toegepast bij psoriasis? *Ned. Tijdschr. Geneeskd.* 128(35):1677, 1984.

7. Petres, J. et al. Der Einfluss von Fumarasuremono-athylester auf die Nucleinsaure-und Proteinsynthese PHA-stimulierter menschlicher Lymphocyten. *Arch. Derm. Forsch.* 251:295-300, 1975.

8. Baron, D. fumaarzuur worden toegpast bij psoriasis (Vraag en Antwoord). *Ned. tijdschr. Geneeskd.* 128(24):1152-1153, 1984.

9. van Dijk, E. Fumaarzuur voor de behandeling van patienten met psoriasis. *Ned. Tijdschr. Geneeskd.* 129(11):485-486, 1985.

10. Kuroda, K. and Akao, K. Reduction by fumaric acid of side effects of Mitomycin C. *Biochem. Pharm.* 29:2839-2844, 1980.

11. Anthony di Fabio, *The Art of Getting Well,* 1988, see http://www.arthritistrust.org.

12. Dr. Jonathan Wrights' *Nutrition & Healing,* 819 N. Charles St., Baltimore, MD 21201.

I also refer the reader to *Townsend Letters for Doctors* article "Immunosuppression of Polyunsaturated Fatty Acids in Autoimmune Diseases, Cancer and Heart Attacks" written by Wayne Martin, published July 1988, p. 271. [*The Townsend Letters for Doctors and Patients* is an informal newsletter available by subscription (for those interested) by writing to *Townsend Letters for Doctors*, 911 Tyler Street, Port Townsend, WA 98368.]

Psoriasis and Liver Sclerosis

The Case of Christopher Salvadore del Rio

Dr. Catherine Russell, Guadalajara, Mexico, describes a "most pathetic psoriasis patient that, through 20 years of cortisone treatment, had reached the point of sclerosis." Traditional physicians had told him "We can't do anything more for you. Just go home and die."

Christopher's niece described her uncle's condition to Dr. Russell, as Dr. Russell loved to get so-called hopeless cases.

Dr. Russell obtained fumaric acid esther as recommended by Helmut Christ, M.D. of Bisingen, Germany, starting Christopher on that substance as well as saturating him with vitamin C to negate the effects of the cortisone. She also addressed Christopher's obvious liver problem. As she didn't know about the benefits of milk thistle extract for the liver at the time, Dr. Russell addressed Christopher's sclerosis problem with homeopathic medicine, B complex.

Christopher's psoriasis and liver sclerosis were totally cleared up, based on laboratory tests made at the same location that had been administering his cortisone shots. The liver cleared up in about 2 years.

Pyrithione Zinc

Used effectively for more than 10 years in Europe is Pyrithione Zinc, chemically a 2% spray of $C10H8N2O2Zn$, or bis-[1-hydroxy-2(1H)-pyridinethionato-O,S]zinc. The spray substance consists of 2 mgs per milliliter (2mg/ml) of pyrithione zinc. Sprayed twice a day over the skin provides what appears to be permanent cure, even for the worst cases, according to reports by several medical doctors, doctors of osteopathy, and chiropractors. At most 1 to 2 cans are required to bring relief.

Successful clinical trials have been carried out in Spain and Argentina, according to a report by medical journalist, Morton Walker, D.P.M. as published in *Townsend Letter for Doctors and Patients*, January 1997, page 58.

This substance, Skin-Cap Spray, can be ordered via Progressive Laboratories, Inc., 1701 W. Walnut Hill Ln., Irving, TX 75038; (800) 527-9512.

Staphylococcus Antibody/Complement

This Christmas (1998) one of us (Anthony di Fabio) spent with friends watching the application of specifically prepared antigen/complement materials from bovine colostrum, the cow's first milk on calving (See our "Universal Oral Vaccine," http://www.arthritistrust.org).

"What I personally observed was a kind of Christmas miracle. Nowhere had I ever read or heard of Psoriasis being related to staphylococcus, other than an associated infection. Here's what I observed:

"A patient had gross, raised blotches of skin Psoriasis that would not heal no matter what treatments were tried.

"A liquid preparation of staphylococcus antibody/complement was taken orally, 1 teaspoon each hour, and a cotton ball was also used to wipe the mixture on the Psoriasis blotches. The wiping on of the liquid was done every time itching occurred, and also occassionally throughout the next days. Also the oral treatment of the liquid was continued each hour.

"Within minutes (literally) of the first wiping the blotches began to disappear. Within a day, all blotches were reduced in size. Within two days, only the longest standing, and grossest blotches remained.

"Finally, all marks were gone! What a great Christmas present!"

Dr. Jonathan Wright got the following letter from Dr. Steven Smith who founded Loma Lux Laboratories. He'd received it from a Tahoma Clinic client who wanted to let him know how his psoriasis responded to Loma Lux's nickel bromide product, Psorizide Forte. This was published in the April 2004 issue of *Nutrition & Healing*.

Dear Dr. Smith:

I would sincerely like to compli-ment your company and your Psorizide Forte. I believe that this treatment saved my life.

I had been suffering from moderate psoriasis for many years when it rather suddenly took a turn, for the worse. The psoriasis had gotten so severe that the only untouched area of my body was my face. The skin on the bottom of my feet and hands begin peeling off My scalp, legs, arms and back were also severely affected. The plaques must have covered 80 plus percent of my body. Then my ankles began to swell up like watermelons and my thighs were beginning to also swell. 1 was in such had shape mentally and physically by this point, I thought that I was going to die.

1 had been seeing an M.D. dermatologist who had prescribed Triamcinolone, a synthetic cortisone ointment. The ointment started losing its effectiveness with time and I was getting worse daily. I then went to be treated by Dr. Jonathan Wright, M. D., in Renton. Washington. He recommended Psorizide Forte to treat my psoriasis. The day after I started taking [it] my psoriasis started getting better. Within a week my normal skin began returning.

Today, which is about six weeks since I began using Psorizide Forte I have only small remnants of psoriasis left. I look and feel normal again and I feel so fortunate that I found this product I have since been telling all of my doctor friends and anyone with psoriasis about my remarkable recovery and where to get your product

—Dr. L. P, Seattle, WA

Jonathan V. Wright, M.D.: Thanks to Dr. L.P for sharing your experience. Nickel still tends to get a bad rap for triggering skin irrita-tion, but, ironic as it seems, when it's combined with bromide and taken in tablet form, nickel can be a very effective psoriasis treatment.Like anything else, this therapy doesn't work every single time, but in many of the patients I've treated, the psoriasis disappears completely. Other times, it's substantially improved. It's worth trying, as the quantities of nickel and bromide required are quite low and adverse reactions are few.As a *Nutrition & Healing* subscriber, if you'd like to read more about this therapy, see the October 2002 by visiting www.wrightnewsletter.com. Jonathan Wright is not involved financially with the Loma Lux Corporation or Dr. Stephen Smith.

Reprinted from *Nutrition & Healing*. Subscription available from Reader Services Department, 819 N. Charles St., Baltimore, MD 21201; tel. (203) 699-3683.

Boron, Also a Necessary Supplement

Anthony di Fabio & Rex E. Newnham, Ph.D.,D.O., N.D., Gus J. Prosch, Jr., M.D.

Boron was not generally recognized as a necessry dietary supplement until Dr. Newnham circled the earth twice measuring the amount of boron eaten at various places and comparing this quantity against incidence of arthritis.

Boron is produced almost entirely by cosmic rays and therefore is found in relatively low abundance on earth, although some locations, like Turkey, have large deposits.

The primry use of elemental boron is to make boron filaments which are used in a manner similar to carbon fibers. Boron is used on an industrial scale as an additive to glass fibers. Boron is also used as fertilizers in agriculture and other miscellaneous uses. Boric acid is mildly antimicrobial, and used as a natural antiseptic.

Since the pioneer work of Dr. Newnham, more and more recognition is being given to the use of boron as a necessry human supplement, one that can also improve the health and nutritional value of foods.

In 1986 The Arthritis Trust of America   received information on Boron and Arthritis from Rex E. Newnham, Ph.D., D.O., N.D. of Leeds, England.

Dr. Newnham demonstrated demographic evidence for the usefulness of Boron in treating or preventing Rheumatoid Arthritis and Osteoarthritis. His article follows:

"In countries where there are minimum amounts of available boron in the soil there is much more arthritis. In most developed countries there are about 20% of people with some musculo-skeletal disease, which is generally arthritis. In places where there is more than usual boron in the soil there is much less arthritis.

"Jamaica and Mauritius have more than usual arthritis, and there is very little available boron in their soils. Most or all of the food and other crops show severe boron deficiency in these soils. Soil or plant analyses in these countries support the visual signs of deficiency.

"Fiji is another tropical sugar producing country, and there the Indians have much more arthritis than the Fijians. The Indians eat mostly rice which is a monocotyledon plant, and these require much less boron than do the dicotyledons. The Fijians eat mostly starchy root vegetables, which are dicotyledons. Actual figures were not available.

"There is an area in Northern Thailand where there is a considerable boron deficiency, and Professor Jack Loneragan of Murdoch University is supervising work that will rehabilitate this soil. It has also been established from Thais who live in the USA that there is considerable arthritis in these parts of the country, but there has so far been no cooperation with the university or the Health Department in Bangkok. No visit is planned unless there can be some cooperation.

"Dr. Bridges-Webb recently completed a survey in southern Australia which showed that about 20% of the population suffered from a musculo-skeletal disease, and this is typical of the people in the other Western cultures[1].

"Israel is an advanced country that has less than 0.5% arthritis, according to a survey conducted by Professor Bentwich[12]. It is interesting to note that there are no known shortages of boron in their soils. The soils of the Jordan Valley even have excess boron, so much so that in places only the very tolerant date palm will grow.

"At Carnarvon in Western Australia there was 0.35 ppm of boron in the water supply. This was reduced to 0.2 ppm a few years ago because there was some toxicity to legume crops. In this tropical environment the transpiration rate is high so that all minerals are soon concentrated in the plant. A survey was conducted there in 1981 which revealed that there was only 1% arthritis in that community. It was even found that some people went there from 1000 miles away so as to enjoy the good climate and get rid of their arthritis. It was the good water more than the climate that was the important factor in their health. Similarly in New Zealand there is a place called Ngawha, where spa pools contain 300 ppm of boron. This is a well known curative pool for arthritics[2].

"Over 60 years ago Dr. Herbert, the government balneologist, or specialist on spa water treatment, recommended certain pools as beneficial for arthritis. All of these had a high boron content, but he did not know what the reasons for their curative properties were[3]. It is now being shown that it is the high boron content of the water. People used to bathe in these waters and they also drank some of the water.

"Professor O.L. Meyers recently supervised a survey in South Africa that showed how the Xhosa tribal people had 2% Rheumatoid Arthritis in their native state, but when the same people went to the big cities, they soon developed the prevalance for arthritis as was shown by the rest of the city population[4]. This is assumed to be about 20%. An experiment was devised to give the reason for these rather startling figures.

"In 1985 efforts were made to collect samples of mealies or maize or corn from the native gardens and from commercial farms.

"It took until 1986 to collect all the required samples. The Xhosa people live in Transkei, and one cannot just go there and get cobs of mealies. A pharmacist from Uitenhage tried and failed to get any on his first effort. Later he did get some, from some sort of stall. A Xhosa man from Durban who goes home to Transkei every month got some samples grown from truly native gardens. These were analysed by Professor Verbeek in the Department of Chemistry, University of Natal in Pietermaritzburg, (Republic of South Africa[5].

"See Table I, Analysis of Mealies From Various Sources. Of the four samples shown in Table I and collected in Transkei, the first two came from

154

land that had never had chemicals added, it was truly a native garden. Information about the last two from Transkei is being obtained. Transkei is the traditional home for the Xhosa tribe.

"This table supports the hypothesis that was made four years ago in Aberdeen in which the boron intake of national groups was estimated on the grounds of observation of deficiency symptoms of foodstuff and on what analysis had been done. This is shown in the following table[6]: "See Table II, Daily Boron Levels in Food, by National Groups From this table it is seen that 5-6 mg of boron each day is sufficient to maintain good health without arthritis. In 1967 Ploquin published an article 'Boron in Foodstuffs'[5] and he shows how the boron content of some common foods will vary from 1 to 150 ppm, depending on the variety and the soil, but especially the fertilizer treatment of the soil. Some of the old crushed rock fertilizers had sufficient boron, but the newer synthetic types contain none. Crops will remove from 30 to 300 g of boron per hectare. Grains remove the least while fruit trees and Cruciferae remove the most. Most commercial crops are grown with fertilizer, and this means the minimum of boron, but those grown on gardens that have never had fertilizer, but to which all wastes are returned, have the most. The South African work shows this very well.

"Ploquin did produce the table III. Three additional columns have been added which will give nearer to the actual quantity consumed by the average person in America, England or Australia, New Zealand or South Africa in 1986[5]. See Table III, Ideal Amounts of Foodstuffs Consumed per Week

"The revised daily intake of boron is below 2 mg as is consumed by some people in the English speaking countries. Most ingest only 1-2 mg daily. There are large numbers of people who eat what is often called junk foods, with well over the average for sugar, hamburger type meat meals, fried meat and eggs. Most of their calories come from sugar and fat with no fruit or vegetables. As fruit accounts for 65% of the revised boron intake, and fresh fruit and vegetables for 72% of Ploquin's figure, people who eat this junk food will ingest less than 2 mg boron daily, probably less than 1 mg.

"Ploquin does show that those who drink half a litre of wine each day will take in much more boron, but that is more of a European habit, and those who eat much fast food or take away foods and junk foods will have much less.

"In 1979 there was a report of Dr. Rex E. Newnham claiming that 'Boron Beats Arthritis'[8]. It was the first paper linking boron with arthritis and much work has been done since then. It is very interesting that boron compounds in concentrations as low as 0.0005M will inhibit bacteriophages and protozoa, this was reported by Zittle in 1951[9]. Other microorganisms are destroyed by higher concentration. This [may] give a reason for the success of boron supplements in alleviating rheumatoid arthritis. Nielsen has shown that boron seems to be able to effect calcium and magnesium metabolism in the rat[10]. This agrees with Loughman's work in which he showed that boron acted as a membrane catalyst to allow other ions to pass into the cell[11]. On this basis boron will allow ATP (adenosine tri-phosphate) to enter cells of worn-out cartilage or collagen, so as to give energy for cell division, and thus to repair tissues, and so to overcome the effect of arthritis.

"There is increasing evidence that boron is an essential trace element for both man and animal. It does influence calcium and magnesium metabolism, and this is possibly through the parathyroid gland[10]. It does alleviate and seems to cure arthritis either by acting [against whatever organism may cause Rheumatoid Diseases] and/or as a membrane catalyst that permits repair of damaged cartilage and collagen.

"It has been shown by Professor Jeffries, an orthopaedic surgeon at Otago Hospital, New Zeland, that patients who had been taking the boron supplement had harder bones than the normal arthritic patient. This supports the work of Nielsen that boron does influence calcium metabolism. We must get more evidence on this and then it will probably be shown that lack of boron is one of the main causes of osteoporosis.

Dr. Newnham's hypothesis is making headway via physicians and vitamin research organizations. His Osteo-trace[TM], B-Alive, or Bone Salts tablets have also helped the elderly, in Still's Disease, Juvenile Arthritis, and Lupus, especially in its severe form of Systemic Lupus Erythematosus. Infants do require a reduced dose of 1/4 to 1/2 tablet twice daily

Other products, such as Vitamin Research Products of Mountain View, California, also recommend and sell Boron and also Biotech, P.O. Box 1992, Fayetteville, AR 72702.

It is interesting and helpful to compare Jeff E. Young's, (M.S.) article with Newnham's. I quote from Vitamin Research Products' nutritional newsletter, Volume 3, Number 5, August 1988:

"BORON

"Boron — Becoming Recognized as an Essential Mineral
Part 2 of 2 Parts

"We have heard of the importance of micro-essential minerals such as manganese, molybdenum, selenium, and vanadium. We know that calcium is required for sound bones. Now research shows that boron may play a key role in the retention of calcium. But, what is boron? The latest study conducted by the U.S. Department of Agriculture indicated that within 8 days of supplementing 3 mg. of boron, a test group of postmenopausal women lost 40 percent less calcium, one-third less magnesium, and slightly less phosphorus through their urine. These are the minerals which make up our bones.

"Each day the women took a 3 mg. boron supplement in the form of sodium borate. They retained an average of 52 mg. more calcium which is equal to a gram of calcium every 20 days. The body contains roughly 1,100 grams of calcium, so over a period of several years, that's a significant savings in calcium.

"The absorption of calcium into our body is a very complicated process. it requires sex hormones, especially estrogen. This is the reason why menopausal women, whose ovaries are no longer producing estrogen, have a hard time absorbing calcium. Even though many are taking a calcium supplement, most of the supplemental calcium is wasted through urination. Currently, estrogen replacement is the only proven treatment for Osteoporosis, the brittle bone disease that affects millions." [See *Chelation Therapy*[13] as well as *Prevention and Treatment of Osteoporosis*[14]; also note that, according to Gus Prosch, Jr, M.D., calcium should always be taken with an equal amount of magnesium, and both should be in a form that is bio-available: *Proper Nutrition for Rheumatoid Arthritis,* all at http://www.arthritistrust.org.]

"After the exciting discovery of calcium retention by a small boron supplement, a question arises. How can boron make such a dramatic difference? The answer is found in the blood serum of the experimental subjects. Researchers have discovered that the blood level of the most active form of estrogen — 17-beta estradiol — DOUBLES to the level found in women on estrogen replacement therapy; that's a fifty percent increase over the pre-study levels! Also, the blood levels of testosterone — a male hormone and precursor of estradiol — MORE than doubled.

"The researchers suspect that the body needs boron to synthesize estrogen, vitamin D, and other steroid hormones. It may also protect these hormones against rapid breakdown. Another study further substantiated this theory. A group of chickens were fed with a low vitamin D diet which normally would have stunted their bone growth. However, this phenomenon had been halted by the boron supplement, and the chickens were growing normally.

"Osteoporosis affects as many as 15 to 20 million older Americans predominately women. Each year Osteoporosis contributes to about 1.3 million fractures (primarily in the hip, spine and wrist) in people 45 years old and over. This costs an estimated $3.8 billion annually [paid] to the medical industry.

"Calcium supplement sales are at an all-time high as women try to prevent bone loss. Unfortunately, only a certain type of bone, the cortical.

Since boron is rich in fruits and vegetables, the finding also indicates that vegetarians should have a much lower occurence of osteoporosis. On the contrary, Eskimos, who eat almost no fruits and vegetables, have a very high incidence of bone demineralization, even during their youth. Excessive phosphorus, which is found in meat, also causes detrioration of bone (but that's another story)." [Consider the impact on health of carbonated drinks with their high and, for some, continuous intake of phosphorus: Ed.]

"Table I
Average Boron Content in Different
Food Groups

Food Group	Boron (ug/g dry weight)

157

Cereals	0.6-2.3ug
Meat	0.1-0.3ug
Fish	0.1-0.9ug
Dairy Products	0.1-1.5ug
Vegetable foods (fresh)	1.1-41ug
Vegetable foods (canned)	0.4-2.0ug
Fruit	0.8-3.8ug
Other	2.6ug"

[Dr. Newhham says thatYoung has provided these figures as average boron contents of certain food groups; and that "it would be much more meaningful if the maximum and minimum figures were also given. We should aim to get quality in our food, rather than a large quantity of mediocre food. Processed foods, freezing, canning do reduce the mineral contents. Even home cooking will reduce the mineral content if the cooking water is discarded."]

"Table II

Boron Content in a Serving

(mg. Boron per 100 ml).

(3-1/3 fluid ounces or 0.42 cup)

or 100 gr. (3-2/3 ounces, dry weight)

Apple sauce, bottled	0.279mg
Grape Juice, bottled	0.202mg
Apple Juice, bottled	0.188mg
Peaches, canned	0.187mg
Broccoli, frozen flower	0.185mg
Broccoli, frozen stalks	0.089mg
Cherries, frozen	0.147mg
Pears, canned	0.122mg
Carrots, canned	0.075mg
Green beans, frozen	0.046mg
Orange juice, frozen	0.041mg
Lettuce, iceberg	0.039mg
Noodles, egg	0.037mg
Cornflakes, fortified	0.031mg
Bread, white enriched	0.020mg
Ice cream, vanilla	0.019mg
Potatoes, canned	0.017mg
Chicken breast, ground	0.005mg
Coffee, freeze dried	0.005mg
Rice, Minute	0.003mg
Milk, 2% fat	0.002mg
Beef, ground round *	Not detectable
Cheese, cheddar or cream*	Not detectable
Eggs, frozen	Not detectable

Sugar, granulated Not detectable

* [These vary from Table I and so supports the need for maximum and minnimum values alongside average figures: Ed.]

[Dr. Newnham says, "There are 5 drinks and 20 foods in the above list. Normal people do not eat this much in a day and the total boron intake is [about] 1.7 mg. The only fresh and unprocessed food is the lettuce. When the frozen foods are thawed in the manner done by most people, much of the mineral content is lost."]

Table 3
Food With Highest Level of
Boron (In ug/g Fresh Weight)

Soy meal	28ug
Prune	27ug
Raisin	25ug
Almond	23ug
Rosehips	19ug
Peanut	18ug
Hazel nut	16ug
Date	9.2ug
Honey	7.2ug
Wines	8.5ug
Raisin	25ug

"Nature normally supplies boron in boric acid complex with sugar, polysaccharides, adenosine 5-phosphate, pyridoxine, riboflavin, dehydroascorbic acid and pyridine nucleotides.

"Postmenopausal women, aged 48 to 82 were equilibrated with a low boron diet for 119 days. When they were given 3 mg of boron as a supplement, their calcium excretion through urine decreased, and estradiol (estrogen) and testosterone in their blood serum increased significantly.

Furthermore, the responses were not temporary: The beneficial result of boron supplementation seems to last for as long as the boron supplements are given.

"When the diet of the subjects contained adequate magnesium, the effects of boron became less significant. The reason is not yet fully understood.

"Even though there currently are no definitive answers for the total role of boron, the scientists who discovered the boron/calcium/estradiol connection suggest that boron may be crucial for the addition of the hydroxyl (OH) group onto the hormones and vitamin D. The presence of hydroxyl groups make a big difference in their hormonal characteristics. The differences between testosterone and estradiol (estrogen) are mainly determined by a single hydroxyl group.

"Actually, vitamin D behaves more as a hormone, rather than as a vitamin. The vitamin D which we get from food or from dietary supplementation is not fully activated. It requires a conversion in the liver, and also another conversion in the kidney in order to become fully active. This fully active vitamin D is called 1 alpha, 25 dihydro-cholecalciferol. People with a poor liver and/or kidney function are at a higher risk of getting Osteoporosis. As the name of the active vitamin D implies, dihydro means two hydroxyl groups contained in each vitamin D molecule. They make a big difference when it comes to biological activity.

"In excess, boron is harmful to plants, livestock and humans. Boron inhibits many enzymatic activities with harmful effects. These enzymes include zanthine oxidase, alcohol dehydrogenase, alkaline phosphatase, catechol oxidase, polyphenol oxidase, tyrosinase, peroxidase, IAA oxidase, phosphoglucose isomerase, phosphaglucomutase and phosphorylase (which inhibits starch synthesis). Enzymes are the machinery of metabolism. When one or more enzymes are hindered by toxic substances, the result can be fatal.

"How much boron is toxic? We have discussed the estimation of boron requirement, which is about 2 mg per day (0.705 ounces). Researchers found the lowest reported lethal dose of boric acid is about 45 gr. (1.6 ounce) for an adult and 2 gr. (0.705 ounces) for an infant." [This ends Young's paper. Dr. Newnham shows that 6 mg per day of boron (.213 ounces) is necessary for good health: Ed.]

Additional Information

Since Dr. Newnham's paper was sent to our physicians in 1986, there has been considerably more research performed on the effects of boron in various forms of arthritis.

Gus J. Prosch, Jr., M.D., until his retirement, was asked to review an article by Dr. Newnham entitled "Boron and Arthritis: Is There a Connection?" I have abstracted some of Prosch's comments in review of this article:

"Dr. Newnham's findings and research, if eventually conclusively proven, will serve to explain and possibly verify with further research, certain unexplained observations I have made in my own private practice when treating numerous patients with Rheumatoid Arthritis, Osteoarthritis and Osteoporosis.

"In treating arthritic and osteoporotic patients, I consistently observe better results when I supplement the diet of these patients with either Calcium Orotate or Calcium Aspartate along with Norwegian Cod Liver Oil — which I feel is the best source of natural Vitamin D3. The D3 more efficiently helps regulate the excessive excretion of calcium than the more commonly used synthetic vitamin D2. I've noticed that using Calcium Carbonate or other forms of calcium do not give the same consistent results as in the orotate or aspartate forms. Dr. Hans Neiper claims the orotate and aspartate forms of calcium carry the mineral directly into the cells to be utilized more efficiently. I have often wondered why the more common forms of calcium do not perform as well as the orotates and aspartates.

"Dr. Newnham states that the parathyroid gland contains more boron

160

than any other tissue in humans. Boron enhances parathormone activity which is the prime organ controlling bone mineralization. Dr. Newnham's research makes me now consider that if arthritic patients are deficient in boron, there is a strong possibility that the parathyroid bone mineralization effects are not functioning efficiently. By supplementing these patients with boron, could the patients be given regular forms of calcium such as calcium carbonate and would they receive the same benefits as by using the orotates and aspartates?

"Dr. Newnham's article also stimulated my imagination concerning the possible imbalance of certain anabolic hormones in arthritics as well as the known deficiencies in osteoporosis patients such as 17- beta estradiol and testosterone. I have previously noted further improvement in treating many arthritic patients and in nearly all osteoporosis patients when I supplement these patients with small amounts of these anabolic hormones. Dr. Newnham further documents a previous study by Nielsen and Hunt which proved that a boron supplemented diet with post-menopausal osteoporosis patients markedly reduced their urinary excretion of calcium and magnesium as well as greatly elevated the serum concentrations of 17-beta estradiol and of testosterone. The increase in the serum concentration of these anabolic hormones may eventually prove, with further research, to be the reason many arthritic patients respond in a more positive manner to any therapy when they are given the hormones. It is obvious why osteoporosis patients respond better when given these hormones.

"Dr. Newnham's article confirmed other observations I have noted in treating arthritic patients. For the past five years I have been a dedicated proponent of [The Arthritis Trust of America Foundation treatment program]. Provided I adequately supplement the patient's diet with various nutritional suplements, I have experienced a consistent eighty percent remission rate in these patients

. . . . I have noticed that approximately sixty-five percent of Rheumatoid Arthritis patients and twenty-five to thirty percent of osteoarthritic patients undergo the Herxheimer reaction when treated with [The Arthritis Trust of America Foundation medications and The Proper Nutrition for Rheumatoid Arthritis]. (Also see The Herxheimer Effect[15])

"Dr. Newnham has in his research verified the fact that arthritic patients undergoing treatment with Boron supplementation often experienced the Herxheimer reaction and the reaction is always a good prognostic sign."[In Dr. Newnham's article], considerable evidence presented is strictly demographic in nature and this type of evidence [is not conclusive]. As I read the article a second time, the demographic studies took on an entirely different importance to me and I found the accumulated information extremely interesting. All in all, I feel that Dr. Newnham did a remarkable job in collating and presenting this information . . .

"[Dr Newnham's] article has some deficiencies and inadequacies but the merit and reasoning of the article far outweighs the negative points. It is definitely not an illogical hypothesis and the theory presented certainly does not conflict with present day thinking and especially from a nutritional standpoint. . . I believe the article will motivate further research from the published findings."

Rex Newnham, D.O., Ph.D., N.D.[16], states: "As we use more and more superphosphate on our food crops the availability of soil boron is decreased. It is estimated that most people in western societies ingest less than 2 mg boron daily. This is based on the analysis of school meals in the U.S.A.[17], but analyses earlier in this century put the figure at 8 mg[18].

"The prevalence of arthritis seems to follow inversely the availability of boron in the soil. Jamaica has least boron and 70% with arthritis.

"Mauritius has very little and has much arthritis. Northern Thailand is very short of boron and has much arthritis but no figures are available. In Fiji the Indians have much more arthritis than do the Fijians, and the reason is that Indians eat mostly rice while Fijians eat mostly starchy root vegetables. Monocotyledons have much lesser need for boron than do the dicotyledons.

"The Theory Behind Boron Metabolism

"Based on work done at Oxford in the Agriculture Faculty[19] it is believed that at the cellular level mineral metabolism is similar with both plants and man. If this can be relied on, then boron is a membrane catalyst which allows various ions to pass through the cell membrane, particularly phosphates to support synthesis of ATP. This will give energy for efficient repair. It is obvious that in Osteoarthritis the cartilage is worn out, if it is because it lacks the necessary energy for cell division, it explains the action of boron. Then in Rheumatoid Arthritis there is an autoimmune reaction for no known reason. It is suggested that the reason is that certain collagen fibres are overage and cannot repair themselves,due to lack of energy-rich compounds within the cells."

In an article entitled "Prevention is Better Than Cure — The Sad Story of Arthritis and Osteoporosis" by Rex E. Newnham, Ph.D., D.O., N.D., Newnham has said, "It has been said that if we grow old enough then we will all get arthritis. Old enough is generally in the fifties or sixties, but some survive to the eighties or nineties without any arthritis. In recent years, especially in some countries there are growing numbers of young children who develop juvenile arthritis or Still's desease; and some of these are even too young to walk. Just recently a case was brought to my attention of a young girl aged 9 months, but she was crying much and was evidently in pain, then it was noticed that some of her joints were swollen and red. This was juvenile arthritis and we were able to cure her in 2 weeks using mineral nutrients. The orthodox method would have been to give her pain killing drugs, in fact these are used for all arthritis.

"In America there are Poison Control Centres where every case of poisoning is reported, and it is seen that analgesics or pain killing drugs are

162

responsible for many deaths each year. The latest figures show that these have died from taking analgesics in recent years as shown in brackets: 22 in 1983, 52 in 1984, 87 in 1985, 82 in 1986, 93 in 1987, 118 in 1988, 126 in 1989, a total of 580 in 8 years and the numbers seem to be increasing as time goes on. There is not much hope for arthritics here.

"The latest of these analgesics are called NSAIDS or Non-Specific Anti-Inflammatory Drugs [also Non-steroidal Anti-Inflammatory Drugs] but they will induce stomach bleeding and ulcers. The Food and Drug Administration admits that these drugs cause 200,000 cases of gastric bleeding each year and many of these have to be hospitalised. Probably 2,000 of these die each year and these drugs are mainly used for rheumatoid arthritis. We badly need some good preventive for this disease.

"All our chronic diseases seem to be increasing and this is a bad effect of modern medical methods. Acute diseases can generally be relieved, or at least the severe symptoms are covered up, but there is evidence that sometimes when the cause is not corrected the trouble goes deeper only to be manifested later in some other chronic disease. This is well seen when people have a number of dental fillings, but then the metals in their mouth set up an electrical discharge and the people complain of allergies, pains that are difficult to diagnose, digestive problems, multiple sclerosis, myalgic encephalitis, even heart problems have all improved when these toxic metals were properly removed from teeth. Yet most people accept these fillings as normal.

"There is osteoporosis which is another bone disease in which calcium is constantly lost, it attacks women after menopause and men after age 70. One can see old men and women who are hunch backed and stooping for very age. This is due to collapse of vertebrae. It is generally associated with much pain and inability to do necessary tasks. The bones are weaker and will break more easily, especially at the places where there is more tension, such as the hips and the wrist. This means that there are many old ladies filling hospital beds for 3 or 4 months at a time while their hips heal and they are taught to walk again.

"Thirty [now fifty: Ed.] years ago it was discovered that arthritis was associated with a dietary deficiency of the mineral boron. This mineral is present in all good soils, in fact plants will not grow without it. Some parts of the world have more boron than others and less arthirits too. The land of Israel has more boron than is usual in the waters of the Jordan river and the underground water, which is used for irrigation, has 0.2 parts per million boron. Israeli people have about 10 mg a day of boron in their diet and in that whole land, according to professor Bentwich of the Kaplan Hospital and Hebrew University, who did a survey that showed there was only 0.35% of the people with rheumatoid arthritis; and he estimated that a similar number had osteo arthritis a total of 0.7%

"In Britain, U.S.A., Australia, New Zealand and South Africa people have from 1 to 2 mg boron a day in their diet on the average, yet there is 20% of the population with arthritis. There are isolated areas in some of these countries where there is more than average boron in soil or water, such as at Carnarvon in Western Australia where only 1% of the people have arthritis, and Ngawah in New Zealand where nobody has arthritis but people go there to enjoy the spas that are rich in boron.

"In the last 15 years something over 500,000 people have used a boron food supplement tablet so as to get rid of their arthritis. They take 3 tablets a day while they have arthritis and in about 1 to 3 months they can get rid of all the pain, swelling and stiffness. Those who have rehumatoid arthritis generally experience an early aggravation when there is more pain. This is called an Herxheimer reaction and is a good thing as it shows the remedy is working, but they must persevere and in another 2 or 3 weeks all the pain and swelling and stiffness has gone. Then they revert to one tablet a day for a maintenance dose so that they can avoid any more arthritis.

"The American Human Nutrition Research Center has shown that a similar boron supplement will reduce the daily loss of calcium by nearly 50% and this would mean that victims of osteoporosis would live longer and be free of pain and discomfort. This is partly brought about by raising the levels of sex hormones present in the blood. Some of the women in the American trial were using HRT or Hormone Replacement therapy, and the blood levels of these hormones was the same as that of those who were using the boron supplement. HRT has the disadvantage that there can be a higher risk of breast or endometrial cancer. The boron treatment has no such risk as the hormones are made by the body and there is no synthetic material introduced to the body.

"In the mid 1980s a double blind hospital trial was conducted in Melbourne that showed these boron tablets were very efficacious and quite safe. The authorities were looking for ways to stop the use of a boron supplement and did many pathological tests which all proved the complete safety of this supplement. Since then there have been many other boron tablets on the market, and some use different compounds of boron which have never been proven, so it is best to use those brands that have been proven in such a way.

"The reason for the lack of boron in some soils is largely that they have had too much soluble fertilizer applied in recent years, and this in turn inhibits the uptake of the trace minerals such as boron. Farmers have to use methods that will ensure a quick return so they use these fertilizers, but the real quality of the produce suffers. The country where this is seen at its worst is Jamaica, where sugar has been grown for 200 years and the growers started using soluble chemical fertilizer in 1872. The soils are quite worn out and so are the people; 70% of them have arthritis and even the dogs in Kingston are limping. Most British and American soils have three times as much available boron in the soil as is found in Jamaica. A second consideration is above average rainfall leaches boron from soils.

"Fruits and vegetables are the common foods which are rich in boron; honey is also a good source. But these foods should be organically grown. A

164

good apple can have 20 mg boron, but an ordinary apple grown with fertilizer can have as little as 1 mg boron, or maybe less. The same applies to certain other fruits.

"So it seems that the taking of boron should be the first thing to do to prevent or cure this disease."

Sources

Apparently also boron stimulates in a positive way, hormonal factors for both men and women, resulting in healthy bones.

Aging factors, of course, are also involved in Osteoarthritis, and for that reason various treatments aimed at improving metabolism and the general ability to repair oneself, are obviously in order.

At the time this article was written, the following sources for useable boron were valid.

Vitamin Research Products, (1-800-VRP-24HR: toll free number) sells a new Boron Formula which contains Boron (from boric acid) 3 mg; Calcium 60 mg (from Calcium Ascorbate and Calcium Citrate); Magnesium 30 mg (from magnesium oxide); and Vitamin C (from calcium ascorbate) of 90 mg.

Gus Prosch, Jr., M.D. ordered for his patients Boron Citrate from Bio-Tech (1-800-345-1199 toll free telephone; in Arkansas 1-501-443-9148).

References

Newnham Bibliography

1. Bridges-Webb C. *Medical Journal of Australia.* Sept. 6, 1975. 377-378.2. *Ngawha Domain Baths Analysis.* Government Geological Survey. 2nd Sept. 1960.

3. Herbert. *The Hot Springs of New Zeland.* 1922.

4. Meyers O.L., Dyanes G., & Beighton P. "Rheumatoid Arthritis in a Tribal Xhosa Population in the Transkei", Southern Africa. *Annals of the Rheumatic Diseases*, 1977, 36, 62-65.

5. Ploquin J. "Boron in Foodstuffs. *Bull de la Societe Scientifique d'Hygiene Alimentaire*, 55, (1-3), 70-113, 1967.

6. Newnham R.E. "Boron is Essential — It Corrects and Prevents Arthritis". *Trace Elements in Man and Animals.* TEMA5 1984, p. 839.

7. Jalkanen S., Steere A.C., Fox R.I., Butcher E.C. "A Distinct Endothelial Cell Recognition System That Controls Lymphocyte Traffic Into Inflammed Synovium". *Science*, 233. 1 Aug. 1986. p. 556.

8. Newnham R.E. "Boron Beats Arthritis". *Australian & New Zealand Association for Advancement of Science.* 1979.

9. Zittle C.A. "Reaction of Borate with Substances of Biological Interest". *Advances in Enzymology* Vol. 12, 1951. Intersience.

10. Neilsen F.H. *Trace Elements in Human and Animal Nutrition*, Vol. 2. 5th Ed. Mertz W. Academic Press, NY, 1986. p. 420-427.

11. Parr A.J. & Loughman B.C. "Boron and Membrane Function in Plants". *Metals and Micronutrients: Uptake and Utlization* by Plants. Robb & Pierpont. Academic Press. 1983. Chap. 6.

12. Bentwich Z. & Talmon Y. *Prevalence of Rheumatoid Arthritis in an Israeli Population.* Hebrew University. 1980.

Arthritis Trust of America Bibliography

13. Anthony di Fabio, *Chelation Therapy*, The Rheumatoid Disease Foundation, 7111 Sweetgum Road, Fairview, TN, 1992.

14. Anthony di Fabio, *Prevention and Treatment of Osteoporosis*, The Rheumatoid Disease Foundation, Op.Cit,1989.

15. Paul K. Pybus, *The Herxheimer Effect*, The Rheumatoid Disease Foundation, 5106 Old Harding Road, Franklin, TN 37064, 1992; Anthony di Fabio, *The Art of Getting Well*, Op. Cit., 1988.

16. Rex E. Newnham, D.O., "Boron in Medicine — Update" *The Journal of the Academy of Rheumatoid Diseases.* Volume I, Number 2, p. 23-27, 13-630 Mountain View Road, Desert Hot Springs, CA 92240..

17. Murphy, E.W., Watt, B.K. & Page L., "Regional variation in Vitamin and Trace Element Content of Type A School Lunches", *Trace Substances in Environmental Health IV.* Univ. of Missouri. 1971. p. 194-205.

18. Weir, J.R. & Fisher, R.S., *"Toxicologic Studies of Borax and Boric Acid".* Toxicology and Applied Pharmacology 23. 351-364. 1972.

19. Parr, A.J. & Loughman, B.C., "Boron and Membrane Function in Plants". *Metals and Micronutrients: Uptake and Utilization by Plants.* Ch. 6, 1983. Academic Press.

Boron in Medicine — Update

Rex E. Newnham, Ph.D., D.O., N.D.

(Formerly published in The Journal of the Rheumatoid Disease Foundation, *Volume 1, Number 2)*

History. Boron as the sodium salt has been used by man for over 2500 years as a flux for welding gold and as an embalming agent by the Egyptians. As supplies became easier to get, namely from Italy, boric acid and borax became increasingly used as a mild antiseptic, especially for eyes and burns.

For the last 200 years, boric acid has often been used as a food preservative, but this use has been recently stopped because it tended to disguise food that was unfit for use as being in a reasonable condition for use. People must have ingested considerable quantities without any ill effect during this period. Much has been used as a simple home remedy for stings and burns, and as a powder to prevent rash.[1]

Antipathogenic Action. Boric acid and borax in a 2-3% solution will prevent the growth of most bacteria and will kill many fungi. A 1.5% solution has some stimulating effect on phagocytosis *in vitro,* but at 2% this ceases.[6]

Biochemistry.[10] Borates are active complexing agents for diol groups particularly in secchorides, and in some of the B-vitamins and ascorbate and can inhibit certain enzyme reactions. They can reverse gel formation.

Pharmacology. These substances are readily absorbed by damaged skin and by mucous membranes. 50% of borate is eliminated via the kidneys in the first 12 hours, and 90% of the remainder is gone within a week, in all but extreme doses.[7]

Borates are slightly astringent and will tend to allay the pain of burns and

166

wounds. If the dry powder is introduced to the nose, it can bring on sneezing and lacrimation[.6]

Toxicology. These substances are not dangerously toxic, but large doses can be dangerous. The LD-50 for borax is 5.33 g/Kg for guinea pigs, and 2-3 g/Kg for Swiss mice. But for boric acid, it is greater than 4.1 g/Kg for mice.[9]

Rats and dogs were fed a diet containing 52.5, 117, 350, 525, and 1750 ppm boron as borate and as boric acid for up to 38 weeks. In this period, reproductive studies were possible. Only the highest level was there any toxicity with congestion of the kidneys, liver, small gonads, thickened pancreas, and a swollen brain. Even at 525 ppm, there was no adverse effect. Rats ingesting 350 ppm boron for 2 years showed no histologic changes at necropsy.[9]

Some workers have shown that 3 g boric acid or 5 g borax have no effect on the adult human, while others have reported symptoms at 1-2 g per day.[2] No one is likely to take too much in their food even if they do use a supplement that has only a few mg per tablet. Greater absorption is likely to come from a mouthwash or if a borate is applied to damaged skin.

Extensive laboratory studies on both man and animal have not shown the exact role of boron in their metabolism. Patients have been given 10 g/day for extended periods and were still excreting boron after 7 weeks. The LD-50 for the dog is 1 g/Kg and these dogs developed a violet red skin color with persistent vomiting, diarrhea, and meningismus. Acute intoxication can include hypothermia, depression, and ataxia.[5]

With daily doses of 100 mg/Kg, it takes 18 days for the dog to reach a plateau in boron excretion.[5]

The literature from 1848 to 1948 contains data of 86 cases of borax-boric acid toxicity and 42 of these died. Some were given doses of over 100g, yet many had no real confirmation of the cause of death. One 2 day old infant died and this was blamed on the mother who cleansed her nipples with a boric acid solution. A proper autopsy and analysis should have been used to prove the cause of death. Many of the deaths were due to absorption of borax/boric acid through damaged skin. Granulating skin will readily absorb these substances and so will mucous membranes.[5]

The acute toxic dose for an adult is from 20 to 60g in a single dose, but infants have died with 5g, yet others lived after being given 9g boric acid. There is a great individual variation with these substances. A 50% plasma — Ringer's solution IV is the best antidote and will increase the LD-50 for mice by 250%.

The Position in Australia. In 1981 or soon after, the various states scheduled boron compounds in any concentration, and this is an extreme case of bureaucracy because an apple can contain over 10 mg of elemental boron. Many fruits and vegetables contain over 50 ppm boron and when these are grown on a really good soil, they will have up to 160 ppm boron. Should these foods be scheduled?

Yet at the same time, a mouth-wash containing 68% borate was acceptable for OTC (Over The Counter) sales. A good mouthwash with this substance would put many mg of boron into the blood. To become dangerous, the solution would have to be held in the mouth for many hours. Strong solutions or the powder when introduced into other body cavities have proved fatal. That legislation was introduced because a product called Bor-ex containing 5% boron was having remarkable results with both rheumatoid and osteo arthritis. Without advertising, the sales of this product went from zero to 10,000 bottles a month in 5 years. No unwanted side-effects were noticed during these 5 years.

A properly organized trial of Bor-ex was being carried out in one of the country's bigger hospitals. This started 3 years ago, but very regrettably was still not completed at the time of writing this report.

Carnarvon has 0.2 ppm boron in the water supply and people do go there from 1000 miles away in the Southwest to enjoy the good climate and get relief from their arthritis. It is really the good water and not the good climate that helps them. Yet some people in Carnarvon never drink local water. A survey was conducted there in 1981 that brought these facts to light.

The Position in the Rest of the World. West Germany stopped the use of boron compounds in medicine three years ago on the assumption that there were other drugs that would do everything that boron would do and that they would do it better.

In many other countries, a boron supplement is being used as a food supplement, and no claims are made, but satisfied users soon tell other people who need it. Over 250,000 people have used this supplement, and it corrects between 80 and 90% of all arthritis. No untoward side effects have been noted, but there are some useful side-effects, such as would be noticed if boron were the limiting factor in a person's well-being. Cardiopathies have been corrected, vision has been improved, psoriasis has been much improved, balance has been corrected. Arthritis in horses, cattle, dogs, deer, and goats have all been corrected.

As we use more and more superphosphate on our food crops, the availability of soil boron is decreased. It is estimated that most people in western societies ingest about 2 mg boron daily. This is based on the analysis of school meals in the U.S.A,[3] but analyses earlier in this century put the figure at 8 mg.[9]

The prevalence of arthritis seems to follow inversely the availability of boron in the soil. Jamaica has the least boron and 70% with arthritis. Mauritius has very little and has arthritis. Northern Thailand is very short of boron and much arthritis, but no figures are available. In Fiji, the Indians have much more arthritis than do the Fijians, and the reason is that Indians eat mostly rice while Fijians eat mostly starch root vegetables. Monocotyledons have a much less need for boron than do the dicotyledons.

The Theory Behind Boron Metabolism. Based on work done at Oxford in the Agriculture Faculty[4] it is believed that at the cellular level mineral metabolism is similar with both plants and man. If this can be relied on, then boron is a membrane catalyst which allows various ions to pass through the cell membrane, particularly phosphates to support synthesis of ATP. This will give energy for efficient repair. It is obvious that in osteo arthritis the

168

cartilage is worn out, if it is because it lacks the necessary energy for cell division, it explains the action of boron. Then in rheumatoid arthritis, there is an autoimmune reaction for no known reason. It is suggested that the reason is that certain collagen fibers are overage and cannot repair themselves, due to lack of energy-rich compounds within the cells.

Other Boron Compounds. Boranes are hydrides of boron and are very toxic. They are used as solid rocket fuels and can be used to prevent bacterial decontamination of diesel fuel.

Boron analogues of many of the amino acids have been made and tested in North Carolina. The original research was to find carcinostatic compounds of boron, but some of these are also anti-arthritic, anti-inflammatory, anti-tumor and anti-hyperlipidemic in their action on test animals. The amino carboxyboranes are relatively non-toxic, but the cyano boranes are very toxic. More will be heard about these compounds.[7]

Some of the analogues of amino-acids have an LD-50 of 1800mg/Kg so they do not present any problems.

The Future of Boron. When the aforementioned trial is completed, it is likely that many people will require the boron supplement so as to relieve their arthritis and the health departments [Australian] over-reaction will have to be reversed. Farmers will also have to look more to quality instead of quantity, and will have to add trace elements to their soil so as to give good quality crops.

Bibliography

1. Fisher, R.S. Boron — its occurrence in nature, foods, and humans. *Dept. of Medicine, Univer. of Maryland*; 1959.

2. Levinskas, G.J. *Metallo-Boron Compounds and Boranes*. Ed. Adams, R.M. Interscience Publishers, New York; 1964: Ch. 8.

3. Murphy, E.W., Watt, B.K., & Page, L. Regional variation in vitamin and trace element content of type A school lunches. *Trace Substances in Environmental Health* IV, Univ. of Missouri; 1971: 194-205.

4. Parr, A.J. & Loughman, B.C. *Boron and Membrane Function in Plants. Metals and Micronutrients: Uptake and Utilization by Plants.* Academic Press; 1983: Ch. 6.

5. Pfeiffer, C.C. & Jenny, E.H. The pharmacology of boric acid and boron compounds. *Bulletin of National Formulary Committee* xviii: 57-80; 1950.

6. Solis-Cohen. *Pharmacotherapeutics*. 1928: 583-585.

7. Spielvogel, B.F. *Synthesis and Biological Activity of Boron Analogues of the Alpha Amino Acids and Related Compounds*. Duke University. Durham Press: 119-129.

8. Underwood, E.J. *Trace Elements in Human and Animal Nutrition*. Academic Press; 1971: 434-436.

9. Weir, J.R. & Fisher, R.S. Toxicologic studies of borax and boric acid. *Toxicology and Applied Pharmacology* 23: 351-364; 1972.

10. Zittle, C.A. *Reaction of Borate with Substances of Biological Interest. Advances in Enzymology*, vol. 12, Interscience Publishers; 1951.

Cure Systemic Lupus Erythematosus and Progressive Systemic Sclerosis
by
Anthony di Fabio & Ronald M. Davis, M.D.

Introduction

When discussing the more than 100 named diseases that the Arthritis Trust of America calls "Rheumatoid Disease" one begins to understand that Rheumatoid Arthritis is not just a disease in the joints, but rather a systemic disease. That is, depending upon where in the body a disease manifests itself that location often determines the name of the disease. Lupus Erthematosus and Scleroderma are two among the one hundred named Rheumatoid diseases and Ronald Davis, M.D. is the one doctor who discovered that he could heal some of his patients afflicted with these two types of rheumatoid disease.

Lupus Erythematosus and Scleroderma are classified as vascular diseases, along with polyarteritis nodosa, and some other diseases, but Lupus and Scleroderma also have one other thing in common — they can be treated in a similar manner with equally good results!

Lupus Erythematosus is a chronic, nontuberculous disease of the skin marked by disklike patches with raised reddish edges and depressed centers, and covered with scales or crusts. These fall off, leaving dull-white scars.

Scleroderma is a disease of the skin in which thickened, hard, ridged, and pigmented patches occur. During the course of the disease, the connective tissue of the skin layer beneath the epidermis (corium) and the subcutaneous structures are increased and a "hidebound" condition results.

The ordinary form of Scleroderma begins in middle life, and is often considered, by traditional medicine, as incurable.

According to Richard A. Kunin, M.D., "Systemic Lupus Erythematosus is the classic example of an immune system turning against specific cells in the body in joints. The immune complexes formed when antigen from cells combines with antibodies from immune cells and then circulate until the spleen and kidney can excrete them. Along the way these may deposit in various tissues, causing secondary inflammatory disorders such as nodules and inflammation of the skin and kidneys. The spleen is hard-pressed to digest and excrete all of these complexes and the overload can deposit in the kidney causing great damage. In fact, this overload is the most serious complication of Lupus and a frequent cause of death."[10]

The Case of Suzie White

Suzie White 40 years-of-age, had a 2 to 3 year history of finger stiffness and pain and swelling (edema) of toes and the fingers. She also had marked sensitivity to the sun, with mild to moderate butterfly lesions across her nose and cheeks.

The Houston Medical Center (Texas) diagnosed Suzie's condition as Systemic Lupus Erythematosus. She was advised by that center to take gold

shots, and the other traditional palliative and damaging treatments.

Instead, under the care of Ronald M. Davis, M.D.,[20] Suzie decided to try intravenous EDTA (ethylene diamine tetracetic) chelation therapy and DMSO (Dimethylsulfoxide).These infusions also included magnesium sulphate, sodium bicarbonate, Vitamin C, pyridoxine, B-complex, dexpanthenol, and Vitamin B12.

Oral metronidazole and allopurinol — following The Arthritis Trust of America/The Rheumatoid Disease Foundation treatment protocol as described in "The Roger Wyburn-Mason, M.D., Ph.D. Treatment for Rheumatoid Disease," http://www.arthritistrust.org.

She was very lax about taking her intravenous infusions and would come in weekly until she began feeling better, and then she'd wait 2-10 weeks before coming in again. Despite this laxness, Suzie did very well and became free of symptoms.

One year and eight months after starting her treatments with Dr. Davis, Suzie was given 2 hydrogen peroxide intravenous infusions (0.03%) within 2 hours of one another. She has been free of symptoms for the past 3 years.

Dr. Davis says, "As you can see, the anti-amoebic regimen is included in my treatment protocol. I believe this to be most important in treating these diseases. It is amazing how these patients respond to "The Roger Wyburn-Mason, M.D., Ph.D. Treatment for Rheumatoid Disease," http://www.arthritistrust.org.

What is Systemic Lupus Erythematosus?

Systemic Lupus Erythematosus is an inflammatory connective tissue disorder of unknown cause occurring chiefly in young women, and also in children and older adults. According to Alan Gaby, M.D., the word "lupus" is latin for "wolf," and erythematosus means "redness," together the terms represent or refer to the red lesions appearing on the face and that resemble a wolf's bite.[17]

Historical Identification

Kaposi first recognized skin and visceral involvements in 1872; Osler described skin lesions (polymorphic) in conjunction with arthritis and kidney failure by the early 1900s. In 1920-30 Systemic Lupus Erythematosus was identified as a distinct disease. It is now recognized as a disease entity that evolved from a group of clinical manifestations that include characteristic pathological and laboratory findings.

Historically there have been two definitions: Cutaneous Systemic Lupus Erythematosus, and Systemic Lupus Erythematosus. This distinction is no longer felt to reflect two different diseases.

Distribution of Systemic Lupus Erythematosus

There may be as high as 1 per 100,000 among family members of those afflicted.

The prevalence among African-American, American-Indian and several Asian groups is higher than among Whites. Black females have a higher incidence rate of 7 to 8 per 100,000, as compared to 2 to 3 per 100,000 among White females.

The ratio of female-to-male is approximately 10 to 1, although this ratio is less likely in childhood when the disease occurs prior to puberty.

Both pre-puberty and postmenopausal groups reflect a ratio of 2:1 to 3:1.

Clinical Symptoms

Anemia; fever; hair loss; headaches; high blood pressure; inflammation of lung lining; inflammation of membrane surrounding heart; joint pain; kidney problems; sensitivity to light; skin lesions, including characteristic "butterfly" redness of skin over cheeks and bridge of nose; symptoms vary according to organ affected. Systemic Lupus Erythematosus manifests itself through body fluids (humoral) and cellular abonormalities and through tissue destruction in many different organs.

As this disease progresses, the afflicted may find that it has been diagnosed differently over time.

It may also be defined as a Mixed Connective Tissue Disease involving arthralgias or arthritis, swollen hands, inflammation of muscles (myositis), capillary congestion and swelling (Raynaud's phenomenon), gastrointestinal problems (esophageal hypomotility) and lymph system (lymphodenopathy). These characteristics are also accompanied by certain positive laboratory findings (high titers of antibodies to ribonucleoprotein). (See *Soft Tissue Arthritis: Bursitis, Fibromyalgia; Fibromyositis; Fibrositis; Rheumatism* and *Arthritis: Osteoarthritis and Rheumatoid Disease Including Rheumatoid Arthritis,* http://www.arthritistrust.org; also at Kindle at Amazon.com, bookstores and at arthritistrust.org)

As these characteristic symptoms often overlap in Systemic Lupus Erythematosus, the term "Mixed Connective Tissue Disease," drops out, and the terms "Systemic Lupus Erythematosus," or "Progressive Systemic Sclerosis," are applied more frequently.

Diagnosis Criteria

Because there are so many clinical manifestations and expressions of this disease, diagnoses can often challenge the clinician. No single finding or test result will confirm the presence or absence of this disease, but rather, accurate diagnosis lies with comparison against a pre-established set of criteria, as defined by the American Rheumatism Association[1]. Any four or more of the eleven criteria presented, either in succession, or simultaneously, constitutes the basis for positive diagnosis.

Eight of these criteria include a history and physical examination which includes cheek rash, disc-like rashes, photosensitivity, oral ulcers, arthritis, inflammation of lung or heart membranes, kidney involvement, and nerve involvement with seizures or psychosis.

Two more criteria involve routine laboratory analysis supplying further evidence of involvement of various organs, as well as a complete blood count to identify various blood disorders.

One criteria requires more sophisticated laboratory tests, for antinuclear antibodies.

Other tests may be used to screen out additional diseases, such as for syphilis.

Onset of Systemic Lupus Erythematosus

Systemic Lupus Erythematosus may begin abruptly with fever, simulating acute infection, or can develop insidiously over many months or even years, with only occasional flare-ups of fever and discomfort.

Any organ that has been affected may also present with symptoms unique or characteristic to that organ.

As many as 90% of the patients complain of joint symptoms that range from intermittent to acute, single joints to many joints, some for months or even years before other manifestations occur.

The characteristic "butterfly lesion," or "erythema," is one of several skin appearances. Others include disc-shaped lesions, and other forms on the face, exposed areas of the neck, upper chest and back and other areas exposed to light. These lesions may join one another, making the skin worse in appearance (edematous).

Ulcers may appear in the central portion of the hard palate near the junction of the hard and soft palate, the cheek and gum mucosa and the anterior nasal passage. Blistering and ulceration are otherwise rare.

During active phases of the disease, loss of hair may occur.

Redness, swelling and reddish-purple lesions may show around the sides of the palms with extension of fingers, around the nails, and at the palms of the fingers.

Small blood vessels or the lymph system may be affected by inflammation, resulting in purple patches on the skin.

Sensitivity to light occurs with about 40% of the patients.

After long-standing disease, joint deformity, without joint erosion, is common, particularly deviation of the fingers and dislocation of certain finger joints (proximal interphalangeal).

Inflammation of the lining of the lungs may occur recurrently.

Bacterial or viral pneumonia is common.

Inflammation of the lining of the heart is often present. Heart problems, usually found after autopsy, have occurred in as many as a third of the cases.

A generalized glandular problem will occur particularly in children, young adults and Negroes. Enlargement of the spleen occurs in 10% of the patients.

Involvement of the Central Nervous System causes personality changes such as epilepsy, pyschoses, and organic brain syndrome.

Kidney involvement occurs in the majority of patients, and may progress to a fatal end. Sometimes kidney dialysis is the only way to keep a patient alive.

Survival Outcome

The outcome of this disease depends mostly upon which organs of the body are affected, and how deeply. Patients with localized skin symptoms usually have a significant chance of long survival, while patients with kidney and brain involvement may have intermittent relapses, and still others may have prolonged remissions. Although the survival rate is mixed, according to the above-described organ deficiency situations, the survival rate is about 70%, with infection and kidney failure being leading causes of death.

Genetic Marker

Identical twins have a higher incidence of Systemic Lupus Erythematosus than do non-identical twins.

There appears to be a multi-gene influence on those with the disease. Those with a deficiency of certain substances in the blood (complement) and certain gene markers (HLA-DR2, HLA-DR3, HLA-B8, others) seem to have a higher incidence of the disease.

Other Causations

As with the other 100 or so Rheumatoid Diseases, Systemic Lupus Erythematosus may be considered to have multiple causes (as described in (*"Arthritis: Osteoarthritis and Rheumatoid Disease Including Rheumatoid Arthritis,"* http://www.arthritistrust.org at Kindle at Amazon.com, bookstores and at arthritistrust.org) and probably should be treated in various ways, including proper nutrtional support.

Alan Gaby, M.D. reports on Nurses' Health Study that appears to show a strong relationship between Systemic Lupus Erythematosus and the use of estrogen therapy, suggesting that, at least in part, it is hormone-dependent.

Beginning in 1976, 69,435 postmenopausal nurses were followed for 14 years. To shore up the hormone-dependency link, Gaby explains that "First, the incidence of Systemic Lupus Erythematosus in adults is 8 times greater for women than for men. Second, Systemic Lupus Erythematosus patients of both sexes have abnormalities of estrogen metabolism. Third, women with Systemic Lupus Erythematosus have low plasma androgen (sex-hormone) levels.

"It should be pointed out," Gaby says, "that most estrogen prescriptions are for horse estrogen (Premarin), which differs substantially from the homones secreted by the human ovary."[11]

According to A.V. Costantini, M.D.,[14] a list of diseases wherein fungal forms of microorganisms have been found include the following: atherosclerosis, cancer, AIDS, diabetes mellitus, Rheumatoid Arthritis, SjÖgren's syndrome, Systemic Lupus Erythematosus, Gout, Crohn's disease, multiple sclerosis, hyperactivity syndrome, infertility, psoriasis, cirrhosis, Alzheimer's disease, Scleroderma (Progressive Systemic Sclerosis), Raynaud's disease, sarcoidosis, kidney stones, amyloidosis, vasculitis, and Cushing's Disease.

Dr. Costantini, believes that the concept of "auto-immune" diseases contains a fatal flaw, because no successful species can develop a system of defense which attacks itself.

Antibodies that are measured in the blood stream and which imply an autoimmune condition are actually antibodies against "ubiquitin," a substance that is present in many species including that of fungi.

Traditional Treatments

Treatment must be individualized depending upon the location of problems or the severity of them. For purposes of treatment, the disease is classified as "mild" or "severe."

Mild disease is characterized by fever, arthritis, inflammation of the lining of the lungs or heart, and rashes.

Severe life-threatening disease involves anemia, massive heart and lung involvement, significant kidney damage, acute inflammation of the vascular system in the extremeties or gastrointestinal tract, Central Nervous System disorders and formation of purple patches on the skin and mucous membranes (thrombocytopenic purpura).

Mild Disease

Analgesics and Non-Steroidal Anti-Inflammatories

Salicylates (aspirin) are used to control the pain and fever.

Other non-steroidal anti-inflammatory drugs are also used, such as indomethacin or ibuprofen. Ibuprofen can be given for those who do not tolerate aspirin.

Anti-malarials

Anti-malarials, such as hydroxychloroquine or cloroquine, may also be used to control rashes or mucous membrane lesions.

Cortisone

Cortisone, taken orally in the form of prednisone, may be added to the regimen to control the symptoms of arthritis and muscle pain (polymyalgia).

Phenylbutazone

Sometimes phenylbutazone is alternated with the aspirin.

Severe Disease

Corticosteroid Therapy

Immediate corticosteroid therapy, usually in the form of oral predisone, is administered, which becomes the mainstay of the treatment.

The other analgesic and anti-inflammatory drugs are not used, because they have become, or are, ineffective.

In Both Mild and Severe Disease

After symptomatic inflammation is under control, minimal dosages of cortisone are used. Usually the dosage is decreased little by little.

Response to therapy is determined by relief of symptoms and signs, or improvement in other laboratory tests.

Infections are treated vigorously, usually with some form of antibiotic.

The usual measures for combating heart failure and kidney problems are employed, including kidney dialysis, if necessary.

Close medical supervision is extremely important during surgical procedures and pregnancy.

There must be concerted effort to eliminate emotional stress, physical fatigue, any implicated or unnecessary drugs, and excessive sunlight exposure.

What's Wrong With Traditional Treatments?

As is true for other rheumatoid diseases, traditional treatments primarily address symptoms and not their causes, and many of the traditional treatments have adverse side-effects.

Most important of all critical comments, there is no attempt to step outside traditional regimens that are doomed in advance to failure, insofar as bringing about health remissions or cures.

Mild Disease

Analgesics and Non-Steroidal Anti-Inflammatories

Aspirin and non-steroidal anti-inflammatory Drugs (NSAIDS) are useful for temporarily alleviating symptoms but do not address the causation of Systemic Lupus Erythematosus. Their extended usage, however, can result in several serious problems.

Salicylates, for example, can erode the lining of the stomach, leading to bleeding ulcers and other gastrointestinal problems. Enteric coated and buffered aspirin is of little use except for those who have peptic ulcers or hiatus hernia.

Sustained-release tablets might provide longer relief for some patients, and may help an individual through some intolerable pains.

Indomethacin has both analgesic and anti-inflammatory properties, and, unlike corticosteroids, has no effect on pituitary or adrenal glands.

Adverse effects of the usage of indomethacin are headache, dizziness, lightheadedness and gastrointestinal disturbances such as nausea, loss of appetite, vomiting, epigastric distress, abdominal pain and diarrhea.[5] Gastrointestinal bleeding may also result from its use.

Indomethacin should not be given to a patient with active peptic ulcer, gastritic, or ulcerative colitis, conditions which can easily accompany a number of Rheumatoid Diseases.

Occasionally fluid retention is a problem.

Central Nervous System effects may be transient and disappear altogether on continued usage with dose reduction, but occasionally they are of such severe nature that therapy must be discontinued altogether.

Patients who show signs of Central Nervous System symptoms should not operate automobiles or other hazardous equipment.

Other nonsteroidal anti-inflammatory drugs such as ibuprofen can be given for those who do not tolerate aspirin. Although less of a gastrointestinal irritant than aspirin, it can produce gastric symptoms and gastrointestinal bleeding.

As the major share of pharmaceutical drug research — which is also the dominant share of arthritis research — is aimed at relieving symptoms for arthritics — not in achieving cures — there are always new analgesic, non-steroidal anti-inflammatory drugs being huxtered as "break-throughs." None of these help our bodies to heal.

Anti-malarials

As with phenylbutazone, hydrooxychloroqiune should be taken under close medical supervision as it may create irreversible retinal degeneration. With its usage, repeated eye tests are required by an opthalmologist before and every 2 to 3 months during treatment.[5]

There are also other serious effects involving the Central Nervous System, neuromuscular reactions, skin, blood, and gastrointestinal effects.

Cortisone

Although relief is nearly instant, on use of "cortisone," it doesn't halt the progression of the disease. Cortisone (prednisone) merely suppresses the symptoms or "clinical manifestations," acting at the microscopic level. It inhibits the early phenomena of the inflammatory process which includes swelling, blood clotting, capillary expansion, and capillary proliferation, fibroblast proliferation, deposition of collagen tissue and later scar tissue formation, and migration of white blood cells into the inflamed area and phagocytic activity.

All of the described functions which are inhibited by the use of cortisone are required by the human body for growth and repair of tissue.

Cortisone impairs wound healing and provides the grounds for predisposition to infection. It has major effects on the monocyte/macrophage systems, preventing the release of a substance that aids in fighting infection, Interleukin I.

Phenylbutazone

Phenylbutazone cannot be considered a simple analgesic, but should be used under careful medical supervision. It's usage can result in serious side affects of anemia and loss of certain leukocytes (agranulocytosis). Through it's use, there is an incidence of 2.2 deaths per 100,000 exposures from the above named conditions. The risk increases with age and long-term usage, especially women, to 6.5 deaths per 100,0005.

Other side effects include gastrointestinal, skin, heart, kidney and other serious effects.

Phenylbutazone has an anti-inflammatory effect but it also has severe toxic effects, including peptic ulcer, sodium and water retention, inflammation of the skin (dermatitis), inflammation of the mouth (stomatitis) and decrease or disappearance of certain leucocytes from bone marrow (agranulocytosis).

Severe Disease

Antibiotics

The use of antibiotics may sometimes be necessary, but its continued use will kill off the intestinal microflora required for good health, and will open the way for organisms-of-opportunity, such as the yeast/fungus *Candida albicans*. (See "The Good Guys Bacteria — Lactobacillus acidophilus & Bifido bacterium," at http://arthritistrust.org)

The effects of an overgrowth of intestinal fungal candidiasis will create additional physical problems, as well as mimic many other physical ailments.

One problem further that Candidiasis creates is an increasing number of food allergies which not only create their own brand of ailments, but can also mimic other physical problems, including this one. (See "The Truth About Allergies & Alcoholism, at http://arthritistrust.org)

Corticosteroids

Large doses of corticosteroids results in a deficiency of lymphocytes in the blood, leading to lymphopenia. Large leucocytes, called "monocytes," show an impaired ability to kill invading microorganisms.

Corticosteroids interfere with a variety of functions, not mentioned here, and the result of all of the adverse phenomena is an increased incidence of infection usually controlled by cellular immunity, which means an increase in infections of mycoplasm, yeast/fungal, bacterial, protozoal, and so on.

The list of microorganisms resulting from the use of corticosteroids resembles the agents to which patients with Hodgkin's disease or acquired immune deficiency syndrome (AIDS) are vulnerable.

Steroids are also widely used in organ transplants involving kidney, heart, liver and bone marrow. In part, subsequent infections that are news-media-wise blamed on infections after transplantations are a direct result of use of the corticosteroids as well as other immunosuppressive drugs.

Other Necessary Treatments

Combating emergency kidney problems — as with the use of kidney dialysis — and other system problems, may, however, be very necessary expedients, but should not be considered as life-long limitations.

Alternative Treatments for Systemic Lupus Erythematosus and Progressive Systemic Sclerosis

Anti-Amoebic (Anti-Microbial) Treatments

Gus J. Prosch, Jr., M.D.[15] uses The Arthritis Trust of America/The Rheumatoid Disease Foundation recommended treatment with beneficial results. ("The Roger Wyburn-Mason, M.D., Ph.D. Treatment for Rheumatoid Disease," http://www.arthritistrust.org or go to Amazone.com and search for any books by Anthony di Fabio.)

Anti-Fungal, Anti-Mycoplasmic Treatments

According to Dr. Costantini,[15] by treating various so-called auto-immune diseases with anti-fungals, including Systemic Lupus Erythematosus, the disease can be halted.

Among the traditional antifungal drugs are found lovastatin, griseofulvin, ketoconazole, neomycin, fibrates, tetracycline and others, some of which may also be effective against Lupus. However, these should all be administered by a health professional, with due consideration for their adverse effects, including that of killing off beneficial microbes — *Lactobacillus acidophilus* — in the intestinal tract.[14] (See "The Good Guys Bacteria — Lactobacillus acidophilus & Bifido bacterium," at www.Arthritistrust.org and also at Kindle.)

Boron

The Case of Johnny Reebuk

Dr. Rex E. Newnham, N.D., D.O., Ph.D.[13] describes an old soldier who was being treated for Systemic Lupus Erythematosus in Brisbane Veteran's Hospital, Australia, but was not being helped by traditional treatments.

Johnny's main symptoms were pains in the muscles and joints with some red blotches on the skin. He came to Dr. Newnham for help, and was given Osteo-Trace® tablets containing 3 mg of boron, and also a zinc supplement for his skin. Within 2 months Johnny was very much better, and he continued the treatment for another 3 months. Two years later, he was still well. (See Boron, Also a Necessary Supplement, at www.arthritistrust.org and also at Kindle.)

Chiropractic

A case of Systemic Lupus Erythematosis is reported by Paul A. Goldberg, M.P.H., D.C.,[18] graduate of Bowling Green State University, Life College and the University of Texas Medical Center Graduate School of Public Health. Dr. Goldberg holds degrees in preventive medicine, nutrition and chiropractic, and was Professor of Clinical Nutrition, Gastroenterology, and Rheumatology at Life College in Marietta, Georgia. He also operated The Goldberg Clinic in Marietta, Georgia.

The Case of Cathy Huxoll

Cathy Huxoll, 29-years-of-age, had a 10 year history of severe fatigue, joint pains, skin problems, and immune dysregulation. She'd been diagnosed with Systemic Lupus Erythematosus, and undergone years of corticosteroid and methotrexate usage. Cathy said her condition was "desperate" and she was on the verge of suicide.

Cathy's husband, a medical physician, tried to dissuade Cathy from consulting with a Chiropractor as they had "nothing of any usefullness for her condition outside of the drugs that she was already taking."

When Cathy appeared in Dr. Goldberg's office she appeared weak, pale and had very poor muscle tone. She'd also had been convinced over the years that her condition was permanent and would only get worse in time, something of a self-fulfilling prophecy.

Dr. Goldberg worked to convince her that she could be optimistic, although recovery might be slow and difficult.

Cathy was anemic, low in amino acid levels, had abnormal bowel flora and was on a diet of refined carbohydrates, coffee, and fast foods. She had numerous food and inhalant allergies. Blood sugar levels were erratic and there were multiple vitamin and mineral deficiencies along with general body toxicity.

Cathy was placed on a dietary reform with elimination of allergens and refined carbohydrates. Specific supplements were given to assist in removing toxic minerals. She was advised to avoid future dental silver/mercury amalgams and to consider replacement of those she had with composite fillings. An amino acid blend was constructed based on her laboratory findings. She was advised to eat whole foods, and provided with other supplements to improve functioning of her body as a whole and the immune system specifically. Acupressure was employed, and the patient began training in meditation and relaxation disciplines.

Cathy's first several weeks were rough. She missed the stimulation of her coffee and junk foods and suffered withdrawal symptoms as she avoided her food allergens. Within two months she began to notice improved energy and a decrease in muscle and joint pain. Her skin began to improve and her color became more healthy. Encouraged by the improvements, the patient doubled her efforts and continued to reap health rewards. Cathy gradually ceased taking steroids and methotrexate.

Four years later Cathy is pursuing a nursing career and enjoys good health and freedom and has only occasional mild joint discomforts which she describes as "very minor in nature."

Diet

As with virtually all health conditions the "cave man" diet is recommended, at least modified as best possible, as discussed in the "Proper Nutrition for Rheumatoid Arthritis," (http://www.arthritistrust.org and at Amazon.com, bookstores and at Kindle.). Additional suggestions from *Alternative Medicine: The Definitive Guide*[3], include (1) avoid overeating, (2) limit cow's milk and beef products, (3) increase green, yellow and orange vegetables, consume non-farmed cold water fish several times a week, (4) avoid alfalfa sprouts or tablets which contain L-canavanine sulfate which can aggravate Lupus, (5) avoid L-tryptophan supplementation, that might promote autoimmune processes.[3]

One should also assess and treat for candidiasis, food allergies and chemical sensitivities.[3]

Enzyme Therapy

Enzyme supplementation, along with proper diet, may be very important for properly digesting food, and for eliminating the inflammatory immuno-complexes that always accompanies Systemic Lupus Erythematosus. (See "Systemic Enzyme Therapy," http://www.arthritistrust.org and also Kindle at Amazon.com, bookstores and at www.arthritistrust.org.)

Dr. Catherine Russell,[21] Guadalajara, Mexico, describes a problem in Mexico which has also long been a serious problem in the United States. Because the Mexican economy has been poor, and although Dr. Russell does not charge much, it's much easier for Lupus patients to get free shots of damaging cortisone, with immediate pain relief, than it is to persist through constructive change of diet, supplements and other remedies. In the United States, it's easier for patients to get "free" or "cheap" treatments through a Health Maintenance Organization or health insurance, where ineffective treatments are dictated by costs, traditional medical practices and insurance dictums, rather than what is necessary for individualized wellness.

Those with Systemic Lupus Erythematosus who stay with Dr. Russell will be given megadoses of vitamin C to assist in getting them off of cortisone (which takes about one month), proteolytic enzymes, B complex, the whole nutritional supplement range and, depending upon where the pain is, she will use intraneural injections and homeopathic remedies. (See *Intraneural Injections* at Kindle at Amazon.com, bookstores and at arthritistrust.org.)

Fasting

Joel Fuhrman, M.D. reports that "Having fasted over a thousand patients with various diseases I can say without hesitation that fasting is very often the only avenue that a patient can use to establish a complete remission.

"This is especially true with autoimmune illnesses like lupus where it is almost impossible to shut off the hyperactive immune system with nutritional modifications alone, without total fasting.

"[The] failure to understand the benefits of fasting, stems from a narrow perspective, viewing fasting as merely a means to enhance detoxification, ignoring the other pathophysiologic mechanisms involved in most chronic degenerative diseases. The body clearly has the mechanism to adequately handle the removal of endogenous wastes generated in the fasting state. In fact, fasting has been shown to improve or normalize abnormal liver function."

It is adviseable to refrain from the use of drugs and other chemical exposures during fasting.

Herbs

According to Burton Goldberg's *Alternative Medicine: The Definitive Guide*3, "Mix equal parts of the tinctures of the Chinese herbs *Bupleurum falcatum*, licorice, and wild yam. Take one teaspoonful of this mixture three times a day. Drink an infusion of nettle twice a day. In addition, as this autoimmune condition can manifest with a range of symptoms, this should be treated with the relevant herbs as they arise: Echinacea, goldenseal, pau d'arco, red clover."[3]

Hormonal Replacement Therapy

A proper functioning hormonal system is a requisite for good health, and often a deficiency in thyroid will accompany Systemic Lupus Erythematosus. (See "Thyroid Hormone Replacement Therapy: Cutting the Gordian Knot," http://www.arthritistrust.org.)

Mineral Infrared Therapy

Dr. Tsu-Tsair Chi has reported on an infrared cermic-coated device that has beneficial effects in strengthening the immune system, decreasing pain, unblocking lymph channels, increasing circulation, and providing lacking trace elements. The Mineral Infrared Therapy device is worth trying for Systemic Lupus Erythematosus.[12] (See *Arthritis: Little Known Treatments*, Amazon.com, bookstores and www.arthritistrust.org or at Kindle .)

Nutrition and Supplements

According to Jonathan Wright, M.D., world reknown nutritionist from Kent, Washington, (1) Vitamin B6 as high as 500 mg three times daily can be very useful in reducing symptoms; (2) more than 80% of Lupus sufferers are lacking in hydrochloric acid, and need supplementation; (3) all Lupus patients have food allergies, and will improve when this condition is handled; (4) more than 50% of women have dehydroepiandrosterone (DHEA) and testosterone levels lower than other women, and they need these deficiencies replaced via hormonal therapy.[3]

Other supplements may include vitamin C and bioflavonoids, proteolytic enzymes (away from meals on empty stomach), digestive enzymes with meals if necessary, calcium/magnesium, zinc, essential fatty acids, amino acids such as L-cysteine, L-methoionine, L-cystine, beta-carotene and vitamin A, vitamin E (1,500 I.U. daily), garlic capsules, vitamin B complex, vitamin B5, vitamin

B12 intramuscular injection (1,000 mcg intramuscular two times weekly), and selenium.[3]

The Case of Angela Boynton

When Angela Boyton, 34-years-of-age, sought out the assistance of Jonathan V. Wright, M.D.[17] for her lupus, she was determined to avoid damaging, traditional treatments, and to do whatever necessary to get well. She'd already read up on books about nutrition and had a pretty good idea about the so-called "cave-man" diet, as reported "What's Right/Wrong About Nutritional Guidelines?" At Kindle or Nook) having restocked her kitchen with whole foods, whole grains and eliminated flour, artificial flavors, colors, preservatives, sugar, artificial sweeteners, hydrogenated or partially hydrogenated oils, and she used practically no canned stuff. She also had worked up her vitamin C intake to "bowel tolerance level."

Angela was on the right track, but Dr. Wright restricted her diet even further, adding in precautionary laboratory tests and additional supplements.

A 24-hour urine test was made for excess oxalate because occasionally the excess is associated with taking large amounts of vitamin C, and can contribute to stone formation which might damage the kidneys. "As you know," Dr. Wright cautioned, "kidneys are a potential weak point in lupus. . . . Since 1973, I've only seen oxalate kidney stones associated with high-quantity vitamin C twice." (See "Linus Pauling, PhD was Right as Explained by Dr. Robert F. Cathcart "at Kindle.)

Dr. Wright agreed that permanently eliminating non-foods — foods that have been processed, packaged or otherwise treated after leaving the garden — was an "absolutely necessary step for optimal health."

Dr. Wright also eliminated 100% of Angela's wheat, oats, barley, rye and any other grains that might contain gluten and gliadin, proteins found in all grains except corn and rice.

Food sensitization tests were made and, where possible, a desensitization program was begun. Dr. Wright explained that "people who have lupus, ulcerative colitis, Grave's disease, juvenile diabetes, vitiligo, and several other 'autoimmune' diseases very frequently share tissue types (genetic markers: HLA types B8, DR3, and DR4) that are also common to celiac disease, the disease caused by gluten and gliadin. . . . The folks with lupus I've worked with have found it very important, along with permanent elimination of cow milk and diary products."

As stomach acid and pepsin are usually low in people with lupus, tests are made for these two, and where required, hydrochloric acid and pepsin capsules are supplemented.

Also Dr. Wright would inject many of the nutrients such as B-vitamins and minerals.

B6 is given, 500 mgs three times a day, because almost "all the drugs that can cause lupus and lupus-like symptoms severely inhibit enzymes that depend on B6," which also, as a side bonus, inhibits the formation of oxalates.

At least one teaspoon of flax-seed oil, along with gamma-linolenic acid

(GLA) should be taken daily. "Primrose, black currant and borage oils are all good. Make sure there's a total of 240 mgs GLA daily." (See "Essential Fatty Acids are Essential," http://www.arthritistrust.org and Kindle.)

As the name "primrose," for example, is not a controlled name, and some unscrupulous packagers use soy-bean oil instead of the proper oil, be sure that you purchase from a reliable dealer, or purchase the brand recommended by your health care provider.

Angela was advised to take 800 units of vitamin E to help the metabolization of essential fatty acids and also to take 30 mgs daily of zinc (picolinate).

As Angela felt that she was sensitive to the vitamin E she'd already taken, Dr. Wright said that he would either desensitize her, or help her find a form with which she was not sensitive.

Angela could not quite understand why she would need hormone treatment at her age (34), but Dr. Wright explained that it wasn't female hormones that the lupus patient might lack, but rather the important precursor, DHEA (dehydroepiandrosterone) and the male hormone, testosterone, as these two are usually of lower-than-normal levels in lupus sufferers. More tests, of course, were to be made to ascertain facts.

Dr. Wright reports that "It's been nearly seven years since Mrs. Boynton's first visit. Although it took her over a year and a half to get all these factors under control and working for her, she's been symptom free for the last five years."

Richard A. Kunin, M.D. Treatments

Richard A. Kunin, M.D. controls inflammatory responses by use of Omega-3 essential fatty acids, such as those found in cod liver oil and a good grade of flax oil. "Anti-histamines, including certain bioflavonoids, offer additional anti-inflammatory benefits. Vitamin E, selenium and vitamin C also can be very helfpful if used promptly, so as to minimize joint deformity. Doses as low as 40 mg per day can take the heat out of the tissues if the support nutrients are given. Vitamin A is the most important of the vitamins, since it is so often depleted in people with relapsing auto-immune disease — healing and repair require vitamin A, which is depleted in many people who have been ill or have had infections."[10]

Oxygen Therapies

A modern pioneer in a method of treatment centuries old, Charles Farr, M.D., Ph.D.,[9] of Oklahoma City, Oklahoma, was able to prove that the good effects from the use of hydrogen peroxide intravenous infusions were due to its ability to stimulate oxidative enzymes, returning them to normal.

Other scientists and researchers had long ago proven that hydrogen peroxide used both internally and externally can kill foreign microbial agents and, in fact, our macrophages — an important part of our defensive system against infection — routinely manufacture and use hydrogen peroxide to kill microbial agents.

Dr. Farr, and other physicians, use hydrogen peroxide for a wide range of health conditions, among which are AIDS, arthritis, cancer, candidiasis, chronic fatigure syndrome, depression, Systemic Lupus Erythematosus, emphysema, multiple sclerosis, varicose veins and fractures.

According to Dr. Farr, many other conditions besides these will also be benefited.[3]

There is also ozone therapy and photophoresis applicable to treating many conditions. (See "The Miracle of Hydrogen Peroxide Therapy at Kindle.)

Qigong for Arthritis

The balancing of the distribution of biolectrical energy to body parts in need can be an important therapy.[16]

Roger Jahnke, O.M.D., Santa Barbara. California, has successfully treated a number of Systemic Lupus Erythematosus patients. Using Chinese medicine, including acupuncture, herbal supplements, and Qigong, his patients have been able to solve this degenerative problem.[35

See Roger Jahnke, O.M.D., books, *Qigong: Awakening and Mastering the Medicine Within, The Self Applied Health Enhancement Methods*; tape, *Deeper Relaxation for Self Healing*, Health Action, 243 Pebble Beach, Santa Barbara, CA 93117; Dr. Yang Jwing-Ming, *Qigong for Arthritis*, also see http://www.arthritistrust.*The Remarkable Ronald B. Davis, M.D. Treatment*

The Case of Maria Aladante

Maria Aladante, 37 years-of-age, was diagnosed as having Systemic Lupus Erythematosus at a Houston, Texas medical center. Pain in her hands and fingers kept her from performance of her duties as a court reporter.

When she came to Ronald M. Davis, M.D.[20] she was given the same treatment as described for Suzie White at the beginning of this article.

Within twenty intravenous infusions Maria began regaining the use of her hands and fingers. SjÖgren's syndrome — a marked drtyness of all mucous membranes resulting from deficiency of glandular secretions in the throat, salivary glands, upper respiratory tract, sweat and stomach glands — also began to resolve.

With continued intravenous infusions and physical therapy, Maria returned to her court reporter functions, with no restrictions, and she has remained medication and symptom free.

The Case of Alice Wilson

Alice Wilson, 65 years-of-age, was diagnosed with Systemic Lupus Erythematosus at a medical school near Ronald M. Davis'[20] office, and placed on traditional treatments of cortisone, cytotoxic drugs and so on.

Dr. Davis used essentially the same treatment as already described for Suzie White, with alternation between EDTA/DMSO and hydrogen peroxide intravenous infusions.

Response was immediate and Alice has done well, currently off all medications except aspirin and tylenol for mild pain. Alice has returned to all normal activites and no longer suffers from Lupus symptoms.

Universal Oral Vaccination

Early research with Rheumatoid Arthritis and "Rheumatism," involved staphylococcus and streptococcus killed organisms injected as antigens, the successful results thus strongly supporting the infectious nature of Rheumatoid Arthritis. As many forms of Rheumatoid Disease seem to have an infectious and/or allergenic component, such as Ankylosing Spondilitis, Candidiasis, Crohn's disease, Fibrositis, Fibromyalgia, food allergies, rhinitis, and so on, this form of protection may be not just all-inclusive, but also cheap and all-important.

Drs. H. Hugh Fudenberg and Giancario Pizza,[22] using a substance related to the "immune milk" derived from a cow (as reported elsewhere) — dialzyable leucocyte extract/transfer factor — "13 of 34 patients improved considerably, despite the fact that they received only two injections the first week and one injection weekly for one month, then one injection monthly for the following five months." (See "Universal Oral Vaccine," http://www.arthritistrust.org and also at Kindle.)

References

1. *Textbook of Internal Medicine,* J.B. Lippincott Company, East Washington Square, Philadelphia, PA 19105, 1989.

2. *The Merck Manual of Diagnosis and Therapy*, 13th Edition, Merck, Sharp & Dohme Research Laboratories, Division of Merck & Co., Inc., Rahway, N.J.

3. Burton Goldberg Group, *Alternative Medicine: The Definitive Guide*, Future Medicine Publishing Co., Puyallup, WA, 1994.

4. Ronald Davis, M.D., "A Treatment for Scleroderma & Lupus Erythematosus," Supplement to The Art of Getting Well, The Arthritis Trust of America/The Rheumatoid Disease Foundation, 7376 Walker Road, Fairview, TN 37062, 1989; also Permission to republish portions granted to *Townsend Letter for Doctors*, 911 Tyler Street, Port Townsend, WA 98368, December, 1989, p. 625.

5. *Physicians' Desk Reference*, Medical Economics Co., Inc., Oradell, N.J. 07649, 1989.

6. Efrain Olszewer, M.D.,Fuad C. Sabbag, M.D., Alan Rory Zapata, M.D., *DMSO (Dimethylsulfoxide) Treatments in Arthritis*, Supplement to The Art of Getting Well, The Arthritis Fund/The Rheumatoid Disease Foundation, 5106 Old Harding Road, Franklin, TN 37064; also see Pat McGrady, Sr., *The Persecuted Drug: The Story of DMSO*, The Nutri-Books Corporation, Box 5793, Denver, CO 80217, 1981; Mildred Miller, *A Little Dab Will Do Ya! DMSO: The Drug of the 80's*, Quality Advertising Co., Degenerative Disease Medical Center, Las Vegas, NV, 1981.

7. Anthony di Fabio, "Chelation Therapy," Supplement to The Art of Getting Well, The Arthritis Trust of America/The Rheumatoid Disease Foundation, 7111 Sweetgum Road, Fairview, TN 37062, 1993.

8. Dr. Paul K. Pybus, *The Herxheimer Effect*, Supplement to The Art of Getting Well, The Arthritis Fund/The Rheumatoid Disease Foundation, 7111 Sweetgum Road, Fairview, TN 37062, 1991.

9. Charles Farr, M.D., Ph.D., "Hydrogen Peroxide Therapy," Supplement

to the Art of Getting Well, The Arthritis Trust of America/The Rheumatoid Disease Foundation, 7111 Sweetgum Road, Fairview, TN 37062, 1992.

10. Personal letter from Richard A. Kunin, M.D.

11. Alan R. Gaby, *Townsend Letter for Doctors*, August/September 1995.

12. Dr. Tsue-Tsair Chi, N.M.D., Ph.D., *Mineral Infrared Therapy*, Chi's Enterprises, Inc., 5465 E. Estate Ridge Rd., Anaheim, CA 92807, 1933.

13. Personal communication with Rex E. Newnham, D.O., N.D., Ph.D. November 6, 1995.

14. A.V. Constantini, M.D., *The Fungal/Mycotoxin Connections: Autoimmune Diseases, Malignanacies, Atherosclerosis, Hyperlipidemias, and Gout*, Keynote Speaker, American Academy of Environmental Medicine, Reno, Nevada, 1993.

15. Personal interview with Gus J. Prosch, Jr., M.D., November 22, 1995.

16. Jwing-Ming Yang, *Arthritis — The Chinese Way of Healing and Prevention,* YMAA Publication Center, Yang's Martial Arts Association (YMAA), 38 Hyde Park Avenue, Jamaica Plain, Massachusetts 02130, 1991.

17. Alan R. Gaby, M.D., "Commentary," also Jonathan V. Wright, M.D., "Treatment of Lupus."*Nutrition and Healing*, C/O Publishers Mgt. Corp., PO Box 84909, Phoenix, Arizona 84909, Volume 2, Issue 12, December 1995.

18. Personal communication with Paul A. Goldberg, M.P.H., D.C.

19. Personal interview with Roger Jahnke, O.M.D.

20. Personal correspondence with Ronald M. Davis, M.D.

21. Personal interview with Dr. Catherine Russell.

22. H. Hugh fudenberg, Giancarlo Pizza, "Transfer Factor 1993: New Frontiers," *Progress in Drug Research*, Vol. 42, Birkhauser Verlag Basel (Switzerland), 1994.

23. Joel Fuhrman, M.D., "Fasting and Detoxification," *Townsend Letter for Doctors & Patients*, April 1996, p. 84.

Progressive Systemic Sclerosis
(Scleroderma)
by
Anthony di Fabio & Ronald M. Davis, M.D.

The Case of Mrs. Rodriguez

This fifty-five year old Mexican lady had tightness and swelling of her face, hands, arms and feet. Her symptoms had begun approximately one year prior to coming to Ronald Davis, M.D.[18] of Seabrook, Texas, for treatment.

She'd had surgery on her right wrist for Carpal Tunnel Syndrome, and was supposed to have the other wrist operated on, too, but since she had not improved from the first surgery, it was decided not to operate on her other wrist.

Mrs. Rodriguez had difficulty moving hands and fingers, the fingers being fixed in a mild degree of flexion. She was unable to close her fists.

The skin of her hands and arms was darkened and very firm and painful to touch. Her feet and toes were similar to the hands, as the toes could not be moved, and were swollen. The skin of her feet and legs, to her knees, was darkened similar to that of her arms.

The skin on her arms and legs had a glistening, shiny, slick appearance.

She was successfully treated by The Arthritis Trust of America/The Rheumatoid Disease Foundation so-called "anti-amoebic" therapy, as well as dimethylsulfoxide intravenous (DMSO) infusions[4,5] with intravenous ethylene diamine tetracetic acid (EDTA) therapy and hydrogen peroxide intravenous infusions.[3,4,5,6] (See "Hydrogen Peroxide Therapy" and "Chelation Therapy," http://www.arthritistrust.org also at Kindle.)

What is Progressive Systemic Sclerosis?

Systemic Sclerosis (Scleroderma) is a thickening of the skin by formation of fibrous tissue, and by changes in internal organs that accompany the thickening tissue changes.

Causation of Progressive Systemic Sclerosis

The cause of this disease is considered to be unknown, but it is considered probable that some form of skin (endothelial) injury starts the sequence of events that results in multiorgan involvement.

According to A.V. Costantini, M.D.,[12] a list of diseases wherein fungal forms of microorganisms have been found include the following: atherosclerosis, cancer, AIDS, diabetes mellitus, Rheumatoid Arthritis, SjÖgren's syndrome, Systemic Lupus Erythematosus, Gout, Crohn's disease, multiple sclerosis, hyperactivity syndrome, infertility, psoriasis, cirrhosis, Alzheimer's disease, Scleroderma (Progressive Systemic Sclerosis), Raynaud's disease, sarcoidosis, kidney stones, amyloidosis, vasculitis, and Cushing's Disease.

Distribution of Progressive Systemic Sclerosis

Scleroderma is four times more commen in women than in men, and is found in all racial groups and all geographic regions.

Perhaps 12 persons per million per year are diagnosed with this disease, but many investigators feel that the frequency is greater, as it is often misdiagnosed as Raynaud's disease, a condition that involves capillary congestion and swelling especially of the extremities.

Disease onset is greatest between ages of 25 and 50, although all age groups can be affected.

Clinical Symptoms

Initial symptoms: capillary congestion and swelling, especially of the extremities (Raynaud's phenomenon); gradual thickening of the skin of fingers; joint inflammation, several (polyarthralgia); muscle weakness, indistinguishable from polymyositis (sclerodermatomyositis); segmented cellular death and inflammation of small and medium arteries and deficiency of blood in tissues supplied by these arteries (polyarteritis); visceral disturbances;

Progression of Disease: dilation of capillaries form tumor cells which Tend to form blood and lymph vessels on fingers, face, lips and tongue; face becomes masklike; other vascular, liver and lung problems may occur; skin becomes taut, shiny and pigmented; subcutaneous calcifications develop, usually on fingertips and over bony eminences; symmetric hardening of skin, possibly confined to fingers or other remote body parts.

The best survival outcome is for children, where statistics indicate a survival rate of 90% over ten years or more, although they often develop inflammation of arteries (arteritis) involving the gastrointestinal tract.

Initial Diagnosis

The most common symptom, in 70% of patients, is "Raynaud's phenomenon" which involves capillary congestion and swelling of the extremeties, along with a gradual thickening of the skin of the fingers.

More than one joint may become painful, known as "polyarthralgia."

In some cases there is a muscle weakness, as the predominant feature, and this characteristic is indistinguishable from a condition called "polymyositis," although when found in Scleroderma it is given the name of "sclerodermatomyositis."

Thickening and hardening of the skin, due to collagen tissue accumulation in the lower part of the skin (dermis), tends to be symmetric and may be confined to fingers or distant parts of the upper extremeties; or, the hardening can affect almost all of the body.

Progression of the Disease

As the disease progresses, the skin may become taut, shiny, and over pigmented.

The face becomes masklike.

Small tumors (angiomas) may appear on the fingers, face, lips and tongue.

Calcifications may develop below the skin more commonly in women, usually on the fingertips and over bony eminences.

Biopsies will show increased collagen fibers beneath the skin, along with

188

thinning of the outer skin (epidermal) layers, and certain kinds of atrophy. Swelling of the fingers, while painless, may be accompanied by symptoms of morning stiffness, joint pains (arthralgia), and Carpal Tunnel Syndrome.

Internal organs will also lose their proper functioning, usually paralleling observable skin changes. Changes may restrict themselves to a cluster called the CREST Syndrome, named after the characteristic symptoms of calcinosis, Raynaud's phenomenon, esophageal dysfunction, sclerodactyly (fingers and toes), and telangiectasia (dilation of capillaries and minute arteries, forming a variety of tumors), all names given to various ones of the above described symptoms.

Other visceral changes develop, which characteristically include organ changes caused by vascular deficiencies of the lung and liver.

Joints and tendons become painful due to friction rubs, particularly of the knees and through the tendon sheaths. (See *Soft Tissue Arthritis: Bursitis, Fibromyalgia; Fibromyositis; Fibrositis; Rheumatism* and *Arthritis: Osteoarthritis and Rheumatoid Disease Including Rheumatoid Arthritis*, http://www.arthritistrust.org or at bookstores and at Amazon.com and at Kindle.)

Flexion contractures occur at the fingers, wrists, and elbows resulting from fibrosis of the synovium and the tissues surrounding joint structures.

Ulcers may become common, especially at the fingertips and overlying finger joints.

Esophageal dysfunction is the most frequent visceral change, including difficulty in swallowing (dysphagia) and acid return flow (reflux)

Decreased mobility of the small intestine may also be associated with malabsorption resulting from anaerobic bacterial overgrowth. (Anaerobic bacteria are those that can live in an oxygen-free environment.) There may also be degeneration of the mucosa, and entry of air into the submucosa of the intestinal wall.

Large-mouthed sacs develop in the colon and ileum where muscle tissue atrophies.

Fibrosis of the lungs causes defective gas diffusion. Inflammation of the lining surrounding the lungs and heart may also occur.

Heart arrhythmias and nerve conduction disturbances and other cardiac abnormalities may occur. Cardiac problems tend to develop and can reach heart failure.

Severe kidney disease may develop.

Rheumatoid Factor (RF) tests are positive in a third of patients. Antibody tests (serum antinuclear or antinucleolar antibodies) are positive in 60%.

Patients with Scleroderma will often have mixed connective tissue disease, and will show clinical and blood tests of Scleroderma as well as muscle inflammation (myositis), anemia, abnormal lowering of white blood cell count (leukopenia) and other positive signs of Systemic Lupus Erythematosus.

Clinical changes are sometimes very slow, the progress of the disease becoming unrecognizable from year to year.

A medically defined "generalized" condition of the disease involves assessment of the presence of skin thickening on the chest and abdomen.

A medically defined "limited" condition involves skin changes to sites such as the wrist, ankles and clavicles.

After a long period (ten years) an improving medically defined "generalized" disease or a medically defined worsening "limited" disease becomes undistinguishable.

Early deaths usually involve, bacterial infections, pneumonia, malignancy, or heart involvement.

Associated Conditions

Associated medical conditions depend upon organs affected, and the symptoms produced by the specific organ dysfunction. Certain organs — endocrine glands, gastrointestinal tract, kidneys, and lungs — occur frequently, with corresponding difficulties.

Generally there may also be joint pains (arthralgias), Carpal Tunnel Syndrome, congestive heart failure, thyroid deficiencies (Hashimoto's thyroiditis), inflammation and degneration of connective tissue (Polymyositis), malignant tumors (neoplasms), deficiency in secretion of tears (SjÖgren's syndrome), Raynaud's phenomena, Rheumatoid Arthritis, and Systemic Lupus Erythematosus.

Traditional Treatments

No traditional treatments have been shown to be effective.

Corticosteroids are used to alleviate symptoms.

As with Rheumatoid Arthritis, various forms of D-penicillamine and cytotoxic immunosuppressive drugs — such as methotrexate — are used.

Feeding problems are usually addressed by advising the patient to take small feedings, more frequently.

Tetracycline and other broad-spectrum antibiotics are used to suppress the intestinal microflora, to hopefully alleviate symptoms of intestinal malabsorption.

Physiotherapy is used to preserve muscle strength, but is ineffective in preventing joint contractures.

What's Wrong With Traditional Treatments

No traditional treatment attempts to step outside of known, already failed modalities.

Corticosteroids

The most dramatic, short-lived relief may come from corticosteroids, drugs that dramatically relieve pain, swelling, and heated joints for a short period. When first discovered, it was hailed as the panacea for the arthritic, and then it's many damaging effects became known.

Steroids, or their analogs (triamcinolone hexacetonide; prednisolone tertiary-butylacetate) were, and are, given orally, as prednisone, by injection into the joints themselves (intra-articular), or at specific sites, especially near connections of tendons, ligments, and other locations near joints.

Although corticosteroids dampen down the clinical symptoms and permits temporary freedom of movement without pain, their usage is, or should be,

190

restricted because of many damaging side effects.

D-Penicillamine

D-penicillamine is, at best, a routinely used "experimental drug," and has never been shown to heal anyone, or bring about any kind of remission.

Immunosuppressive Drugs

Usage of cytotoxic drugs such as methotrexate is an attempt to change the course of an immune system presumed to have gone awry.

These are drugs that are routinely used in the treatment of cancer, usually also vainly so, and also for the suppression of the immune system during and following transplanted organs.

Tetracycline

The continued usage of antibiotics, including tetracycline, for the purpose of controlling unwanted organisms-of-opportunity in the gastrointestinal tract, is doomed to long-term failure for at least two reasons: (a) the usage of antibiotics itself, destroys the "good guys" microflora, *Lactobacillus, acidophilus*, so necessary to human digestion and nutrition, thus allowing organisms-of-opportunity to take root in the mucosa of the intestinal tract, thus appearing to require more administrations of antibiotics; (2) there is no attempt during administration of antibiotics to replace the "good guys" *Lactobacillus, acidophilus* microflora. (See "The Good Guys Bacteria — Lactobacillus acidophilus & Bifido bacterium" at Kindle)

In the presence of renal or liver dysfunction, particularly in pregnancy, 2 grams or more taken daily intravenously has been associated with deaths. Even oral dosages can be damaging.

There are many additional adverse effects possible when using tetracycline, including gastrointestinal, skin, hypersensitivity reactions, and blood.[9]

Small Feedings, Taken Frequently

While small feedings, frequently taken, may be a necessary evil, there is apparently no attempt to correct the situation that makes this evil necessary, nor to guide the patient through a truly constructive dietary regimen.

Non-Traditional Treatments

Anti-Amoebic (Anti-Microbial) Treatments

Gus J. Prosch, Jr., M.D.,[13] Birmingham, Alabama, reported that he effectively treated his Scleroderma patients exactly the same way as he does his Rheumatoid Arthritis patients. (See "The Roger Wyburn-Mason, M.D., Ph.D. Treatment for Rheumatoid Disease," http://www.arthritistrust.org or at Kindle.)

Anti-Fungal, Anti-Mycoplasmic Treatment

According to Dr. Costantini,[15] the concept of auto-immune diseases contains a fatal flaw, because no successful species can develop a system of defense which attacks itself. "No species of life can make an antibody against itself; particularly causing fatal disease such as Scleroderma."

Antibodies that are measured in the blood stream and which imply an autoimmune condition are actually antibodies against "ubiquitin," a substance that is present in many species including that of fungi.

"Scleroderma responds well to the antifungal agent griseofulvin."

It has also been reported that colchicine is a good anti-mycotoxin, which may be one of the reasons why Gouty Arthritis responds to administration of colchicine. (See "Gout is Curable," at www.arthritistrust.org or see Kindle.)

Other possible antifungal antibiotic agents have similar action to colchicine. Reported by Dr. Costantini are also lovastatin, griseofulvin, ketoconazole, neomycin, fibrates, tetracycline and others, some of which may also be effective against Scleroderma. Care must be taken that these are administered under the supervision of a health professional, and that *Lactobacillus acidophilus* replaces the intestinal microorganisms bound to be destroyed.

Boron

The Case of Sister Theresa

Sister Theresa, suffering from Progressive Systemic Sclerosis, lived in a retirement convent in Pietermaritzburg, South Africa. She was very stiff and unable to handle stairs properly. In order to go downstairs she had to sit on each step and bounce down to the next on her buttocks. "It was truly a traumatic process," Dr. Newnham[11] reports, "to see her go downstairs."

Sister Teresa was given boron tablets with 3 mg of boron in the form of Osteo-Trace®, and in three months she could walk up and down stairs properly.

She is now 84-years-of-age. (See "Boron Also a Necessary Supplement" at www.arthritistrust.org or at Kindle at Amazo and at bcom, bookstores.)

Detoxification and Nutritional Support

According to Mark Davidson, D.O., N.D.[15] (also trained in Chinese medicine and acupuncture), an ideal clinic would address the whole person, not just components that make up the person. Dr. Davidson says that "So many people say they've got the cure, they've got the whole picture. I tend to see little parts of a puzzle. You get a better picture when you get more viewpoints. ... We look at the patient's physical, emotional, electromagnetic, biochemical and spirtual being, using a team of experienced practitioners, each contributing their health expertise in a particular area but applying it in such a manner that the whole individual is treated."

The Health Regeneration Clinic near Waynesville, North Carolina, handles all forms of degenerative diseases, including arthritis and cancers. The following is a brief description of their treatments:

• The patient is placed in an environment conducive to peace and serenity surrounded by woods and forests with pure water, fresh air, bio-dynamic gardens, and a spring-fed, solar-heated swimming pool.

• Dr. Davidson, and the other health-care professionals, believe that how a person thinks influences their emotions and physical conditions. "In treating degenerative problems, our emphasis is on our modern way of life. Change of habits and patterns that get to the core of things. If you can advise people on how to handle stress factors in their life, relationship factors, communication skills, work problems, you're looking at a multi-factorial approach in dealing with stress." If a person's beliefs, thoughts and emotions are chaotic, scattered, or confused, they will have a difficult time healing. "The physical problem is the end-stage of unresolved, strong emotions." Staff members help clients confront the issues that they need to address. (See "Stress," http://www.arthritistrust.org or at Kindle.)

• As most people with chronic illness have major toxicity problems, usually stemming from the bowels, Dr. Davidson believes that cleansing of the bowels is of primary importance. This is done by means of fiber, herbs, enzymes and nutrients, plus colonic irrigation. Dr. Davidson says that "Usually toxicities found in the gallbladder, liver and kidneys are cleared only through proper bowel cleansing." (See "The Truth About Allergies and Addiction," at www.arthritistrust.org or at Kindle.)

Ozonated colonics and other forms of cleansing will also rid the burden of parasites, of which there are many forms. "This is an important factor, as is getting rid of the lining of the small bowel, because behind the lining you'll usually find a lot of parasites: worms, amoeba, flukes and so forth." See *Tissue Cleansing Through Bowel Management,* by Bernard Jensen)

"We also flush out the liver and gallbladder with the use of herbs, nutrients, acupressure, acupuncture, shiatsu; Japanese "finger pressure"), Swedish massage, and by stimulating the lymph system. People who finally deal with their unresolved anger may have a spontaneous detoxification of their liver and gallbladder."

Body tissues are cleansed by using steam cabinets, Turkish baths, herbs that cause sweating, ozonated baths, all of which help toxins to come through the skin. Homeopathic remedies and herbs help to speed up the metabolism and therefore also help detoxification.

• After the bowel and organs are detoxified, Dr. Davidson starts giving the right nutrients, preventing additional toxicity from entering into tissues, liver and gallbladder from poor food choices."We also educate people. We teach them about water purity, air pollutants and how to find foods low in or free of toxins, so that when they return home, they can continue their process of detoxification."

• As many people develop clogged lymph systems, preventing toxins from being removed from the body, we use lymphatic massage therapy accompanied by a device that combines magnetic therapy with soft laser principles. This is a gentle massage, and it breaks up congealed lymph, permitting the free flow of lymph drainage again. Dry skin brushing is taught, or bouncing regularly on a trampoline-rebounder, as these will also help lymph to drain. (See *Lymphatic Detoxification* and *Lymph Drainage Therapy,* http://www.arthritistrust.org and at Kindle.)

• "Most chronically ill people have toxin-producing infections," Dr. Davidson believes. "This stems from root canal teeth or previous tooth extractions. As these infections are tied in with acupuncture meridians which pass through internal organs, these organs are also affected. Therefore it's important to clean out pockets of dental infection and 'dead' teeth."

• Uneven bites or malocclusions — where teeth do not match up perfectly — can also affect health. Muscles on one side of the jaw create stress to the cranium, neck and back, producing mis-alignment in the cranial-sacral region, and this can affect many other internal organs.

As mercury amalgam is one of the primary sources of accumulated toxicity and immune suppression, these fillings should be considered for replacement. Such fillings also create unhealthy electromagnetic effects resulting from the chemical/electrical activity of two dissimilar metals (mercury and silver). Like a small battery, a constant current is created from the acid/alkaline pH of the saliva. Current, which creates a flow of electrons, also creates a magnetic field which influences release of certain hormones and neurotransmitters, affecting bodily functions. The electro-chemical action can also disassociate otherwise harmless chemicals, creating a cumulative toxic condition. (See and *Root Canal Coverup*," George Meinig, D.D.S..)

A dentist is provided to assess and to solve these otherwise hidden problems. (See *It's All In Your Head*, Hal A. Huggins, D.D.S..)

Only a biological dentist should address problems of mercury replacement or gum infections!

Although not necessarily related to teeth, geo-magnetic fields (geo-pathic lines) can also influence a persons health, and education is important to avoid certain electromagnetic stress.

• Once there is sufficient metal removed from the teeth, intravenous chelation therapy is used, starting with di-mercapto-propane sulfonate (DMPS), which attaches to and removes bi- and tri-valent metals such as mercury, lead, arsenic, copper, cobalt, chromium, cadmium, and silver. After this, ethylene diamine tetracetic acid (EDTA) is used as a chelator. This substance attaches to the calcium that holds atherosclertic plaques together, allowing them to dissolve and flush from the body, thus opening up as much as 80% of the peripheral circulation, providing improved cellular nourishment and oxygenation. (See "Cleaning Out Your Plumbing — Chelation Therapy," www.arthritistrust.org or at Kindle.)

• Dr. Davidson says that "These approaches must be combined with changes in the person's diet, lifestyle, and nutrient supplementation. One of our prime goals is for people to come to our clinic, learn the techniques, and take them back home to use and to show others. We're not interested in treating diseases, but in building health."

Enzyme Therapy

Enzyme supplementation, along with proper diet, may be very important for properly digesting food, and for eliminating the inflammatory immuno complexes that always accompanies Progressive Systemic Sclerosis. (See "Systemic Enzyme Therapy," http://www.arthritistrust.org. or Kindle.)

Herbs

As reported in *The American Journal of Natural Medicine*, in a study of 13 female patients with Scleroderma, oral administration of 20 mg of *Centella asiatica* (Gotu Kola) given 3 times daily, was very successful in 3, successful in 8, and unsuccessful in only 2 out of 13. "Improvement consisted of decreased skin hardening, reduced joint pain, and improved finger mobility."14

Mineral Infrared Therapy

Dr. Tsu-Tsair Chi has reported on an infrared cermic-coated device that has beneficial effects in strengthening the immune system, decreasing pain, unblocking lymph channels, increasing circulation, and providing lacking trace elements.[10] (See *Arthritis: Little Known Treatments*, Kindle at Amazon.com, bookstores and at www.arthritistrust.org.)

Qigong for Arthritis

The balancing or distribution of biolectrical energy to body parts in need can be an important therapy.[13]

The Case of Carlene Charles

Roger Jahnke, O.M.D.,[17] Santa Barbara, California, has had several cases of Scleroderma. Carlene Charles, in her early 30s, was one of his most brilliant patients, as she stated up front that she was going to have a team of health care providers, and that she was not going to buy in on the idea that Scleroderma was going to kill her.

"Her physician, who is a reasonable primary care provider, encouraged her to follow her desire to use Chinese medicine, herbs, acupuncture, etc.

"After about four years Carlene arrested her disorder. There was a point where her mouth and her face began to show Scleroderma signs, and she actually recovered from that — both face and feet actually recovered from moderate stage Scleroderma signs, however her hands only partially recovered.

Ronald Davis, M.D. Remarkable Alternative Treatment

More on Mrs. Rodriguez

When Mrs. Rodriguez came to Dr. Davis for help — as reported at the beginning of this chapter — she had all the symptoms of Progressive Systemic Scleroderma, a disease that Dr. Davis had previously treated successfully, just as he had treated Rheumatoid Arthritis and Systemic Lupus Erythematosus successfully.

Medications taken by Mrs. Rodriguez under traditional treatments were 2 tablets of acetaminophen with codeine, 4 tablets 6 times per day; 1 tablet of Tylenol, 500 mg each 4 hours, 1 250 mg tablet of Pen V-K each 6 hours; Procardia caps, 10 mg 3 times each day; 250 mg tablet of hydroxyzine 4-6 hours as needed with itching; 250 mg Cuprimine capsule 2 times daily; 400 mg Ibuprofen capsule 3 times daily; 10 mg Flexeril 1 tablet 2 times daily; 300 mg Tagamet 2 tablet 3 times daily; 150 mg Zantac 1 tablet 3 times daily.

Mrs. Rodriguez had difficulty moving her hands and fingers, the fingers fixed so that she could not close her fists.

Skin on the hands and arms were darkened and very firm and painful to touch.

Feet and toes, similar to her hands, could not easily be moved, and were swollen.

As described in the section on Systemic Lupus Erythematosus, Dr. Davis started the patient with (1) The Arthritis Trust of America/The Rheumatoid Disease Foundation's recommended anti-amoebic treatment, and also began (2) dimethylsulfoxide intravenous (DMSO) infusions[4,5] with intravenous amino acid ethylene diamine tetracetic acid (EDTA) therapy.[3,4,5,6] (3) Dr. Davis also later administered intravenous infusions of hydrogen peroxide (H2O2).[8]

Only a moderate Herxheimer[7] effect (organism die-off effect) was noted on the first two medications of the anti-amoebics, and was hardly noticeable on the next four treatments. (See The Healing Fever — The Herxheimer at www.arthritistrust.org or at Kindle.)

Intravenous infusions of dimethylsulfoxide intravenous (DMSO)[4,5] with intravenous ethylene diamine tetracetic acid (EDTA) therapy[3,4,5,6] was begun at the same time as the anti-amoebic therapy.

After the first month, hydrogen peroxide (H2O2)[8] was used in place of the dimethylsulfoxide intravenous (DMSO)[4,5] with intravenous ethylene diamine tetracetic acid (EDTA) therapy.[3,4,5,6]

Mrs. Rodriguez's improvement was quite evident during the following year. Her hands, arms, feet and legs began to soften within the first week of treatment.

She felt that the hydrogen peroxide (H2O2) made her "itch on the inside" of her hands, arms, and feet, but the next day after the infusion she felt much better results than she had with the intravenous therapy of dimethylsulfoxide(DMSO) accompanied by intravenous ethylene diamine tetracetic acid (EDTA).

Her condition continued to improve after and between treatments, even when she went 2 to 3 months without treatment.

She had a total of 80 ethylene diamine tetracetic acid (EDTA) with dimethylsulfoxide(DMSO), and 30 hydrogen peroxide (H2O2) infusions.

The skin of her face, arms, hands, legs and feet is now normal in appearance in texture, and she no longer has fatigue and malaise, and her energy and activity levels are normal. She has normal function of her hands and fingers, and is without pain.

The Case of Mrs. Devin

Ronald M. Davis, M.D. of Seabrook, Texas, was approached by fifty year old Mrs. Devin who had been in good health two years prior to to her present health problems, although she'd had the usual childhood illnesses. There were no prior adult illnesses and no surgeries, no history of tuberculosis, diabetes, cardiovascular disease, or hypertension.

She first began to notice a sensation of swelling and tightness of the skin of the face and extremities. These symptoms rapidly progressed to the point of rendering the patient unable to walk, or to do daily household work, as hypertension and headache were early symptoms.

In a year-and-a-half, the condition of the patient deteriorated from mild stiffness of the joints and tightness of the skin, to complete immobilization, with loss of the use of her extremities and loss of flexible facial characteristics. Her fingertips felt coldness and pain.

Mrs. Devin was diagnosed as suffering from Progressive Systemic Sclerosis, a disease that Dr. Davis learned can be successfully treated using the same treatment he had developed for Systemic Lupus Erythematosus.[4]

She had tightness and hardening of the skin of the body, deformities of the hands, arms, legs and fingers, with an inability to walk, progressive kidney failure, nausea, headache, and fatigue.

One night Mrs. Devin awakened with a sensation of smothering and chest tightness, so she was rushed to the local hospital emergency room, where she was found to have a blood pressure in the range of 200/110. She was given anti-hypertensive medication, and remained on this drug until her final treatments with Dr. Davis.

Kidney involvement was extensive, necessitating dialysis (peritoneal), which she was doing at home with her husband's assistance. She was also under the care of a rheumatologist and The Texas Kidney Institute at Hermann Hospital in Houston.

Mrs. Devin was unable to perform ordinary household tasks or even to walk as her legs and feet had become stiff and immobile.

Throughout the inevitable progress of her disease under the care of traditional practitioners, she was placed on Compazine, 25 mg tablets 4 times daily for nausea, 2 Dialome, 3 times per day; 1 Capoten 75 mg, 2 times daily; 5 mg prednisone 1 time daily, 0.1 mg Catapres, 1 time at bedtime, and kidney dialysis with 1 liter of solution 4 times daily.

She had been on antihypertensive medications for over one year, and on dialysis for nearly nine months when Dr. Davis first saw her in his office.

During the treatment administered by Ronald Davis, M.D., she responded immediately, and improved continuously. Although it took a year to bring about nearly a complete cure of Mrs. Devin's condition, Dr. Davis' treatment was essentially simple, relying on two parts, as follows: (1) The Arthritis Trust of America/The Rheumatoid Disease Foundation recommended treatment for Rheumatoid Disease; (2) intravenous dimethylsulfoxide (DMSO) infusions[6] with intravenous ethylene diamine tetracetic acid (EDTA) therapy.3,7 (See "The Roger Wyburn-Mason, M.D., Ph.D. Treatment for Rheumatoid Disease," http://www.arthritistrust.org and Kindle.)

The first treatment used was 300 mg of allopurinol by mouth three times per day for 7 days, simultaneously with 500 mg of metronidazole, two tablets A.M. and P.M. (2 grams per day) for two consecutive days a week for six weeks.

It's now been several years since her last treatment. She has full use of her kidneys without dialysis, and was last reported walking about Alcatraz Island on vacation with her husband.

Ronald Davis, M.D., Seabrook, Texas, says, "I truly feel that in order to get complete cure of these rheumatoid diseases, the anti-amoebics must be used."

Under this "anti-amoebic" treatment, the patient experienced a severe Herxheimer reaction, including increased nausea, headache and rather severe joint pains, as well as increased muscular aches and pains.[9] Moderate relief of these symptoms was obtained by increasing the prednisone by one tablet on the Herxheimer days.

A rather severe Herxheimer continued throughout the six weeks of treatment.

Intravenous treatment using dimethylsulfoxide intravenous (DMSO) infusions[4,6] with intravenous ethylene diamine tetracetic acid (EDTA) therapy[3,4,7] was begun, and continued periodically for the next two years, gradually tapering off in frequency of administration.

In summary, Dr. Davis uses The Arthritis Fund/The Rheumatoid Disease Foundation's treatment protocol for Rheumatoid Disease (including for Rheumatoid Arthritis), as a starting point, and follows up with intravenous infusions of either (1) ethylene diamine tetracetic acidEDTA/ dimethylsulfoxide (DMSO a strong anti-oxidant); and/or (2) hydrogen peroxide infusions.

Dr. Davis reports that he has had "four cases of Scleroderma which were arrested and all symptoms of SjÖgren's syndrome (dryness of mucosal secretions) reversed," using the same protocol as described in this section and the sections on Systemic Lupus Erythematosus and Rheumatoid Arthritis.

"Mrs. Devin is free of symptoms after 8-1/2 years from her last treatment. At last contact, the only medication she is taking is Capoten and Norvasc for residual hypertension. Her kidneys still function well.

"The treatment we use for Rheumatoid Arthritis, Systemic Lupus Erythematosus and Progressive Systemic Sclerosis (Scleroderma) works well in arresting the progress of the diseases as well as reversing most of the skin and organ changes.

"We have had no untoward effects with these treatments except for the pungent odor the patients gets (temporarily) from the DMSO intravenous infusions.

"Sometimes the Herxheimer reaction is severe, but not to the extent that requires discontinuing therapy.

"There have been no untoward effects from the EDTA intravenous infusions, since the dosage is calculated [according to proper standards], given slowly, with close monitoring of blood pressure and blood sugar.

"No patient, to this point, has failed to respond to this therapy." (See "Mycoplasma Experiments," http://www.arthritistrust.org, *and Arthritis: Little Known Treatments*, at www.arthritistrust.org and at Kindle.)

Cooperative Assistance in
This Remarkable Alternative Treatment
Ronald Davis, M.D. received cooperation and assistance in bringing about this remarkable change with the help of Dr. Katy Thompson of the Texas Kidney Institute at Hermann Hospital, Houston, TX, Dr. Stanley Jacobs of

the University of Oregon, and also from Charles H. Farr, M.D., Ph.D. of Oklahoma and Garry Gordon, M.D. of Arizona.

Reported by Julian Whitaker, M.D., Stanley Jacob, M.D., world authority on the use of dimethylsulfoxide (DMSO), and one of the national advisors to the Scleroderma International Foundation states that DMSO "is the treatment of choice for both Scleroderma and Raynaud's phenomenon and is beneficial for Rheumatoid Arthritis."[16]

Universal Oral Vaccination

Early research with Rheumatoid Arthritis and "Rheumatism," involved staphylococcus and streptococcus killed organisms injected as antigens, the successful results thus strongly supporting the infectious nature of Rheumatoid Arthritis. As many forms of Rheumatoid Disease seem to have an infectious and/or allergenic component, such as Ankylosing Spondilitis, Candidiasis, Crohn's disease, Fibrositis, Fibromyalgia, food allergies, rhinitis, and so on, this form of protection may be not just all-inclusive, but also cheap and all-important.

Injecting known, specific allergens or antigens into the cistern (base of teat) of a cow just prior to calving produces protective substances that are curative.

This form of treatment has been shown to be effective with a wide variety of ailments including Rheumatism, Rheumatism, coughing, respiratory problems, sore throat, skin conditions, acne blemishes, upset stomach, cold and flu, diarrhea, and impetigo.

Drs. H. Hugh Fudenberg and Giancario Pizza,[20] using a substance related to the "immune milk" derived from a cow (as reported elsewhere) — dialzyable leucocyte extract/transfer factor — "excellent results were obtained ....in 3 cases with Scleroderma, with complete recovery in 2 and considerable improvement in the third." (See *Universal Oral Vaccine*, http://www.arthritistrust.org or on kindle.)

References

1. *Textbook of Internal Medicine,* J.B. Lippincott Company, East Washington Square, Philadelphia, PA 19105, 1989.

2. *The Merck Manual of Diagnosis and Therapy*, 16th Edition, Merck, Sharp & Dohme Research Laboratories, Division of Merck & Co., Inc., Rahway, N.J, 1992.

3. Burton Goldberg Group, *Alternative Medicine: The Definitive Guide*, Future Medicine Publishing Co., Puyallup, WA, 1994, 2002.

4. Ronald Davis, M.D., "A Treatment for Scleroderma & Lupus Erythematosus," Supplement to The Art of Getting Well, The Arthritis Fund/ The Rheumatoid Disease Foundation, 7111 Sweetgum Rd, Fairview, TN,1989; also permission to republish portions granted to *Townsend Letter for Doctors*, 911 Tyler Street, Port Townsend, WA 98368, December, 1989, p. 625.

5. Efrain Olszewer, M.D., Fuad C. Sabbag, M.D., Alan Rory Zapata, M.D., *DMSO (Dimethylsulfoxide) Treatments in Arthritis*, Supplement to

The Art of Getting Well, The Arthritis Fund/The Rheumatoid Disease Foundation,7111 Sweetgum Road, Fairview, TN 37062; also see Pat McGrady, Sr., *The Persecuted Drug: The Story of DMSO*, The Nutri-Books Corporation, Box 5793, Denver, CO 80217, 1981; Mildred Miller, *A Little Dab Will Do Ya! DMSO: The Drug of the 80's*, Quality Advertising Co., Degenerative Disease Medical Center, Las Vegas, NV, 1981.

6. Anthony di Fabio, "Chelation Therapy," Supplement to The Art of Getting Well, The Arthritis Trust of America/The Rheumatoid Disease Foundation, 7111 Sweetgum Road, Fairview, TN 37062, 1993.

7. Dr. Paul K. Pybus, "The Herxheimer Effect," Supplement to The Art of Getting Well, The Arthritis Trust of America/The Rheumatoid Disease Foundation, 7111 Sweetgum Road, Fairview, TN 37062, 1991.

8. Charles Farr, M.D., Ph.D., "Hydrogen Peroxide Therapy," Supplement to The Art of Getting Well, The Arthritis Trust of America/The Rheumatoid Disease Foundation, 7111 Sweetgum Road, Fairview, TN 37062, 1992.

9. *Physicians' Desk Reference*, Medical Economics Company, Inc., Oradell, NJ 07649.

10. Dr. Tsu-Tsair Chi, N.M.D., Ph.D., *Mineral Infrared Therapy*, Chi's Enterprises, Inc., 5465 E. Estate Ridge Rd., Anaheim, CA 92807, 1993.

11. Personal communication with Rex E. Newnham, D.O., N.D., Ph.D. November 6, 1995.

12. A.V. Constantini, M.D., *The Fungal/Mycotoxin Connections: Autoimmune Diseases, Malignanacies, Atherosclerosis, Hyperlipidemias, and Gout*, Keynote Speaker, American Academy of Environmental Medicine, Reno, Nevada, 1993.

13. Jwing-Ming Yang, *Arthritis — The Chinese Way of Healing and Prevention*, YMAA Publication Center, Yang's Martial Arts Association (YMAA), 38 Hyde Park Avenue, Jamaica Plain, Massachusetts 02130, 1991.

14. Gotu Kola (*Centella asiatica*) for Scleroderma, *The American Journal of Natural Medicine*, Vol. 2, No. 9, IMPAKT Communications, Inc., November 1995, p. 16; from Sasaki S., et. al: Studies on the mechanism of action of asiaticoside (Madecassol) on experimental granualtation tissue and cultured fibroblasts and its clinical application in systemic scleroderma. *Acta Diabetologica Latina* 52:141-50, 1972.

15. Personal interview with Mark Davidson, D.O., N.D.; also see "Wellness: Why You Need Detoxification and Nutritional Support," *Alternative Medical Digest*, Issue 8, Future Medicine Publishing, Inc., Puyallup, Washington 98371.

16. Julian Whitaker, M.D., "DMSO Update," *Health & Healing*, Phillips Publishing, Inc., 7811 Montrose road, Potomac, MD 20854, December 1955.

17. Personal interview with Roger Jahnke, O.M.D.

18. Correspondence with Ronald M. Davis, M.D.

19. Personal interview with Dr. Catherine Russell.

20. H. Hugh fudenberg, Giancarlo Pizza, "Transfer Factor 1993: New Frontiers," *Progress in Drug Research*, Vol. 42, Birkhauser Verlag Basel (Switzerland), 1994.

A Treatment Protocol for Scleroderma & Lupus Erythematosus
by
Anthony di Fabio and Ronald B. Davis, M.D.
Sources are given in references.
Permission to republish also granted to *Townsend Letter for Doctors*,
911 Tyler Street, Port Townsend, WA 98368, December, 1989, p. 625

The case that follows applies to Lupus Erythematosus and Scleroderma. As it was for the most part written by Ronald Davis, M.D., it may be difficult for the lay person to read. I have placed in bold type the salient features of the case log so that, if you prefer, you may scan through the record easily.

If you are also a victim of one of these terrible scourges, you will most likely wish to present this article to your doctor. They will have no trouble reading Dr. Davis' notes, and will understand fully.

Lupus Erythematosus and Scleroderma are classified as vascular diseases, along with Polyarteritis Nodosa, and some other diseases, but Lupus and Scleroderma also have one other thing in common — they can be treated in a similar manner with equally good results!

Lupus Erythematosus is a chronic, non-tuberculous disease of the skin marked by disklike patches with raised reddish edges and depressed centers, and covered with scales or crusts. These fall off, leaving dull-white scars.

Scleroderma is a disease of the skin in which thickened, hard, ridged, and pigmented patches occur. The connective tissue of the skin layer beneath the epidermis (corium) and the subcutaneous structures being increased, a hidebound condition results. The ordinary form begins in middle life, and is often incurable.

The above is according to *The American Illustrated Medical Dictionary* (W.B. Saunders).

The Arthritis Trust of America/Rheumatoid Disease Foundation is proud and happy to bring to you a wonderfully successful case history of Scleroderma developed by Ronald M. Davis, M.D.

The total case history will be reproduced here for those who wish to follow it in detail.

To summarize, this is a report of a case of severe progressive systemic sclerosis in a forty-nine year old white female, who was in good health two years prior to being seen in Dr. Davis' office. In a year-and-a-half, the condition of the patient deteriorated from mild stiffness of the joints and tightness of the skin, to complete immobilization, with loss of the use of her extremities and loss of facial characteristics. Kidney involvement was extensive, necessitating peritoneal dialysis, which she was doing at home with her husband's assistance. During the treatment to be described below, she responded immediately, and improved continuously. It's now been over a year since her last treatment. She has full use of her kidneys without dialysis, and was last seen walking about Alcatraz Island on vacation.

Indeed, her quality-of-life is vastly improved! If she is not cured, then she enjoys an extended remission of all symptoms!

Treatments used were two of our recommended Rheumatoid Disease medications, intravenous EDTA Chelation Therapy, intravenous DMSO Therapy, and Physical Therapy as could be tolerated by the patient.

Since Lupus Erythematosus and Scleroderma, like Psoriasis, have been virtually intractable by traditional treatments, this single success story bears repeating.

But more than this single success story, Ronald Davis, M.D. states and assures us that he has had similar successes with others using the same regimen.

We consider this a breakthrough of the first magnitude, and worthy of your serious consideration, if you or your relatives or friends suffer from either of the above diseases.

The Reversal of Scleroderma (Progressive Systemic Sclerosis)

Initial History and Physical Examination:
May 22, 1984

Chief Complaint: Tightness and hardening of the skin of the body, deformities of the hands, arms, legs, and fingers. Inability to walk, progressive kidney failure, nausea, and headache. High blood pressure.

History of Chief Complaint: The patient first began to notice a sensation of swelling and tightness of the skin of the face and extremities about the Spring of 1982. These symptoms rapidly progressed to the point of rendering the patient unable to walk, or to do daily household work. Evidently her kidneys had become affected early in the disease, as hypertension and headache were early symptoms. Patient had been on antihypertensive medication for over one year, and on peritoneal dialysis for nearly nine months, when we saw her in our office. She was under the care of a rheumatologist in Houston and The Texas Kidney Institute at Hermann Hospital in Houston.

Past History: Usual childhood illnesses wihout sequelae (sequela: Any lesion or affection following or caused by an attack of disease), no serious adult illnesses, and no surgeries. No history of TB, diabetes, cardiovascular disease, or hypertension prior to the onset of this disease. Patient is allergic to Demerol.

Family History: Essentially noncontributory, there being no history of the rheumatoid diseases, TB, CA, diabetes, or cardiovascular problems.

Medications: Compazine — 25 Mg. tabs 1, four times daily as needed for nausea.

Dialome — 2, three times per day

Capoten — 75 Mg. 1, two times daily

Prednisone — 5 Mg., 1 daily

Catapres — 0.1 Mg., 1 at bedtime

Peritoneal dialysis with 1 liter of solution four times daily (prepared by Texas Kidney Institute at Hermann Hospital, Houston.)

Review of Systems:

HEENT: Patient had begun to notice numbness and coldness of tips of fingers, with a sensation of swelling of hands, fingers, toes, arms, and legs about two years ago. The skin of the face, at the same time, became tight and inelastic making facial expressions and movement very difficult, and eventually impossible. No problems with vision or hearing, but had noticed difficulty swallowing recently.

Chest & Lungs: In late 1982 the patient was awakened in the middle of the night, with a sensation of smothering and chest tightness. She was rushed to a local hospital Emergency Room, where she was found to have a blood pressure in the range of 200/110. She was given anti-hypertensive medication, the blood pressure was reduced, and the symptoms abated. She has had to remain on medication for blood pressure control since.

Gastro-intestinal: Negative except for extreme nausea, which has been present since earliest symptoms began in 1982.

Genito-urinary: Patient is Gravida (was pregnant) 5, Para 5 (had 5 children successfully), abortus 0, stillbirth 0. She has five children living, and in good health. She had been on peritoneal dialysis at Texas Institute for past ten months.

Neurological: Negative.

Skin & Extremeties: This condition began with a sensation of coldness and pain of the fingertips. The fingers and hands soon became stiff and immobile, as did the legs and feet. Within six months, the patient was unable to walk or do ordinary daily tasks. She also complained of severe fatigue during the course of this illness, as she had for several months before the first symptoms had begun. The skin and extremities had become slick, shiney, and very hard to the touch within six months after the onset of the first symptoms. The skin of the face was no different.

Physical Examination:

General: The patient is a forty-nine year old caucasian female of Italian extraction in obvious acute and chronic distress from kidney and musculoskeletal disease. (Blood Pressure 140/90, Pulse 94, Temperature 100, Respiration 20, Height 60", Weight 109#.)

HEENT: Head was normal. Eyes: Sclerae and conunctivae were clear, EOM's (Extra Ocular Movements) intact bilaterally, pupils were equal and equally reactive to light and accommodation. Optic fundi were not examined. Visual acuity was not done. Ears: skin of ears was slick, shiney, and quite tender to touch. Nose: Same. Throat: Throat was clear.

Chest: Lungs were clear to auscultation (listening to lungs) and percussion. The breath sounds were diminished due to shallow breathing from restriction of the rib cage. Heart: Normal sinus rhythm, rate 110 and regular and there were no murmurs.

Abdomen: Thin, symmetrical abdomen, without masses, tenderness, or visceromegaly (enlarged organs) to palpation, and the bowel sounds were normal. Rectal and pelvic exams were not done. The catheters for peritoneal dialysis were in place, there was no sign of infection or irritation.

Neurological: Examination was limited due to immobility of the extremities and tenderness of the skin, but no gross abnormalities of the neurological system were noted.

Skin & Extremities: The skin was white and glistening, and appeared to have been stretched tightly over the bony skeleton. The joints at the elbows, wrists, knees, and ankles were difficult to move. The fingers were fixed in flexion and could not be moved at all. She was the classical Maskof face.

Initial Laboratory Data: Hemoglobin 8.4; White Blood Count 7400; Ca++ 9.3; BUN 91; Serum Creatnine 8.3; Glucose 113; Triglycerides 377; Uric Acid 6.6; SGOT 28; SGPT 23; Protein 7.0; Albumin 3.7; Globulins 3.3; LDH 204; Phosphate 4.6; 24 Hr. Creatinine Clearance 7.0; Na+ 140; K+ 5.0; Cl- 100; CO2 24.

Chest X-ray: Negative; EKG: Sinus Tachycardia, otherwise normal Urinalysis: Specific Gravity 1.010; pH 5.0; Protein 1+; Glucose 0; Casts: 2+Red Blood Cell; Bacteria 1+; Red Blood Cell 4-5/high powered field; White Blood Cell 3-4/high powered field.

Impression: 1. Severe Progressive Systemic Sclerosis (Scleroderma).

2. Nephrosclerosis with kidney failure secondary to scleroderma.

3. Severe anemia secondary to 1. and 2.

Treatment Plan: 1. Rheumatoid Disease Foundation therapy. (See The Roger Wyburn-Mason, M.D., Ph.D. Treatment for Rheumatoid Disease, http://www.arthritistrust.org.)

2. Intravenous DMSO therapy

3. Intravenous Chelation therapy (EDTA)

4. Physical Therapy as tolerated by patient

Clinical Course: On May 22, 1984, the Rheumatoid Disease Foundation therapy was begun in accordance with its protocol, which is as follows: Allopurinol 300 mg. by mouth three times per day for 7 days. Metronidazole 500 mg. — Two tablets A.M. and P.M. two consecutive days a week for six weeks. The patient was told to continue all current medicines. She experienced increased nausea and headache, plus she had rather severe joint pains, as well as increased muscular aches and pains. These symptoms were believed to be due to a Herxheimer type reaction, for they were most bothersome following taking the Metronidazole on Tuesdays and Wednesdays. Moderate relief of these symptoms was obtained by increasing the Prednisone by one tablet on these days.

5/29/84: Condition unchanged, patient complaining of increased nausea from the medication and dialysis. Blood Pressure 140/70; Temperature 98.6; Weight 107#.

6/19/84: Patient complaining of worse nausea, with wretching and more joint stiffness. She doesn't feel that she is "getting any better". Blood pressure 140/70, Temperature 98, Weight 106#, Rx — **Take**

Allopurinol 300 mg. 2 times daily for 1 week, and gradually reduce and discontinue Prednisone over the next 3-4 weeks.

7/23/84: **Nausea continues, still feels terrible.** (Blood pressure 140/74; Temperature 98; weight 104#; Rx — **DMSO 5cc in 500 cc D5W [5% Dextrose Solution] Intravenous over 1 hour.**)

7/25/84: **Less nausea today, but really not feeling any better.** Blood Pressure 142/76; Temperature 99; Weight 103#; Rx — **DMSO 5cc infusion #2 no problems encountered.**

7/27/84-8/17/84: **Patient received 5cc DMSO in 500 cc D5W (5% Dextrose Solution) over a 3 hour time span without adverse effects of any sort. Her vital signs remained the same. These infusions were given 3 times weekly.**

8/27/84: **This date I talked with Dr. Stanley Jacobs, M.D. of the University of Oregon regarding his treatment of scleroderma and rheumatoid arthritis with DMSO. He uses 0.5-1.0 cc of DMSO per kilogram of body weight three times weekly. (The DMSO used was Rimso 50, which is 50% DMSO.) Since this patient had been on only 5 cc DMSO per treatment, it was decided to increase her DMSO by 5-10cc per treatment until her maximum dose of 50 Gm. DMSO in 500cc D5W (5% Dextrose Solution) was reached, and then to continue treatments three times per week at that level. She was given 10cc DMSO today in the infusion, without untoward effects.**

9/10/84: **Intravenous #19 to day with 32-1/2cc DMSO.** Blood Pressure 122/70; Weight 105. **Patient appears somewhat improved, as the nausea is mild and intermittent. She seems to be improving and gaining strength weekly. She can now wrinkle her forehead, smile, and walk slowly with assistance.** Serum Creatinine 3.9; Serum Creatinine Clearance 13. **Kidneys are evidently regaining some function.**

9/24/84: **45cc DMSO given today in 23rd treatment. Patient is responding well to therapy, skin is softening, joints are mobile, except for fingers, and she is walking almost normally without assistance.** BUN 57; Creatinine 4.2. Liver function studies were normal. Hb 8.9; White Blood Count 7300. **Patient told to keep taking Fe script (Iron prescription) for low hemoglobin. I talked with Dr. Thompson at Hermann Hospital. She is pleased with patient's progress and said we should continue the treatments, and that she would be happy to continue to assist in the care of this patient.**

9/26/84: **50cc DMSO given intravenous today without side effect except for the garlic-like odor DMSO gives. The patient continues to improve and feel well.** Blood Pressure 122/70; Weight 103#.

10/12/84: **Continues improving, offers no complaints.** Treatment #29 today. Hemoglobin 8.7; Ca 9.4; BUN 48; Creatinine 3.8; Glucose 88; Triglycerides 391; HDL 44.2; Alkaline Phosphatase 46.9; SGOT 16; LDH 90; P 4.8; Cholesterol 314; Uric Acid 3.8; Na+ 156; K+ 4.7; 24 Hr. Creatinine Clearance 13.1; Urinalysis: Specific Gravity 1.010; pH 6;

Rest of Urinalysis negative; Vital Statistics unchanged.

11/27/84: Patient has not had a treatment in one month, so we will go back to 30cc DMSO and go back to 50CC with next infusion. Patient looks great, is walking briskly without any problem, and is free of any discomfort. The skin appears normal and is normal to the touch, having lost its slick, shiney appearance. Hemoglobin 9.6; White Blood Count 6000; Ca 9.2; BUN 51; Creatinine 3.0; Triglycerides 398; Electrolytes and liver tests were normal. **Prognosis now looks good.**

12/22/84: Dr. Thompson discontinued peritoneal dialysis, but left the catheters in place in the event we have to re-institute dialysis. Patient is improving very well at this time, having a lot of energy, and carries out her normal household duties. Fingers are much more flexible and patient can almost clench fists. She has had 39 DMSO infusions to date. Blood Pressure 140/70; Weight 106#; Serum Creatinine 3.0.

1/21/85: Infusion #44, 35CC DMSO. Blood Pressure 160/80; Weight 107#.

1/31/85: Patient complaining of slight headache. Physical exam not remarkable, and I can only explain increase in Blood Pressure by the fact that she hasn't been getting her treatments very regularly. Blood Pressure 160/102; Weight 105#. She was told to increase Capoten from 75 Mg at bedtime, to 50 Mg. a.m. and 75 Mg. at bedtime; Hemoglobin 11.5; White Blood Count 13,900; Normal Differential Urinalysis negative; BUN 57.1; Creatinine 3.0; Na+ 145; K+ 5.0.

2/26/85: Infusion #49, 35cc DMSO. Patient continues to improve, although lab data remain at December 84 levels. **We have started adding 2 cc B6 and 15cc (7.5Gm.) ascorbic acid to each intravenous beginning 2/8/85. No unwanted side effects have been observed.**

3/26/85: 30cc DMSO today in treatment #53. Patient is doing very well, offering no complaints. Hemoglobin 10.9; White Blood Count 6000; BUN 68; Creatinine 3.3; Urine output normal; Blood Pressure 130/80 Weight 101#.

4/25/85: Infusion #57, with 50cc DMSO. No problems. Patient seems to continue improving. Blood Pressure 140/84; Weight 102#; BUN 57.2; Serum Creatinine 2.7.

5/30/85: Infusion #65 today. No DMSO, just 1cc EDTA in 500cc D5W, with 2CC B6 and 15cc ascorbic acid given intravenous over 3 hours. No adverse effects noted. Preinfusion Blood Pressure 140/82. Post infusion Blood Pressure 140/80. Hemoglobin 10.6; White Blood Count 5000; 24 Hr. Creatinine Clearance 21.37; Serum Creatinine 2.7.

6/6/85: Infusion #66 with 50cc. DMSO. No Problems. Blood Pressure 140/80; BUN 48; Serum Creatinine 2.8. **Skin of face, arms, legs, and hands approaching normal. Patient has lost her Mauskopf appearance, and has normal mobility of the facial skin.**

6/10/85: Infusion #67, with 2cc EDTA without problem. Preinfusion Blood Pressure 160/80. Postinfusion Blood Pressure 162/76; Weight

107#. **Patient offered no complaints during, or after infusion.** BUN 45.8; Creatinine 3.0; 24Hr. Creatinine Clearance 21.37; Urinalysis Specific Gravity 1.010; pH 5.0; Protein trace; 1-2 White Blood Count/high powered field.

6/20/85: Infusion #68, 50CC DMSO and 2CC EDTA. Patient complained of nausea, and had one episode of vomiting during the infusion, which she felt was due to the DMSO. Will reduce DMSO to 40CC next infusion. Preinfusion Blood Pressure 160/90. Postinfusion Blood Pressure 162/88; Weight 105#.

7/11/85: Treatment #70 continued with 40cc DMSO and 2cc EDTA — no complaints or problems. Preinfusion Blood Pressure 150/92. Postinfusion Blood Pressure 15/90; Hemoglobin 11.2; 24 Hr. Creatinine Clearance 23.71. **Patient appears and says she feels normal.**

7/22/85: EDTA increased to 3cc, along with 40cc DMSO for infusion #72. Preinfusion Blood Pressure 150/90. Postinfusion Blood Pressure 150/86; Weight 105#. Procedure was tolerated well by patient. BUN 58.7; Creatinine 2.6; Urinalysis: Negative.

7/30/85: For infusion #73, EDTA was increased to 5cc, again with 40cc DMSO. No problems encountered during or after treatment. Pre, and post infusion Blood Pressure 150/86; Weight 106#; BUN 55.4; Creatinine 2.8.

8/19/85: Infusion #74 with 5cc EDTA and 40cc DMSO was well tolerated by the patient, and there were no difficulties during or following the treatment. Preinfusion Blood Pressure 142/90, Postinfusion Blood Pressure 140/90; Weight 105#; BUN 45.7; Creatinine 3.0.

10/18/85: Infusions 74 thru 81 were given with 5cc EDTA only and were without incident. Blood Pressure remained in the 150/84 range, and patient continued to progress very well. Her Weight remained the same, but she was having to diet to keep her weight 105# or below. BUN 41; Creatinine 2.7; Creatinine Clearance 21.

11/5/85: Since it had been almost a month from the last treatment, only 20cc DMSO were given in infusion #82. It was without incident. BUN 47.9; Creatinine 2.4; Creatinine Clearance 28.39; Blood Pressure 142/80; Urinalysis: negative; Weight 105#.

12/11/85: Infusion #83 was with 7cc EDTA, 5cc ascorbic acid, and 5cc (1250Mg) Pantothenic Acid all in 50cc D5W (5% Dextrose Solution) intravenous. This was given in 1 hour, there were no adverse effects, lab values and Blood Pressure readings remained the same.

1/6/86: About middle of December 85, Dr. Thompson removed the peritoneal dialysis catheters, since they had not been used for one year.

7/25/86: Since 2/5/86 patient has received infusions 84-90 on the average of one per month, with no adverse effects. All of these treatments contained EDTA 8cc, ascorbic acid 15cc, in 50cc D5W (5% Dextrose Solution), given in one hour. BUN 48; Creatinine 1.6, Creatinine Clearance 38.66. Infusion #91 was given this date. Blood Pressure 150/90; Weight

110#. **Patient has felt well and has led a normal life for the past six months.**

The patient has not been seen at the Kidney Institute at Hermann Hospital since January 1986 although Dr. Thompson has followed her progress by phone, through my office and with the patient.

Dr. Ronald Davis expresses his heartfelt gratitude to Dr. Katy Thompson of the Texas Kidney Institute at Hermann Hospital, Houston, TX and to Dr. Stanley Jacobs of the University of Oregon for their kind and able assistance and cooperation in the treatment of this patient.

The following two cases are condensations of and the cases just reported. They came from a presentation given by Ronald Davis, M.D. to a medical convention.

The Reversal of Scleroderma Report of Two Cases
September 6, 1994
Ronald M. Davis, M.D.
Seabrook, TX 77586

Description: The procedures used for the arresting of the progress of two cases of severe scleroderma and the return of the patients to near normal health and activity. One patient was treated with intravenous EDTA and DMSO and with oral anti-amoebics, the other patient with intravenous EDTA and DMSO, alternating with intravenous H202, and oral anti-amoebics.

Title: The reversal of scleroderma(progressive systemic sclerosis), report of two cases.

Davis, RM

Abstract: *This is a report of the reversal of two cases of scleroderma, the first case that of a fifty year old white female with severe kidney involvement, treated with intravenous EDTA and DMSO therapy, and Metranidazole and Allopurinol tablets (according to the Rheumatoid Disease Foundation protocol). The second case is of a fifty-five year old Mexican female with early disease, but having rather severe involvement of the hands, face, and arms. She was treated with a combination of intravenous EDTA & DMSO therapy, alternating with intravenous H202 (0.03%). Metranidazole and Allopurinol tablets were also used with this patient. The response of these patients to the described therapies is outlined in this report. Conventional therapies had failed in both patients.*

Scleroderma is among the connective tissue diseases, which include systemic lupus erythematosus, rheumatoid arthritis, polymyositis-dermatomyositis, Sjogrens Syndrome, and mixed connective tissue disease. They are characterized by chronic inflammation, and a dysfunctional immune system, involving joints, serosal membranes, connective tissue and blood vessels in multiple organs (1). Kidneys and lungs are the organs most commonly affected.

The standard treatment for scleroderma consists of large doses of steroids and methotrexate as well as other anti-cancer agents, and gold therapy. These treatments, while at times do offer some relief from the disease, are attendant with unwanted, severe, and sometimes fatal side effects. Death due to the ravages of the disease is the eventual outcome. Although some cases of spontaneous remission have been reported they are very rare.

Case 1: This first case of scleroderma was a forty-nine year old lady who had been told by her rheumatologist at the Houston Medical Center, that there was nothing more he could do for her. The patient was terminally ill and she wanted to take our therapy, as she had been given no hope of recovery.The patient first began to notice a sensation of swelling and tightness of the skin, face, and extremities approximately two years prior to being seen in our office May 22,1984. These symptoms rapidly progressed to the point of rendering the patient unable to walk, or do daily household work. Evidently her kidneys had become affected early in the disease, as hypertension and headache were early symptoms. The patient had been on antihypertension medication for over one year, and on peritoneal dialysis for nearly nine months, before being seen in our office. She was under the care of a rheumatologist in Houston, and the Texas Kidney Institute at Hermann Hospital in Houston.

Medications being taken as of May 22, 1984:

Dialome - 1 t.i.d.

Compazine -25 Mg. tabs i. q.i.d. for nausea.

Capoten - 75 Mg. i. b.i.d.

Prednisone - 5 Mg i. daily.

Catapres - o.1 Mg 1 @ hs.

Peritoneal dialysis with 1 liter of solution(prepared by The Texas Kidney Institute at Hermann Hospital) in Houston.

Physical Examination:

BP 140/90 P 94 T 100/O R 20 Ht 60" Wt 109#

The patients' skin was white and glistening, and appeared to have been stretched tightly over the bony skeleton. The joints at the elbows, wrists, knees, and ankles very difficult to move. The fingers were fixed in flexion and could not be moved at all. She had the classic Mauskopf face.

Initial Laboratory Data:

Hgb. WBC Ca++ BUN Creat. Gluc. Trig. Uric A. SGOT SGPT Prot. Alb.

8.4 7400 9.3 91 8.3 113 377 6.6 28 23 7.0 3.7

Glob. LDH Phos. 24hr Creat Cl. Na+ K+ Cl- Co2

3.3 204 4.6 7.0 140 5.0 100 24

Urinalysis: S.G.1.010 Ph 5.0 Prot. 1+ Gluc. - Casts 2+rbc Bact. 1+ rbc 4-5/hpf wbc 3-4/hpf.

Chest X-ray: Negative

EKG: Sinus tachycardia, otherwise normal.

Impression: Progressive Systemic Sclerosis (Scleroderma) Nephrosclerosis with kidney failure secondary to scleroderm. Severe Anemia secondary to the two conditions above

Treatment Plan:

1. Anti-Amoebic therapy
2. I.V DMSO therapy
3. I.V. Chelation therapy.
4. Physical therapy as tolerated by the patient,

Clinical course: On May 22, 1984 anti-amoebic therapy was initiated in accordance with The Rheumatoid Disease Foundation protocol, which is as follows; Zyloprim 300 Mg t.i.d. for 7 days. Flagyl 500 Mg - two tablets A.M. and P.M. on two consecutive days a week for six weeks(2). The patient was told to continue all current medications. She experienced increased nausea and headache, plus she had severe joint pains as well as increased muscular aches and pains. These symptoms were thought to be due to a Herxheimer type reaction, for they were most bothersome following taking the Flagyl on Tuesdays and Wednesdays.

On 7/27/84 the patient received an IV of 5cc of Rimso 50 (50% DMSO) in 500cc D5W over 3 hr. timespan, without untoward effects(3). These infusions were continued three times weekly, increasing the Rimso 50 by 10cc per treatment until the maximum dose of 50cc of Rimso 50 was reached. This dosage was decided uponfollowing a telephone conversation with Dr. Stanley Jacob of the University of Oregon, this being his protocol for the treatment of scleroderma(8/27/84).

By the fourth month of therapy, the Prednisone had been gradually withdrawn and discontinued, kidneys regaining function and patient able to walk without assistance. Seven months after the initiation of therapy, enough kidney function had returned to allow stopping dialysis. The patient was feeling well and appeared well in all respects. She still had some restriction of motion of the fingers, but was improving steadily, and skin had lost its shiny slick look.

One year after beginning therapy, the patient's condition had improved to the point that it was felt we could begin adding EDTA to the infusions. This was done 5/30/85, at which time 1cc of EDTA was added to the iv as was 15cc ascorbic acid, and 2cc B-6, and given over three hours. No side effects were noted. Pts. Creat. was 2.8, her clearance was 21.7.

The EDTA was gradually increased to 8cc as the patients kidney function continued to improve. She continued improving on treatments monthly until she pronounced herself "cured" on 10/1/87. She has been on only otwo medications since that time, those medicines being Capoten 75Mg i. daily and Catapres 0.1 Mg @ Hs. The patient is leading an active, normal life.

Case 2: This fifty-five year old Mexican lady presented with tightness and swelling of face, hands, arms and feet. Her symptoms began approximately one year prior to coming to our office. She had had surgery on the right wrist for carpal tunnel syndrome in December 1990. She was supposed to have the other wrist operated on too, but since she did not improve after the first surgery, it was decided not to operate on the other wrist. She was being treated at Lyndon B. Johnson Hospital in Houston, Texas.

Medications being taken 8/12/91:

1. Acetaminophen w/codeine #3 2 tabs q 4-6 hrs. prn pain.
2. Tylenol 5oo Mg. 1 tab q 4 hrs.
3. Pen V-K tabs 250Mg. 1 tab q 6 hrs.
4. Cephalexin 250 Mg. caps 1 capsule q 6 hrs.
5. Procardia caps, 10Mg. 1 capsule t.i.d.
6. Hydroxyzine 250Mg. tabs 1 tab q 4-6 hrs. prn itching.
7. Cuprimine 250Mg. caps 1 cap b.i.d.
8. Ibuprofen 400Mg. caps 1 tab t.i.d.
9. Flexeril 10Mg. tabs 1 tab b.i.d.
10. Tagamet 300Mg. tabs 1 tab q.i.d.
11. Zantac 150Mg. tabs 1 tab b.i.d.

Physical Exam:

BP 120/80 P 74 T 99 R 16 Ht. 62" Wt. 178#

Physical findings were limited to the skin and joints. There was difficulty moving the hands and fingers. The fingers were fixed in a mild degree of flexion and patient was unable to close her fists. The skin of the hands and arms, to the mid humerus level was darkened and very firm and painful to the touch. The feet and toes were similar to the hands, as the toes could not be moved, and were edematous. The patient's skin of the feet and legs to her knees was of a darkened color similar to the arms. The skin of arms and legs had a glistening, shiny, slick appearance.

Laboratory Data: Done at LBJ Hosp. 8/12/91

Pulmonary function study was normal.

Blood studies, serum electrolytes, smac 28 were wnl.

Hgb 11.8 Hct 35.6 ESR 50 RA neg ANA Pos 1:320 Speckled pattern

Sjogren Antibodies A and B negative

Scleroderma antibodies Pos 1:640

X-rays Barium swallow negative Chest X-ray Mild cardiomegaly.

EKG Not done

Impression:

1. Progressive Systemic Sclerosis (Scleroderma).
2. Carpal Tunnel Syndrome, secondary to scleroderma,(operated);
3. Anemia, mild, secondary to 1
3. Possible mild asymptomatic cardiomyopathy secondary to 1.

Treatment Plan:

1. Anti-Amoebic therapy
2. I.V. Chelation-Dmso Therapy.
3. I.V. Hydrogen Peroxide Therapy.
4. Physical Therapy as tolerated by the patient.
5.MSM p.o. q.id.

Clinical Course: The anti-amoebic therapy was started on 8/14/91. Moderate Herxheimer reaction was noted on the first two episodes of taking the medication, but was hardly noticeable the next four treatment episodes. At the same time, IV infusions of chelation-DMSO were started and continued three times weekly. There was gradual but quite evident improvement in the patients condition over the next year. In September 1992, iv H2O2 was started three times weekly instead of the chelation-DMSO infusions. 2.5cc of 3% H2O2 in 250cc D5W, with 1.6cc NaHCO3 was the formula used in the treatment(4). This was a 0.03% solution of H2O2 .

The response to this therapy was immediate and dramatic, as the patient began to have softening of the tissues of the hands, arms, feet, and legs almost within the first week of treatment. She stated that the peroxide treatment made her "itch on the inside" of her hands, arms and feet, but the next day after the infusion she felt a lot better. She felt that the peroxide infusions were giving much better results than the chelation-Dmso infusions. Her condition continued to improve with each infusion and between infusions, even when she went 2-3 months between treatments. She has had a total of 80 chelation-DMSO infusions and 30 H2O2 infusions, and her condition is continuing to improve. The skin of her face, arms, hands, legs, and feet is normal in appearance and texture. She no longer has fatigue and malaise, and her energy and activity levels are normal. She has normal function of her hands and fingers, and is without pain.

Discussion: There seemed to be a better response of the second patient to H2O2 therapy than the chelation-DMSO therapy. It is difficult to compare the two cases, for the lady in case 1 was more acutely ill with systemic disease, which the lady in case 2 did not have, however their overall responses to treatment was excellent, albeit quite different. It was the patient in case two's opinion, and my opinion that the H2O2 infusions were superior to the Chelation-DMSO infusions. I shall continue to use both therapies, but will begin with H2O2 infusions, as well as the anti-amoebic therapy in the future.

(Also see "Thyroid Hormone Therapy: Cutting the Gordian Knot," http://www.arthritistrust.org also at Kindle.)

REFERENCES

1. Mukerji Baasanti, Alpert Martin A. Hardin Joe G When the lungs are involved by connective tissue disease. Postgraduate Medicine 1993;94(5):147

2. di Fabio, Anthony, *Rheumatoid Diseases Cured At Last*, Franklin TN,1982, The Arthritis Trust of America/The Rheumatoid Disease Foundation, 7111 Sweetgum Road, Fairview, TN 37062; see http://www.arthritistrust.org.

3. Halstead BW, Youngberg S. The DMSO Handbook Colton CA 1981 Golden Quill Publishers Inc. P.O Box 1278 Colton CA 92324

4.Farr CH Workbook on Free Radical Chemistry and Hydrogen Peroxide Metabolism including protocol for the intravenous administration of hydrogen peroxide Oklahoma City OK 1989 IBOM Foundation P.O. Box 891954 Oklahoma City, OK 73189

5. Cranton EM, Bypassing Bypass Medex Publishers Inc. Ripshin Rd., P.O. Box 44 Troutdale VA 24378-0044 1982

6. Halstead BW The Scientific Basis of Chelation Therapy, Colton, CA 1979 Golden Quill Publishers Inc. P.O. Box 1278 Colton CA 92324

7. Cranton EM A Textbook on EDTA Chelation Therapy J of Adv Med

2(1/2) 1989

8. Douglas WC Hydrogen Peroxide MEDICAL MIRACLE Atlanta GA 1992 Second Opinion Publishing P.O. Box 467939 Atlanta GA 30346-7939

Author: Ronald M. Davis, M.D. 5002 Todville, Seabrook, TX 77586

Acknowledgements:

Stanley W. Jacob, M.D., Oregon Health Sciences Univ. Portland, Oregon who saw the patient in case 1 in consultation in July 1984, and for his assistance via telephone conversations regarding his DMSO protocol.

Charles H. Farr MD, PhD , for the many interruptions in his busy schedule, to assist in the care of both of the patients, with answering questions about protocols of EDTA, DMSO, and H2O2 therapies.

Garry Gordon, MD 5335 Compass, Tempe AZ 85283 without whose help I would probably not have gotten involved in chelation and other alternative therapies.

Katy Thompson, M.D., Texas Kidney Institute, Hermann Hospital, Houston, Texas for her kind assistance and co-operation in the care of the patient in case 1.

Blood Type and its Influence on Diet

by Gregory Kelly, N.D.

All rights reserved by the The Roger Wyburn-Mason and Jack M.Blount Foundation for Eradication of Rheumatoid Disease AKA The Arthritis Trust of America ®

Permission to publish granted by Gregory Kelly, N.,D.

The basic premise of this article is that if you use your blood type as a guide for the daily selection of foods, you will be healthier, you will reach your ideal body weight, and you just might slow the aging process.

With the abundance of diet plans available, an obvious question to ask is, "Which diet should I choose to follow?" The truth is we can no more choose the right diet than we can our hair or eye color. It has already been chosen for us, and the secret of it lies in an aspect of our genetic blueprint known as our blood type. Accordingly, there are no absolute right or wrong lifestyles or diets; there are only right or wrong choices based on each individual's genetic code.

Anthropologists have speculated that blood types historically evolved due to changes in diet, culture, and social conditions. Due to these differing environmental factors, each blood type has particular strengths and limitations. When these tendencies are known and diet is modified to maximize an individuals genetic strengths, it becomes easier to maintain health. So, the first critical component of the blood type diet revolves around the question of which foods your blood type ancestors had available, and thrived upon.

A second critical component of the blood type diet is the idea that some foods might contain substances with opposing blood type activity. Every life form has unique antigens that form part of their chemical signature. Similarly, each blood type possesses an antigen with a unique chemical structure. Blood type antigens are ubiquitous throughout the body and are among the most powerful antigens involved in the process of identification of "friend or foe." When the body senses foreign antigens, antibodies are generated which defend the body against the invaders. The "anti-other-blood" type antibodies are among the strongest antibodies in our immune system. For example blood type A contains the A antigen on cells and correspondingly produces an antibody against blood group B. Blood type B, on the other hand, has the opposite configuration, with a B antigen on cells and production of antibodies against blood type A. Blood type O produces antibodies against the A antigen and the B antigen, while blood type AB produces no anti-ABO blood group activity.

In the case of an inappropriate blood transfusion, these antibodies can generate a life threatening reaction; however, little attention has been shown to these antibodies in other contexts. Fortunately (or unfortunately) many foods have components which might look similar enough to an opposing blood group antigen to generate a mild antibody response. For example, the antibody created by blood type A looks for anything that is B-like, and B-like substances contain a sugar known as galactosamine. So eating foods which contain this sugar might provoke an unwanted immune response.

The last major piece of the blood type puzzle has to do with dietary proteins known as lectins. It has long been recognized that some foods are capable of causing the cells of a certain blood type to agglutinate while having no impact on cells of another blood type. While other foods will actually indiscriminately agglutinate cells of all blood types. These reactions are dependent upon the interaction of human cells with specific lectins found in food.

A lectin can simplistically be defined (note: the actual definition is more complicated) as any compound found in nature, usually diverse protein structures, which can interact with surface antigens found on the body's cells, causing them to agglutinate. Following ingestion of food containing a detrimental lectin, a chemical reaction can occur between the food you eat and your blood or tissues because of these lectins.

As a general rule, blood type O thrives on animal protein and tends to experience a great deal of health problems when they eat a lot of grains and beans. Some specific foods to avoid include wheat, corn, dairy, cauliflower, and oranges.

Type A individuals thrive on a vegetarian diet. Considered to have evolved as a primary blood type to deal with the historical challenges associated with farming and cultivation, blood type A individuals typically do not have the digestive capacity to deal with large quantities of animal protein, but can metabolize a wide range of grains and beans effectively. Soy, lentils, buckwheat, some fish, and plenty of vegetables energizes these individuals.

Blood type B is considered to be the nomad and has the greatest range of food choices. This blood type is typically thrives on most dairy products, and does well on meats like lamb and venison. Although individuals with this blood type have the most dietary flexibility, certain common foods such as chicken and corn can be very aggravating.

Blood type AB represents a merging of Types A and B; blending strengths and weaknesses of these two blood types. Like Type B, AB's require meat protein; but, because of their A-like sensitive digestive tract and naturally low stomach acid, AB's need smaller and less frequent portions. Because of the enigmatic blend of the A and B blood types, type AB individuals tend to have health challenges if they consume foods that are detrimental to either type A's or type B's.

A fuller explanation of the role of blood types and health, as well as comprehensive recommendations of foods to include and omit from your diet based upon your blood type, can be found in the book *Eat Right for Your Type* published by G.P. Putnam's Son's (ISBN 0-399-14255-X.) Information on blood type and diet can also be accessed at Peter J. D'Adamo's, N.D., web-site at http://www.dadamo.com.

Here is how to make Coley's Toxins
by
Wayne E. Martin, B.S.

Wayne Martin was born June 17, 1911 and died May 13, 2006. He was a professional chemist who, during America's great depression era, wanted to be a medical doctor but could not afford medical school. Still his interest in medicine stayed with him until his death.

During the past twenty four years we've been fortunate to have Wayne Martin as one of our most esteemed advisors. Wayne was not just a knowledgeable advisor, but also a fine friend, one who unstiningly gave of his medical knowledge to whomever inquired.

Wayne Martin graduated from Purdue University with a BS in Chemical Engineering in 1933 with major emphasis on biochemistry and bacteriology. Depression years prevented him from obtaining a medical degree, his first love, but did not stop him from a lifetime of interesting synthesis of the world's medical literature, often resulting in discoveries of interesting treatments used today by many complementary/alternative medical practitioners.

His professional work in Chemical Engineering also resulted in remarkable findings results of which are still used by people everywhere. Ninety percent of the beryllium copper alloys used worldwide contain 1.80% of beryllium instead of the more expensive form of 2.2 to 2.5% beryllium set by Germans at the Siemans and Haliske Company. Working at the Beryllium Corporation, Wayne Martin in 1935 discovered that the 1.80% beryllium to copper alloy (Berylco 180) was superior in many ways and less expensive. For more than fifty years automobiles — and you — have used Wayne Martin's beryllium alloy.

Early in World War II, at the Sperry Gyroscope Company, and also as a "dollar-a-year" consultant with The War Production Board (WPB), Wayne Martin developed two National Emergency (N.E.) aluminum casting alloys (319, 380). Ninety-five percent of today's aluminum castings are made of these two alloys. Sixty million pounds monthly of this aluminum alloy is currently used to produce the modern automobile.

At end of World War II, the Beryllium Corporation was stuck with a plant owned by the Atomic Energy Commission for which they wanted a peace-time use. Wayne suggested that it be used to make potassium titanium fluoride. The entire aluminum industry uses it to grain-refine aluminum. After it's return to the Atomic Energy Commission, Henry Kawecki, Wayne's friend, formed the Kawecki Chemical Company to manufacture potassium fluoride, becoming a multimillion dollar firm, all on Wayne's ideas.

In 1950 Wayne Martin helped to place aluminum/magneisum alloy (AL MG 35) for which there was a large market. In 1960 he developed another aluminum alloy (Precedent 71) which, over a period of 20 years, made his employer, U.S. Reduction Company, a great deal of money. (Think of the skin of airplanes, among other uses.)

Wayne retired in 1979, becoming a salesman with The Southern Aluminum Casting Company of Bay Minette, Alabama. Thereafter each retirement has led to further consulting jobs, so he never truly retired.

So why was a Chemical Engineer who invented important metal alloys featured here as a consultant in medicine?

Although the great American depression had steered him elsewhere for survival's sake, he never lost touch with medicine. His enquiring mind synthesized many medical articles and research papers to bring to light remarkable treatments in heart, cancer, and other medical problems.

In one example from years' gone by, in 1963 Wayne organized the Nutrition Research Products Company dedicated to doing something about the 600,000 deaths each year from heart attacks. His idea was carried to The Royal College of Surgeons and The National Heart Hospital in London, England, where Nutrition Research Products Company spent $200,000, and proved that his ideas were effective in preventing heart disease.

Wayne periodically gave himself weak hydrochloric acid shots because he'd learned — long before the advent of antibiotics — that administration of these weakened solutions stimulated macrophage and leucocyte activity, thus killing and/or warding off invasive infections. (See *Three Years of Hydrochloric Acid Therapy*, http://www.arthritistrust.org, "Books and Pamphlets" tab.) His story about the Harvard medical school graduate who became wealthy by specializing in this treatment in Las Vegas, NV was very educational as well as hilarious.

Wayne had a lifetime love affair with the study of problems related to the heart and circulation and also with various types of cancers.

Many years before the expenditure of billions of dollars to "find the cure for cancer," Coley's toxin was bringing about remarkable "permanent remissions." This so aggravated the medical monetary and power structure that the simple mixture was forbidden. Having seen at first hand cures brought about by this mixture in his early adulthood, Wayne could never cease telling about it. Some years ago he invested a good sum of his own money to have the product made in Brazil, thus making it available to any patient who wished to use it.

Again, alas! Tthe long arm of "forbidden medicine" reached into Brazil, and the US supply was again halted.

Nonetheless, Wayne found another way to help cancer patients by publishing the formula for Coley's toxin so that any patient or doctor can make up their own supply, if desired.

But even prior to his publication of Coley's toxin, certain doctor friends began manufacturing their own Coley's toxin and are having great success in bringing about "permanent remissions," among some of their patients!

Wayne Martin's thinking about medical treatment has been frequently reported in *Townsend Letter for Doctors & Patients* (911 Tyler St., Port Townsend, WA 98368-6541; http://www.towsendletter.com). It is there one should go for his many articles.

In his youth, Martin's motorcycle accident resulted in loss of a leg. Phantom pain haunted him for years until he discovered that it could easily and safely be diminished thru the use of ginger.

Martin's recommendations for the safe easing of pain through the use of ginger can be found in our Arthritis Trust of America Summer 2001 Newsletter at http://www.arthritistrust.org, "Newsletters" tab. Some of his writings are also found on the same website under the button "Research "and then "Research Papers and Letters."

Martin was a remarkable human being, one who cared greatly for his fellow man, who gave without concern for rewards, who loved life, and who made each hour, each minute count toward bettering his fellow man.

We are so glad that he passed away peacefully — not in pain or suffering from degenerative disease — just a few months before his 95th birthday! But, we are not at all happy that he passed so early in his life — and we shall sorely miss this intelligent, generous, kind scientific advisor!

Let Wayne speak for us as the following comments also describe how to make Coley's Toxin.

But first a bit of history on Coleys Toxins. Dr. William Coley was a young surgeon in New York City .in 1890, aged 28. The first 110 pages of Stephen Hall's book *A Commotion in the Blood,* Henry Holt and Company New York 1997 is about Coley and Coley's. Toxins. The following story in part is from this book.

In 1890 a young late teen age woman named Bessie Dashiell came to Coley with a painful injury to one hand. She had taken a long trip by rail and had injured her hand in a Pullman car seat. In time the injury proved to be round cell sarcoma.

Coley amputated her hand but the cancer spread throughout her body and she died a horrible death. Coley was shaken by her death and said there has to be a better way to treat cancer, He spent many hours of his spare time going through the records of New York Hospital and he found a clue.

In 1885 a poor German immigrant named Stein had had surgery for round cell sarcoma four times and was considered as being hopeless. At this time he was infected with erysipelas. He nearly died from the infection but the cancer was gone.

Coley then spent many hours in the lower east side ghetto and at last he found Stein — in the best of good health six years later.

Coley then determined to infect late stage cancer patients with erysipelas, He did not have to wait long. The patient was another immigrant named Zola.. The case of Zola was almost the case of Stein. Coley had much trouble getting an infection started with Zola and when he did it was so severe that he feared Zola would die of the infection but as in the case of Stein, Zola went into remission that proved to be a cure.

Coley then began to treat twelve late stage cancer patients by infecting them with erysipelas. With two patients, they died from the infection. With one patient there was an infection with a fever of 105 degrees Fahreheit.

In this case the patient's tumors disappeared but there was a recurrence that caused death. Of the other nine patients, he could not infect them,

Coley then turned to a killed vaccine of erysipelas, killed by heating to 66 degrees centigrade for two hours, This vaccine caused a mild fever reaction but not strong enough to be an anticancer treatment, Coley then added the newly discovered *Bacillus prodigiosus* now called *Serratia marcescens* to the vaccine. It was killed by heating to 66 degrees Centigrade.

This was and is Coley's Toxins. It was injected into a tumor or done as intradermal injections. First the patient was cold followed by a fever of 101 degrees to 104 degrees for a few hours.

The first patient to be treated with Coley's Toxins was a boy. His name was John Ficken. He had a large tumor of malignant sarcoma in the abdomen that had been like a bowling ball. It was considered that the patient was hopeless. On Jan. 24, 1893 an injection of the new Coley's Toxins was done in the tumor, The reactions to the injections were severe chills and fever. The injections were done every other day for .3.5 months. By this time the boy's tumor had decreased by 80 %. Coley stopped treatment then. The boy was gaining back lost weight. The boy was sent home at this time and was traced in 1907 still alive and well. So Coley had a success with his first cancer patient treated with Coley's Toxins..

Coley then started to treat cancer patients with Coley's Toxins with a degree of success. Other doctors were beginning to get Coley's Toxins from Coley. Here will be given a case of success in the treatment of breast cancer, The patient was a 42 year old woman in New Britain, Connecticut, in Oct. 1895. She had a tumor on one breast the size of an orange. She had lost 29 lbs in weight. Her doctor was M. Storrs of the Hartford Hospital.. She was considered as being inoperable. On Dec. 16, 1895, injections were begun with Coley's Toxins.in the tumor. Injections were given every second day. Injections were then changed to one a day. It was thought that her temperature reached 104 degrees. The tumor began to shrink in size and there was much necrotic tissue to be removed from the tumor. By March of 1896 the tumor had disappeared. Most of the treatments had been done at her home. The patient had gained the 29 pounds she had lost. She remained well until her death in 1943 of heart disease at an age of 80.

In Dec. 15, 1894, there was an editorial in the AMA's publication JAMA saying that Coley's Toxins was useless in cancer treatment.

By the spring of 1896, Coley had treated 160 cancer patients with his Toxins. Nearly half of these 160 patients had shown a degree of benefit but with a few of them the results had been nothing short of remarkable.

In 1897 Coley took the post of head of the sarcoma ward at Memorial

Hospital in New York City. Meanwhile the Mayo Brothers had come strong for Coley's Toxins in treating cancer..

Then we must consider Dr. Jam's Ewing. He was a pathologist who came to Memorial Hospital about the same time as Coley. In time he was known to the news media as Mr. Cancer and he developed for Coley and his toxins the most bitter animosity. He thought that the newly discovered radium and the X ray machine was the Utopian cure for cancer.

Ewing attracted the interest of James Douglas CEO of the Phelps — Dodge Corp. Douglas had a daughter with breast cancer. Ewing, Douglas and his daughter went to England were she could be treated with radium. The treatment failed and she died of breast cancer, this after the first breast cancer patient cured by Coley's Toxins as has been reported. in this letter.

Douglas was not swayed by the death of his daughter. He formed a firm for the mining of radium and made a gift of several hundred thousand dollars worth of radium to Memorial Hospital and in return for the gift, Ewing was made medical director of Memorial Hospital. Ewing became Coley's boss and Coley's worst enemy.

For many years Coley could not treat sarcoma patients with Coley's Toxins and he must treat them with radium. For several years Coley's sarcoma patients were treated with radium only and not one of them was helped in the least.

Meanwhile not far from Memorial Hospital one of the most dramatic cures of cancer by Coley's Toxins took place. The patient was an officer in the merchant marine, The time was 1926. The patient had recticulun cell sarcoma, His leg had been amputated at the hip. Three months later there was a metastasis above the umbilicus. One month later there was a fist sized tumor on the amputated stump. One month later the amputated stump was increasing in size.and there was another orange size tumor on the stump.

Coley's Toxins were injected into the stump. There were signs of regression but the reactions were severe and the patient asked for a respite. During the respite the cancer spread at an alarming rate. The stump had increased in size to 30 inches in circumference and the end of the stump had broken down to a great ulcer from which there was a foul smelling discharge. There were several more tumors, in the scalp, verterbrea, and cranial bones.

Injections were begun again in the stump. Large doses of Coley's Toxins were injected every day. The patient suffered from severe reactions but after 28 days the ulcer in the stump healed and the stump had returned to its normal size. All his other tumors had either vanished or were now very small in size. His doctors wanted to continue with the treatment but the patient said that he had had enough. Sixty days later there was no sign of cancer, The patient"lived free of cancer until 1959 when he died of a heart attack.

Dr. Ernest Codman of the Harvard Medical School had for a long time sided with Ewing as saying that Coley's Toxins were useless in the treatment of cancer but in 1935, one year before the death of Coley, he changed his position and said that the use of Coley's Toxins had produced from time to time miracles in cancer treatment. His observation did no good for in 1936 Coley died and for the time Coley's Toxins died with him.

Pages could be written about the miracles in cancer cures by Coley's Toxins. Two of the miracles will be given here.

In 1912 in Kentville, Nova Scotia, there was a 26 year old woman with far advanced renal cell carcinoma. She was taken by auto the 40 miles to a hospital in Halifax. There a surgeon did surgery on her. He took one look and sewed her back up. He felt that she was so hopeless that she would not survive the trip back to Kentville. By then it was understood that an overdose of Coley's Toxins could cause death. Her doctor had some Coley's Toxins and he injected what he thought to be a lethal dose hoping to end her suffering. It was just the right dose to do wonders for her, She was given 18 injections in the buttocks of Coley's Toxins over the next 18 days. And six weeks later she was free from signs of cancer. She was traced 40 years later still free from cancer,

Coley's daughter Helen Coley Nauts founded in 1953 Cancer Research Institute and it has grown large and prestigious. In 1956 she had Coley's Toxins made at the Memorial.

The American Cancer Society was founded in 1913 and has been a bitter enemy of Coley's Toxins.

In June of 1962, an amendment to the Pure Food and Drug act was passed giving great power to our FDA. At this time the American Cancer Society had a list of unproven treatments of cancer and Coley's Toxins was on that list.

The American Cancer Society held that Coley's Toxins had never helped a cancer patient. The act was called the Kefauver-Harris Amendment. It had a grandfather clause that made legal any drug or vaccine that had a record of success before 1962. Aspirin was at once made legal but with the American Cancer Society saying that Coley's Toxins had never helped a cancer patient, Coley's Toxins was declared to be illegal.

With that background will be told an astounding success of treating hopeless cancer with Coley's Toxins. The time was February of 1961. The patient was a retired contractor. The place was the Baptist Hospital in Oklahoma City. The patient had had surgery for colon cancer. There followed a massive reoccurrence. The liver was enlarged and there were metastases in the peritoneum and lungs.

His doctor was tapping and removing two quarts of bloody fluid from the abdomen each day and one quart of fluid from the lungs. every second day. The fluid from both the lungs and abdomen had cancer cells. Death was expected in a week or so.

Intradermal injections in the buttock was started with Coley's Toxins. There was aching and pain. There were shaking chills with fever of 1020. The injections were done for eight days only and then the miracle happened. There was no more fluid in the lungs after 24 hours. After three days, there was no more fluid to be removed from the abdomen. On day eight of the injections, the patient was feeling fine and the injections were stopped. A week later the patient was gaining lost weight and he was sent home. He was alive and well in 1970 nine years later.

Other cancer patients were being treated with Coley's Toxins and showing benefit but their treatment suddenly stopped. After June of 1962.

Now to tell how to make Coley's! Toxins. From 1894 until 1906 Coley's Toxins was made by Dr B.H. Buxton of Cornell University.

He soaked one pound of ground beef over night in 1,000 cc of water. Then he boiled it for one hour and filtered through cotton cloth. Then was added 10 grams of peptone and 5 grams of sodium chloride. Then it was tested with litmus to get the solution slightly alkaline. It was then boiled for one hour. It was filtered through filter paper. Then it was boiled for one half hour on three days in a row. It was then seeded with a live streptocococcus solution and let stand for 10 days. The solution needs a cover but the growth needs air. It should be cloudy. Then a few cc of the live *Bacillus prodigiosus* was added to the solution and allowed to grow for ten days more.

Then it was heated for two hours at 58 degrees C. A bit of thymol was added. The vaccine was stored at 2 to 4 degrees C.

From 1906 until 1920 Dr Martha Tracy who had worked with Buxton changed the way she made the vaccine. She grew the two bacteria separately. Then she did a nitrogen determination on the *B. prodigiosus* and, depending on what she found, she added a certain amount of *Bacillus prodigiosus* to the streptococcus growth. I do not like this way of making the vaccine. If one makes a mistake in doing the nitrogen determination and one gets too much of the *B.prodigiosus*, the vaccine will turn very toxic. Making the vaccine as per Buxton, one will never get a toxic vaccine.

In 1990 I had a call from Don Carrow M.D. in Tampa. wanting to know how to make Coley's Toxins. I sent him the above information, Rather than using beef broth, he used as a broth Difcco AOAC, a product of Difco Laboratories in Detroit. In 1,000 cc of water he added 15 grams of Difco AOAC, 10 grams of Bacto peptone — another Difco product — 5 grams of sodium chloride and 100 grams of glucose. He got the pH to 7.1 to 7.2.

He then added a few cc of live streptococcus solution and let it stand at 36 degrees C for 10 days. Then he got the 1,000 cc to 25 degrees C and seeded it with live *Serratia marcescens* and let it grow for another ten days. It was heated to 65 degrees C for two hours to get a killed vaccine.

222

He then added 0.03 cc per cc of benzyl alcohol.

It was stored at 20 to 40 degrees C. The 1,000 cc was then filtered through a seven micron filter. Care must be taken not to remove the dead bacteria..

He had a cancer patient ready to treat with his Coley's Toxins. She was a 50 year old nurse with non-Hodgkin's lymphoma. She had a tumor under one arm that was the size of a football. He injected his Coley' Toxins into the center of that big tumor with a three inch long needle. Injections were done each day that produced first shaking chills and then a fever of 104 degrees Fahrenheit. I do not know how many injections were given but the tumor was reduced to a flabby bag which was removed by surgery. The bag contained no cancer cells. Dr Carrow reported in 2002 that the patient was cancer free.

Dr. Carrow died in that year. That is why his name is being used, In 1990 he had a problem with the Florida State Board of Medical Examiners. Coley's Toxins was not the problem. I know that he continued to treat cancer with Coley's Toxins but I was not told of the results.

I am now in contact with two doctors. Their names will not be given. One doctor, Doctor X in Ohio wanted to know how to make Coley's Toxins. I sent him the information given in this letter. He made a great lot of some very good vaccine and he sent me the way he made Coley's Toxins.

He got the live *Streptococcus pyolgenes*, ATTC 19615 and the live *Serratia marcescens* ATTC # 13880 from Micro Biologics www.microbiologics.com in the form of Kwik-Stics. For a broth he used the Todd-Hewitt broth. It was obtained as a powder and is used as a 3 % solution. He used 500 cc of water. To it was added 15 grams of the Todd-Hewitt powder and 50 grams of glucose. The flask was plugged with a plastic foam stopper and autoclaved for 15 minutes at 121 degrees C. The broth was allowed to cool and was stored at 40 degrees C for 3 weeks.

The broth was then seeded with the live streptococcus and allowed to grow at 36 degrees C for seven days. The culture was then gotten to 25 degrees C and was seeded with the live *Serratia marcescens* and allowed to grow for seven more days, The culture then was killed by heating to 65 degrees C for two hours. Then 7.5 cc of benzyl alcohol was added. The 500 cc of the killed vaccine was then filtered with a 15 micron filter. It was stored at 40 degrees C ready for use.

I have just talked to Dr.X. He had much to tell of success in treating cancer with the Coley's Toxins he made. He had had what he called two complete remissions of cancer. He has been giving his Coley's Toxins to a doctor friend in Arizona who is having even greater success with it. He reports a breast cancer patient with bone metastases who had great benefit in a very short time.

Now to tell of Dr. Y of Alabama. But first here is some background. As a student at Purdue University, in 1932, I had a professor of bacteriology who thought well of Coley's Toxins and he had exchanged letters with Coley. Coley had sent him the instructions for making Coley's Toxins. That is how I knew how to make Coley's Toxins.

In 1985 I went to Guatemala and found a bacteriologist and gave him $200.00 to make 1,000 cc of Coley's Toxins. Then I found a doctor with a small hospital. He agreed to put American cancer patients in his hospital and to treat them with injections in the vein of Coley's Toxins. They could stay in his hospital for 30 days and get 20 IV injections of Coley's Toxins. The cost to the patient was $1,000.00. Then I put the word out to several doctors. One patient from near Pittsburg came. She was aged 65 and had ovarian cancer.

She was badly swollen in the abdomen and her CA 125 was over 6,000. She stayed in the hospital for 30 days, and had 20 IV injections of Coley's Toxins, She felt much better. The swelling had greatly decreased and her CA 125 had been reduced to just over 2.,000. She needed more treatment but she returned to the USA.

Meanwhile a doctor in the government of Guatemala told the Minister of Health that the American Cancer Society had Coley's Toxins listed as an unproven remedy. Coley's Toxins was banned in Guatemala. I do not know what happened to the patient.

I had about 800 cc of my Coley's Toxins sent to me. About two years ago I gave the 800 cc of Coley's Toxins to Dr, Y in Alabama. He has added a new diminution to the treatment with Coley's Toxins. He will do an IV of Coley's Toxins in his office. He will then show the patients how to do the injections at home as self medication, and send them home with a 20 cc bottle of Coldy's Toxins. He will tell the patient to have rectal suppositories of Tylenol on hand which will terminate a reaction to Coley's Toxins quickly..

The patient is to do an injection at about 8:00 AM. For an hour the patient will feel cold and may shake. Then the fever will come on and the pulse will increase to about 125. The patient is told to check temperature and pulse every hour. If the fever exceeds 104 degrees F or if the pulse exceeds 135, terminate the reaction with Tylenol. This will not happen often. The fever should end by 6:00 PM.

We should be able to do better than Coley did. He did not have Tylenol. He knew that an overdose of Coley's Toxins could cause death so he had to use lower doses than he would like to use. Having Tylenol on hand will permit the use of higher doses.Then, in Coley's time, it was a hard rule that nothing must be put in a vein. Now it is understood that injections of Coley's Toxins in the vein give greater reactions. The injections can be done every day or every second day.

The injections are done for 30 days and then for one week there are no injections and then the injections are resumed.

All these instructions are given to the patient. Some times the treatment need be done for two or three months. By doing the injections at home, the patient can get two months of treatment that could not be had otherwise and the cost is kept down.

Dr Y has had two complete remissions of cancer and two failures.

In 1935 Coley gave a lecture at the University of Glasgow in which he told of treating several hundred cancer patients with sarcoma. Of them, about one third had remissions that left them free of cancer at 5 years.

His daughter Helen Coley Nauts found good records of just less than 1,000 cancer patients who had been treated with Coley's Toxins. Of them about half had remissions that left them free from cancer at 5 years.

Coley' daughter, Helen Coley Nauts, has told me that at Cancer Research Institute it is felt that the main anti-cancer effect of Coley's Toxins is the anti-cancer effect of fever and of interferon and tumor necrosis factor which are increased during the reaction. I sent a FAX to Professor Leo Zacharski M.D Dartmouth Medical School. He said that Coley's Toxins contains some streptokinase. He said he knew of a woman with endometrial cancer with metastases . She had a heart attack and was treated with an infusion of streptokinase. It terminated the heart attack and her tumors showed a marked regression which has persisted for several months. He was hoping to see a trial on treating cancer with an infusion of streptokinase but he suggested that streptokinase in Coley's Toxins was part of its anti-cancer effect.

I also mde contact with Dr. S. Moncada, Medical Director of the Wellcome Research Laboratories. He said that in the fever reaction to Coley's Toxins or in an infection of erysipelas., the arginine to nitric oxide pathway is activated for the production of nitric oxide which has a strong anti-cancer effect.

I have told in this letter of three doctors who are having some success in treating cancer with Coley's Toxins.

It is hoped that a few doctor readers of this letter will want to make Coley's Toxins and treat some cancer patients with it.

Wayne Martin BS ChE

Copper Therapy for Rheumatoid Disease
by
Seldon Nelson, D.O. and Anthony di Fabio

As has happened to so many of our (Arthritis Trust of America) founding doctors, they've passed along ahead of me. I (di Fabio) suppose I should be grateful that I'm still here to tell some of their story.

I met Seldon at a medical conference held in a modern hotel in New Orleans. We met in the middle of a large room, shook hands and began talking.

The night before I had been walking on — I think — Bourbon street. One of the night clubs lining that street had cut out its side wall so that those walking along could see and hear the Dixieland band that was truly whooping it up.

Now I love Dixieland, Ragtime and Classical about evenly, so I stopped to watch and listen. There, in front of me in the middle of the street was a male African-American perhaps of middle age. He was tap dancing to the Dixieland music, but not quite a proper type of tap dance. Perhaps his tap dancing was more of a home made variety.

I was fascinated because I loved every form of dancing, one time during my life dancing fast jitterbug dancing 365 days a year, year in and year out.

I stared hard, and did my best to imitate this person. I lost myself in this serious concentration.

I looked up and surrounding us both was a large crowd of visitors like myself. Quite embarrassed — because I was lower than a novice at this kind of dancing — I quit and went back to my hotel.

Now that's not the story. The story begins here.

When I met Dr. Seldon Nelson out in the middle of this huge, fancy conference room I told him all about my embarrassment in trying to reproduce the African Americans tap dancing and being watched by such a large crowd of visitors.

Seldon looked at me quite seriously and then said, "Oh, you mean like this?" and he begin perfect tap dancing.

Somewhat shocked, impressed and entertained all at the same time I blurted out, "Where did you learn that?"

"Oh, I was a tap dancer before I became a doctor!"

Now I ask you, how many good doctors can say that?

Dr. Nelson wrote that the late Roger Wyburn-Mason of London, England proved that copper is one of the very best compounds to kill the Amoebae thought to be the cause of rheumatoid diseases. These germs seem to play a very important part in causing or complicating the majority of disease I refered to as the Rheumatoid Diseases. Some of these diseases include Rheumatoid Arthritis, Lupus Erythematosis, Scleroderma, Periarteritis Nodosa, Dermatomyositis, Psoriasis, Thyroiditis, Fibrositis, Endometriosis, Erythema Nodosum, Multiple Sclerosis, Myasthenia Gravis, Crohn's Disease, Ulcerative Colitis, some Diabetes and certain forms of Cancer as well as a

226

number of other diseases.

The problem in America is that there are not many medications that will kill the Amoebae effectively. Also some drugs I presently use to kill the amoebae do not kill all of the germs adequately. This is probably due to the fact that certain amoebae seem to be resistant to the presently used medications. The Rheumatoid Disease Foundation (of which I am a founding member) is presently paying for double blind studies on Clotrimazole which is a very effect-ive drug, but it will be at least a year before available. We desperately need more effective medications that will rid the body of those Amoebae that have been resistant to the presently available drugs.

I have known that when germs or organisms that are more complex or more highly developed than normal bacteria or commonly known germs are killed in a patient, certain toxins are re-leased and the body has to get rid of the dead germs. The Amoebae which cause Rheumatoid Disease are highly developed and quite complex as are the germs that cause Syphilis, Leprosy or African Sleeping Sickness. When any of these diseases are effectively treated, the organi-sms are killed and in the process of ridding the body of the dead germs, these patients can develop numerous flu-like symptoms called a Herxheimer Reaction. This is a good reaction in the sense that the body is getting rid of the dead germs. These flu-like symptoms may include temporary increase in joint pains (get worse before getting better), headaches, chilly sensa-tions, low grade fever, nausea, mild diarrhea, aching all over, skin crawling sensations and a general feeling of weakness. These symptoms are temporary and should encourage a patient to realize that he is responding to the treatment.

Copper is a substance that very effectively kills the Amoebae but the problem is that the only available copper for giving patients has been in the form of salts such as copper sulfate. These salts are poorly absorbed in the intestine and commonly cause severe nausea and vomiting. They are therefore not acceptable in the majority of patients. Copper Aspirinate however causes the fewest problems and is quite effective in most patients.

A new method of getting pure copper into the body has recently been developed which appears to be quite effective in killing the Amoebae. This form of copper is much more active than most available salts and since the amount of copper that is effective is only 3-4 times the body's minimum daily requirements of copper, it is totally safe. It is quite effective and easily taken although it causes a Herxheimer reaction in those patients who are infected with the Amoebae. It is taken by placing very tiny granules or beads coated with copper under the tongue for about one minute. The copper is absorbed directly into the blood stream (in the same way nitroglycerine for heart patients does) leaving the tiny uncoated resin granules which can be swallowed or spit out. The Herxheimer reaction usually begins in about four to eight hours, but it has been observed in as little as 10 minutes and as delayed as 3 days, depending on how severely infected with the Amoebae the patient is. The granules are taken twice daily and are taken until the patient does not have any more Herxheimer Reaction to the copper. This usually is six to eight weeks if the patient takes the copper correctly. When no further Herxheimer Reaction is noted this signifies that no more Amoebae are being killed and the patient can stop taking the copper. Patients being treated however, should take the granules for at least six weeks.

For treating most Rheumatoid Diseases the patient should start out by placing 8 granules under the tongue for one minute 3x daily. If the Herxheimer Reaction is tolerable and not severe, the patient can increase the granules by 2-3 each day (making 8-9 granules 3x daily) until a level or number of granules taken 3x daily is reached at which the Herx-heimer Reaction can be comfortably tolerated. The dosage should be increased no higher than 75 granules 3x daily, however. It is very important that the patient increase the number of granules by 2-3 each day until the tolerated level is reached. This will rid the body of the Amoebae much faster. Copper in this form is a nutrient and not a drug.

In treating Multiple Sclerosis, it is very important to follow a different method of taking the granules. <u>The Patient with Multiple Sclerosis should start out by taking only one granule twice daily</u>. I do not want patients with Multiple Sclerosis to have a severe Herxheimer Reaction as this could aggravate their condition. The granules can be slowly increased by adding one granule extra twice daily until a very mild Herxheimer Reaction is noted. The patient should continue this dosage daily until the Reaction begins to go away before increasing the number of granules. If any questions arise or any problems develop, the patient should contact me immediately.

The beauty about this method of treatment is that a patient can regulate the severity of the Herxheimer reaction. A patient should know that the more severe the reaction is, the more Amoeba are being killed and the patient's disease condition should improve faster. Should a patient require doing something one day in which the reaction would make that something more difficult, the patient can simply cut down on the number of granules that day. however it must be emphasized that the patients must increase the daily dosage up to the maximum (30 granules twice daily) and get the Herxheimer Reaction to-get the best results

Should any patient have any questions I urge   patient to call my office or myself at any time. Good luck, God bless you and I'm looking forward to your complete recovery.

Systemic Enzyme Therapy
by
Hector E. Solorzano del Rio, M.D., D.Sc, Ph.D,

People must know that the correct medical name for the therapeutic use of natural enzymes is "Systemic Enzyme Therapy." This means that enzymes flow throughout our body, producing the desired healing effects.

For an accurate description of Systemic Enzyme Therapy, one needs to know a little bit about the structure and function of enzymes, in general.

You must know that without enzymes, there is no possibility of life, in animals, plants or persons. Enzymes are essential for each and every reaction in a living organism.

We could even follow the arising of life on earth, if we think of enzymes that were necessary for the evolution in each stage. Oxygen from the air arose because certain new enzymes were formed by single plants that released oxygen. These plants had learned to produce certain enzymes that separate oxygen from carbon dioxide in the air. Today, we accurately know how this works. Every second we change; every second we become a new human being. This is because more than 2,700 different enzymes act with an incredible speed to keep our vital functions in order.

Since ancient times it was known by Egyptians and the Arabians that there was an invisible force which made all living things shift. It was a mysterious force that transforms one substance into another; milk became a cheese, grapefruit to wine, etc.

Enzymes are catalysts, or rather we should say, "biocatalysts." We are dealing with determined substances whose presence causes the transformation of an organic substance and it also accelerates it, just as a catalyst would do it. Today we know what these enzymes are and how they act.

Catalysts produce, with a small effort, a big effect. Nature can not waste energy. In technical terms, enzymes are albuminoid, macromolecular bodies, with a complex structure and are active biocatalytically speaking. These albumins are made of 20 different amino acids. Each enzyme is specific not only in its substratum (the place where they react) but also in its effect. In 1930 we only knew 80 enzymes. In 1993 we know more than 2,700 enzymes. However, we do not know how many are left to be discovered.

Enzymes are necessary for the adequate functioning of our whole metabolism. In our body, every part of it is related to all the rest; that is, that even one tiny disturbance, biochemically speaking, can result in a complete imbalance. Diseases are the consequence of this disorder.

In biochemistry, when something is designated with the ending "ase," one can almost be sure that we are talking about an enzyme. In the early stage of the discovery of the enzymes, they were known with names that ended usually with an "in," like the well known pepsin and trypsin.

Enzymes are constantly produced within our body. Described in a simple way, there are certain organic molecular pieces that in small quantities are required to form these enzymes. These pieces are the vitamins, minerals and trace elements. Altogether they are called "co-enzymes."

The deficiency of any of these co-enzymes will result in a specific medical condition. For example, vitamin B[1] deficiency will elicit "beri-beri." The vitamin B[12] deficiency causes a special anemia called "pernicious anemia." The same thing happens with deficiency of essential minerals and trace elements. Basically, in these cases, we are speaking of an illness elicited by a disturbance in the enzymatic balance.

These co-enzymes, in fact, are different from the enzymes. It was already said that enzymes are made of albumin and the co-enzymes are not. The enzymes are rather large molecules. On the other hand, co-enzymes are rather small. Enzymes are not consumed in the true sense during their activity, while co-enzymes are consumed in it and they must be replaced through our diet.

To act adequately, enzymes must be exposed to certain physical conditions. Each of them needs a specific temperature and pH, which causes them to have different speeds of action. To have an appropriate idea of the speed, you must know that lysozyme (an enzyme that helps in the elimination of bacteria) produces a change of approximately 30 molecules of substratum per minute, that is, every 2 seconds. On the other hand, the fastest degrader among the enzymes is quite different, it is carboanhydrase, which changes an incredibly 36 millions of substratum in only one minute.

Some enzymes live only 20 minutes and must be replaced by new enzymes of the same type, recently produced. Other enzymes remain active for a period of several weeks before they are eliminated and when they are, they are eliminated because of their age.

At the Program for Studies of Alternative Medicines of the University of Guadalajara (Mexico), we have researched the therapeutic value of these natural proteolytic enzymes in the treatment of acute and chronic clinical conditions. We have had the opportunity of reaffirming that enzymes are catalytically active polymer compounds made of amino acids. They are involved in virtually all of the vital metabolic processes. They set metabolic conversions in track (in train), control energetic processes and regulate syntheses. Without enzymes, nothing goes on at all within an organism.

It is therefore normal to use enzymes for therapeutic purposes. Substitution in intestinal enzyme deficiency conditions is a classical treatment modality that no one would dispute. External use of enzymes for impaired wound healing (e.g. in the presence of varicose ulcers) has been part of the armamentarium of medical practitioners for centuries. Parental lytic therapy with streptolinase or urokinase for cardiac infarct or for vascular occlusions is today standard throughout the world.

Enzymes are very highly substrate specific. Due to their different places of action, it is therefore reasonable to use mixtures of enzymes in the treatment of diseases. One important enzyme is called the hydrolases, which cleave complex compounds (esters, peptides, and glycosides).

There are some substances that are very similar to co-enzymes. They look so similar that our body can not distinguish between them. In fact, our system does not see the difference and tries to use them as real active enzymatic centers. Of course, the enzyme compensated by such substances (not the true co-enzyme) do not work and the biochemical error makes us sick. For example, when poisoning rats, these poisons very frequently contain an aromatic, vegetal substance known as cumarine. The animal and the human organism see the cumarine as if it were co-enzyme vitamin K. This vitamin K has a definitive role in the production of the enzymes necessary for coagulation. If the body receives cumarine, it incorporates it into the enzymes, instead of incorporating vitamin K, and so the necessary enzymes for coagulation stop functioning. The blood liquefies in a way that causes the rats to bleed to their death.

When we get sick, particularly in the case of an infectious disease, our temperature rises. This is an intelligent way by which nature accelerates the activity of our enzymes to try to get rid of the problem.

To bring about certain tasks of great importance within our organism and to keep our system in a perfect equilibrium between too much and too little, the enzymes work most of the time in continuous steps, that is, in what is called "enzymatic cascades." One enzyme activates the next enzyme, and, in turn, that enzyme activates another enzyme, until one last enzyme finally produces the desired effect. This happens due to nature's design to conserve energy, because these small individual steps require much less energy than big complicated ones. On the other hand, nature desires safety, in that our bodies must be sure that these enzymatic cascades are not activated unless really necessary. That is why there are two security systems. If one enzymatic cascade is wrongly activated, there can be dangerous consequences that may lead to death.

The first lock of the security system is to produce new enzymes, but the characteristic of these enzymes is that they are inactive. That is, they will not work until they are activated by certain changes in the structure of the amino acids. Thus, the innocuous enzymes flow all over the lymphatic system and the bloodstream. Whenever the body needs to have a certain effect, a corresponding enzymatic cascade is activated accordingly.

The inhibitors of the enzymes are the second security system. In biochemistry they are so-called "enzymatic inhibitors." These proper enzymatic inhibitors of the organism can avoid the activation of the enzymes when the quantity of enzymes is too large.

Other several substances have been discovered to help to neutralize certain enzymes, and by this means we can intentionally act on the process of metabolism. The most famous drug in the world, "acetylsalicilic acid," (aspirin) works according to this principle. During a very long time, the fact that acetylsalicilic acid neutralized enzymes was unknown. We used the substance as a pain killer simply because we knew it worked. This acid can be stored firmly as a foreign substance in an enzyme with the complicated name of "cyclooxygenase." Cyclooxygenase plays an important role in the processes of coagulation and inflammations. Thus, the acid inhibits the coagulation of blood and then blood becomes more liquid. It also inhibits the processes of inflammations, and this way the inflammations and pains are diminished.

Think about antibiotics, for example, penicillin; or about steroids, that is, cortisone. These substances also are enzymatic inhibitors. What medical science is doing, then, is using this knowledge in the symptomatic treatment of diseases.

Enzymes are widely used in the food industry. Enzymes are essential in the manufacture of beer. But our interest is in three medical fields. So, in this area, enzymes are used in: (1) analysis, (2) pharmaceuticals and, (3) therapy.

Enzymes are very important in paraclinical diagnosis. For example, in the past it took a long time to determine the blood sugar level. Today, we can use a special tape, wet it with some blood or urine, and in 60 seconds know our blood sugar level. What we are doing, is using our knowledge about the way enzymes react.

In the pharmaceutical area, it was already mentioned that many of the drugs used today are in reality enzymatic inhibitors, such as cytostatics, antibiotics, steroids, etc. Everybody knows that these medicines have different adverse side effects. It would be better to help our body to react, instead of inhibiting it.

After many years of experience in analysis and pharmaceutical areas, it was thought that these powerful enzymes could be used in the therapeutic field, too. This way, a new area of enzymatic therapy began. It was applied to allieviate disturbances in the metabolism, that is, impairments in the functions of the organs and to repair genetic faults.

Soon scientists concluded, thanks to these new biochemical tools, that the genetic defects could be corrected or neutralized by means of the application of enzymes. Besides, the genetic defects are enzymatic defects. So far there have been reported in the medical literature more than 150 diseases that are due to enzymatic faults genetically conditioned. This means that the patient's organism does not form a specific enzyme or it manufactures and places a similar enzyme which has only weak activity. This weak enzyme replaces the right one.

An enzymatic defect genetically conditioned is found also especially in certain human races. For example, the black population is affected by an enzymatic defect genetically conditioned that can lead to the so-called anemia of falciform cells, while half of the Japanese people suffer from another hereditary metabolic error. They lack an enzyme, so-called aldehyde dehydrogenase. This enzyme is required to degrade alcohol. This is the reason why Japanese people are more sensitive to drinking alcohol. Most women have the same enzymatic defect.

Some of the enzymatic defects genetically conditioned have different kinds of consequences that are hardly noticed, while others have a remarkable effect in the display of disease.

DIGESTION

We can say that in spite of the different foods we eat, they all are made of carbohydrates, proteins and fat.

To be able to transform these three basic food substances into biochemical substances, so that our body can take advantage of them, we need also three groups of enzymes; the proteolytic, enzymes (proteases), degraders of proteins, the lipolytic enzymes (lipases), degraders of fat and the amilolytic enzymes (amilases), degraders of carbohydrates.

This enzymatic transformation begins in the moment we place a piece of food in our mouth. As always seen in nature, there is an order. Carbohydrates are first degraded, then albumins and finally fat.

But enzymes not only degrade foods. They also play a specific role in the process of absorption of substances. There are several enzymes that are essential as transporters of the nutrient substances.

We can understand now that when we eat too much, we can help our body to digest more easily our foods by taking some medicine, which contains digestive enzymes.

ENZYMES, GREAT HEALERS

When someone gets sick of any disease we can be sure that something is wrong with his/her enzymes. If the enzymes had been able to eliminate the cause of the disease, then the person would not have become sick.

What we logically must do, in almost any disease, is to replace the type and quantity of the required enzymes as soon as possible. Our body will automatically do the rest.

It is so simple, we just take some enzymatic tablets to help ourselves. In emergency situations, we can administer them in great quantities through injections or even rectally.

The defense mechanisms of the organism are fortified by the enzymes. They are important for all the inflammatory processes, they take care to keep a good blood circulation, they help in wound healing of any kind and even in the case of abnormal cells they regulate cellular growth and fight against viruses. These features are impressive. They embrace almost all the conditions which we nowadays call "chronic diseases."

Of course, enzymes can be taken as a preventive measure against many diseases.

One great problem is obtaining an effective formula of enzymes, as some governmental authorities do not permit the use of a mixture of active substances. It is essential to have a mixture, otherwise the therapeutical effect desired will not be produced. In the literal sense, any food has a mixture of "drugs" [or chemicals] such as vitamins, minerals, trace elements, amino acids, etc. And, we combine these more complexly when we combine foods.

There are some monoenzymatic preparations, but their therapeutic effect is very limited. Many studies have been done regarding the effect of an enzyme used alone and also used in a mixture. There is a clear synergistic effect when combined with more than one enzyme. For example, bromelain, we'll say, has an effect factor of 1, but if we combine bromelain with papain — which we'll say also has an effect factor of 1 — the resulting effect will not be their sum of $1+1 = 2$, but rather $1+1 = 3$, or perhaps even $1+1 = 4$. This is due to their natural ability to act synergistically.

In reality, it is difficult to get a monoenzymatic preparation, since, for example, pancreatin itself is composed of at least 12 enzymes.

Enzymes are very safe. A lethal dose (LD-50: the LD-50 is the measure of the dosage necessary to kill off one-half of a trial group of rats, and is a standard used to measure safety of most drugs) could never be found. Rats, for example, were fed with the equivalent of 2,500 tablets for 6 months, with no significant changes and no harmful effects. Horses were also fed with the equivalent quantity of 250 tablets daily for 6 months, too, with no problems. No toxicity has ever been found.

Since enzymes are natural agents, they can be included in the category of the biological response modifiers (BRM). This means that they do not alter the physiology of our body, instead, they just stimulate our bodies to act according to its own inner wisdom. This is really fascinating. Enzymes will work only if they are needed to do so.

Caution must be taken in certain specific cases. Hemophilic patients should not take enzymes. We can say the same thing concerning the patients who have a risk of hemorrhage. The reason is that enzymes liquefy blood and make coagulation slower. In case of pregnancy, we must ponder the risk. But all the studies in animals have demonstrated no teratogenic effect by enzyme mixtures.

Scientific research has proven that enzymes not only have a synergetic effect, as a mixture, but also elicit the same kind of effect when they are combined with antibiotics, sulfonamids, steroids and other drugs or medicines. Regarding synergy with chemotherapy, we have seen an increase in the effect of the chemotherapy from 8% to 40%. This is wonderful, because it means that we can diminish, in certain cases, the dosage of cytostatic medicines without decreasing their therapeutical effect. About 5% of the patients who take enzymatic mixtures will have a mild side effect. It consists simply in a change of the odor in their stools.

Systemic enzyme therapy is a form of therapy that has been taken over from naturopathy. Today it has a firm place in the spectrum of treatment available under the aegis of mainstream medicine — despite all hostilities. Extensive research made this possible.

It has always been believed that enzymes do not reach the whole organism. This is because it is thought that enzymes are not absorbed in the intestines. The reason for this belief is that enzymes are macromolecules. A macromolecule has a weight of at least 1,000. Enzymes have a weight between 16,000 and 60,000 atoms per molecule.

Everybody knows that new born babies get antibodies from their mothers through the mother's milk. These antibodies must cross the barrier of the intestines' walls to reach the lymphatic vessels and the bloodstream. These antibodies are also macromolecules that have a size similar to that of enzymes. The antibodies are also called gammaglobulins. (See "Universal Oral Vaccine," http://www.arthritistrust.org & Kindle.)

Prof. Seifert (Chirurgischen Universitat-Klinik) in Kiel, fed rats and dogs with equine gammaglobulins radioactively marked to demonstrate on a scientific basis the absorption of these macromolecules. These equine gammaglobulins have a molecular weight up to 12,000 atoms; that is, they are extremely large.

These gammaglobulins were absorbed. This means that they arrived through intestines to the blood and could be found all over the organism of the rats and dogs.

Nowadays, there is no doubt about the absorption of enzymatic mixtures.

HOW DO ENZYMES WORK?

It is very important to remember that medicine does not heal, neither does any other remedy. We know that doctors do not, in the strict sense of the word, cure any disease. All of them can contribute through very different ways of supporting the body, but the healing and the maintenance of health is a task done by one's own defense system of the body.

We cannot speak about the treatment of diseases, or detoxification of the organism, without also including the immune system. We begin with grippe and finish with AIDS, and there is nothing that could be done without taking into consideration the field of immunology.

It is difficult to explain in simple words what the immune system is all about, but I will try to make it simple.

The cells, such as bacteria and viruses, are recognized by our body as enemies, that is, as "antigens," but also some other chemical substances and mutated cells act as antigens. In response to the presence of these antigens, our body produces "antibodies." The antibodies that couple with an antigen form an "immune complex." Macrophages are in charge of destroying these immune complexes enzymatically. But these macrophages look for large immune complexes, so sometimes the medium size immune complexes are ignored. These ignored complexes begin to flow through our lymphatic system and blood stream until they finish sticking on a tissue wall, penetrating that tissue. Eventually they are stored there. From that moment on, these immune complexes become pathogenic, that is, they can cause a disease.

During this situation, we also find macrophages less active because the more immune complexes we have, the more inhibited is the activity of the macrophages. We have then arrived at a vicious circle, where one bad situation produces the other bad situation, and that one in turn producing the first situation.

When the number of immune complexes is so high, the second defense system of our body is alerted. The second immune system is called the "complement system." It is also made of a cascade of nine enzymes activated one by one. When the whole enzymatic cascade has been activated, a huge

235

dissolvent activity of albumins begins and this causes an inflammatory reaction. In consequence, the tissue is destroyed and suddenly that which we call an "auto immune disease" arises; the organism attacks itself.

If, for example, the immune complexes are fixed in the renal tissue, then through the activation of the complement system, an inflammation can occur in the kidney, resulting in what we know as glommerulonephritis. In this particular case, clinical trials have been undertaken and so now we know that what the enzymes do is to interrupt the enzymatic cascade of the complement system.

There are many similar diseases elicited by the activation of the complement system. All of them are so-called "autoimmune diseases." Until recently they were considered as incurable diseases, because they could only be influenced medically very little, if any, that is, chronic inflammations of the intestines, such as Crohn's disease or ulcerative colitis. This kind of sickeness is due to the immune complexes in the intestinal tissues.

The interruption of the complement system cascade always works to avoid damage upon ourselves. To achieve this, we dilute enzymatically the pathogenic immune complexes and we activate the macrophages. This way, we are interrupting the vicious circle that leads to chronic degenerative diseases.

Depending on the organ where these immune complexes are fixed is where the disease is produced. For instance, if the lung is involved, then the result is pulmonary fibrosis. If the pancreas is involved, then we will get a pancreatitis, and so on. The list of the diseases of autoagression caused by immune complexes is very long. The type of disease does not depend only on the place where the immune complexes are fixed, but also on the origin of the antigen.

Among the typical diseases of autoagression, we can find chronic articular rheumatism, glommerulonephritis, and ulcerative colitis. The diseases due to virus, bacteria or certain parasites can also lead to autoagression diseases; for example, as in infectious hepatitis, herpes zoster, toxoplasmosis, etc.

Orthodox medicine frequently uses two kinds of remedies. One is the kind of antiinflammatory drugs which only suppress the symptom but not the disease. The other kind are so-called immune suppressors. These drugs weaken the body's own defenses.

More scientists are taking an interest in the biochemical method of systemic enzyme therapy. Enzymes are adequate to dissolve and to eliminate immune complexes. They also stimulate the body's defenses and accelerate inflammatory mechanisms.

In the beginning of the treatment, an apparent impairment may occur, since the enzymatic mixtures can destroy the immune complexes that are fixed in the tissues. So, enzymes take the immune complexes back to the bloodstream. Because of this, there is a greater quantity of circulating immune complexes and this temporary increase can temporarily increase the symptoms in the patient. [See "The Herxheimer Effect" http://www.arthritistrust.org or at Kindle.] However, the enzymes, in a short time period, if they are adminstered in the right dose, will certainly eliminate the titurated immune complexes that have once again entered the blood stream.

During the Second Mexican National Congress on Enzyme Therapy, Dr. Kunze reported fascinating findings of his immunolgical research. He says that there is no disease where the immune system is not involved. Now we know that enzymes can help to avoid the formation of autoantibodies. They can inhibit the production of immune complexes. They are useful in avoiding the activation of the complement. They mediate the action of the citoquines, as well as the fibrin.

Clinical trials have been done on the systemic enzymatic treatment of many, many diseases. There are two main ones to be discussed herein. When one speaks about hope in the case of Multiple Sclerosis, one must be sure of what one is saying. We all know how terrible this disease is. According to the author (Dr. Hector E. Solorzano del Rio, M.D., Ph.D., D.Sc., chairman of the Program for Studies of Alternative Medicines of the University of Guadalajara), it has been scientifically proven that enzymes indeed help MS patients.

The etiology of MS is unknown. We know that there is a demyelinization, that is, the nerve fibers lose their myelin [insulation] and the symptoms arise. There are certain factors that seem to influence the appearance of this medical condition, such as is the case of hereditary factors, dietary factors, etc.

Another factor found in MS patients is a deficiency of unsaturated fatty acids.

One final theory says that viruses can be the etiological factor for MS. Different clinical trials around the world have confirmed that the MS patients have higher levels of circulating immune complexes.

One of my (Dr. Solorzano) MS patients is named Jose. He was 40 years old, in a wheelchair, and desperate. He had received all known orthodox treatments with no results. So, he took the enzymatic treatment. In one month Jose felt more strength in all of his muscles. He could again take care of himself regarding dressing himself. In three months he could walk, but with some difficulty. After six months of enzymatic treatment, he was no longer sick. He is very happy and now lives a productive life.

Hundreds of patients have been treated with enzymatic therapy, with good results, not only in Germany or Mexico, but in many other countries.

It is important to remember that patients also have dietary care, and that they are also given unsaturated fatty acids. Most of them have a deficiency in selenium, and so we prescribe accordingly.

The sooner the patient receives enzymatic treatment, the faster the improvement will be noticed. Of course, if the patient has not taken immune suppressors, then, again, the response will be seen earlier.

We can also talk about a very frequent but not cured disease by orthodox medicine. This is Rheumatoid Arthritis. Its etiology is not yet known. There are many theories. Some scientists say that it is an autoimmune disease.

There are millions of people suffering from Rheumatoid Arthritis.

In this kind of disease we find high levels of circulating immune complexes. So, this points out that we are really dealing with an autoagression disease. Here the immune complexes are fixed in the articular capsule, that is why eventually the joint will be destroyed.

The regular (traditional) medical treatment is a symptomatic one. The patient receives a prescription of antiinflammatory drugs, analgesic drugs, gold, cortisone and in the worst cases, cytostatic drugs; i.e., methotrexate, etc.

All that these drugs provide is temporary relief. They will not stop the arising of immune complexes, except cortisone. Besides the side effects are not mild and innocuous (including the use of cortisone). Sometimes the side effects are quite dangerous.

Some double blind clinical trials have been done in Germany using, on one side, enzymatic mixtures, and on the other side, gold salts. One main study lasted six months. The scientists were surprised when they knew that they got the same good results using any of them. (In a double-blind clinical trial, the doctor does not know which tablets are whose, and neither does the patient). The great advantage was that the enzymes were very much better tolerated and had no side effects. (Rheumatoid Disease Has Been Cured. See any of the Anthony di Fabio books as writer or editor at www.arthritistrust.org, bookstores or on Amazon.com or at Kindle.Ed:)

INFLAMMATION

Enzymes are not antiinflammatory drugs, instead, they promote the inflammation; this is, inflammation is the marvelous response from our body to a noxious stimulus. Most times we look at inflammation as something bad and to be avoided. It should not be so. It is the way our body is trying to get rid of the harmful foreign agents.

The classical signs of inflammation are; pain, tumor, heat and blush. When inflammation ends, the body repairs the area affected. So, if the inflammation finishes sooner, then the repair will begin earlier. That's the reason why enzymes are promoters instead of inhibitors of inflammation.

If we try to think of a disease which has as a feature inflammation, we'll find that such diseases are those that their names finish with "itis." Such as tonsilitis, colitis, otitis, dermatitis, etc. Thus, we can easily conclude that enzymatic mixtures are excellent for any of these "itis" diseases. Enzymes will help our body to heal itself.

In studies made at the University of Guadalajara, I (Dr. Solorzano) has used enzymes not only to treat sports injuries, but also — read this carefully — TO PREVENT them. This means that patients will take enzymes before playing their sports. When they become injured, the injury heals in a significantly shorter time period. Some times it is almost half of the regular time. It's incredible!

One very frequent and elective wound is one made by the surgeon. Although a surgical operation is for the good of the patient, it is still an aggression to our body. Our system will react the same way if it had been produced by any other harmful agent. Those patients who receive enzymatic treatment before and/or after surgery will have some important advantages. They will stay in bed less time, the risk of a thrombosis will be much less, the patients have a better pyschic state, the pains will go earlier. During surgery the operation field will be better. Patients under enzymes will have a better and faster wound healing, and last but not least, they will spend less money because of hospital costs.

The area where enzymes work the best is in vascular diseases, such as thrombosis, phlebitis, and varicose veins. Enzymes avoid the formation of thrombosis. They lower cholesterol levels and triglycerides.

Dr. Inderst (1990) has reported on the effect of enzyme therapy in vascular disease and found that enzymes cause a definite reduction in symptoms (pain, cramps) and a measurable improvement of objective findings (e.g. swelling) even when lymphedema was present for many years.

Until now the treatment of venous and lymphatic vessel diseases, especially when combined with edema, gave insufficient results. Compressive therapy is rejected by many of the patients suffering from these diseases, so it may be necessary to treat the main symptoms with drugs. Systemic enzyme therapy is a proven method; it diminishes the edema, activates the fibrinolytic system, and stimulates cells like macrophages. The pain and the cramps disappear, swelling goes away, and blood flow increases in a short time. The efficacy of certain enzyme mixtures has been tested by double-blind studies.

CANCER

About 100 years ago, a British embryologist, John Beard, decided to treat cancer patients. He knew that the important enzymes are produced mainly by the pancreas. He had a theory about the etiology of cancer, where pancreatic enzymes were involved. He wanted to try some clinical research with terminal cancer patients, so he extracted the pancreatic juice of the pancreas of pigs and calves just born. His solution had then a high concentration of these useful enzymes.

Almost immediately after the extract was ready, he injected it into his cancer patients. These injections were applied slowly intravenously or intramuscular. Sometimes, when the tumor was available near the surface of the body, he injected right into it.

Of course, not all of these treatments were a success, due to the lack of purification of his extract, as it contained strange albumins which in some cases elicited allergic reactions and even some anaphylactic shock. You can easily imagine that this provoked an immediate reaction from his colleagues. He was seen as a quack.

Eventually Dr. Beard had the opportunity to observe how certain tumor masses really disappeared due to the effect of these enzymatic injections. He also noticed how many of his cancer patients survived longer than the expected, according to the orthodox expectancy rates.

He treated a total of 170 patients with this method. In 1907 he wrote a book describing his experiences with these patients. Some patients were totally recovered, some improved, and some lived longer with a better quality of life.

Almost everything about Dr. Beard was forgotten until Prof. Wolf, who had an office in New York, decided to research enzymes. After reading literature that was written and researched on enzymes, Prof. Wolf wanted to continue the study of these wonderful biological agents.

Prof. Wolf noticed that by using purified mixtures of enzymes there were no risks of frequent allergic reactions.

We know that the war against cancer has not been won. Many people around the world die of cancer every day.

There are many non-toxic approaches to treat cancer, but since our aim in this paper is to speak about enzyme therapy, we'll concentrate on how they are beneficial in the treatment of this disease.

Each cancer cell has on the surface of its membrane, specific antigens. It is naturally ideal when the body can recognize these markers — by being released from the fibrin — because the cancer cell can be destroyed after this. Although the cancer cell is destroyed, however, the antigen remains. By means of a change in its membrane, the cancer cell can sometimes throw off its antigen. It seems that cancer cells do this, so that our defenses go in the wrong direction. Regrettably, this trick really works. If the number of formed immune complexes is kept within the normal limits and our defenses are allright, then our macrophages can embrace and dissolve these immune complexes. If the number of immune complexes is superior to the strength of the macrophages, then some immune complexes remain not dissolved in the blood, as well as in the lymph.

By means of a complicated mechanism — we talk about activation and aggregation of thrombocytes — it promotes a greater formation of fibrin, by depositing the not dissolved immune complexes in the tissue. This normally diminishes defenses. And this fact in turn is especially dangerous in the case of an organism threatened by cancer.

The immune complexes can weaken the body's defenses in another way. Too many immune complexes inhibit the activity of the macrophages, which are the main destroyers of the cancer cells. Their capacity to destroy and to clean out the system is paralyzed. Thus cancer cells can grow without being bothered by macrophages.

What the enzymes do to help is that they discover the receptors. Enzymes also facilitate the reaction of recognition. Another important action of the enzymes is to improve immunity, which is done by breaking the circulating immune complexes by activating the natural killer cells and the T-cells, and also by inducing mediators and cytokines, such as TNF, Tumor Necrosis Factor.

Enzymes have the ability to reduce the thick fibrin layer which is abnormally 15 times thicker than normal. By reducing this fibrin layer the stickiness of the cancer cells is also diminished, and by this means we can prevent metastasis.

One advantage of using enzymes is that we can combine them with orthodox treatment, that is, chemotherapy and/or radioactive therapy. As a bonus, the patient will have less side effects by combining these natural enzymes.

The world-famous professor and doctor from Vienna, Dr. Wrba, states that enzymes are a new approach to cancer treatment. There are two main factors in the treatment of cancer cells (1) defense of the host and (2) virulence of the cancer cells. As has been already said, systemic enzyme therapy increases the defense mechanism, that is, improves the recognition reaction of the cancer cells, plus lowers its virulence. In doing so, Wrba feels that this action causes modulation of the cell membrane, uncovers the cell surface and receptors, improves immunity, facilitates the recognition reaction and reduces the stickiness of the tumor cells.

VIRAL DISEASES

Jaeger (1990) investigated the use of hydrolytic enzymes in the treatment of HIV infection and stated that there are increasing indications that autoimmune processes are involved in the destruction of the immune system that is fundamental to the pathogenesis of HIV infection.

According to Jaeger, a number of autoimmune mechanisms have been replicated in the pathogenesis of HIV infection, particularly in the more advanced clinically symptomatic stages of the diseases. Thus, different auto-antibodies and increased levels of circulating immune complexes have been described.

Thus, enzyme therapy becomes an adjuvant form of treatment. As mentioned earlier, the immune complexes can be eliminated by the hydrolytic enzymes. Results indicate that this form of treatment was well tolerated, patients improved in functional ability and also gained weight. The clinical symptoms typical of the HIV infection were reduced.

Kleine (1990) states that in herpes zoster patients there are typical dermatological findings in the distribution area of one or several peripheral nerves. Pain in this area exist almost always, and internal organs may also be involved. The course of the disease is relatively invariable. The nerve pain can out last the cutaneous manifestation for a long time (post zoster neuralgia). Elderly people and those who are immunodeficient due to diseases or drugs are especially at risk. Systemic enzyme therapy represents a new principle of therapeutic action. The studies indicate a positive influence of the enzymes on the acute form of herpes zoster as well as on the complications.

SUMMARY

Enzyme therapy has long been part of the methods of treatment of traditional medicine. Meanwhile, enzymes have even become one of the most innovative and expanding drug groups, and systemic therapy with proteolytic enzymes has become an important method of treatment in natural medicine.

There is hardly any regulatory system in our body which does not depend on enzymes. Enzymes control coagulation and fibrinolysis, inflammation and complement activity, phagocytosis, wound healing and tissue regeneration as well as the specific and non-specific defense systems. Here the enzymes function as biocatalysts.

The idea of supporting the weakened or stressed human body in fighting disease by administering enzymes seems very reasonable. After all, the structures and various functions of some 2700 enzymes have already been discovered in the human organism.

The most important enzymes used in therapy are hydrolases, which split ester, peptide and clycoside bonds by introducing a water molecule.

The tasks and goals of enzyme therapy are manifold. Enzymes are used to support the body in stress situations, such as chronic or acute inflammations, digestive disorders, vascular or malignant diseases. A further field of application for enzymes is substitution in enzyme defect disorders. The classical examples of this are pancreatic insufficiency or blood clotting disorders due to deficient clotting factors.

Each enzyme has different effects. It is therefore reasonable to use combinations of enzymes to ensure a sufficiently broad spectrum of effects and via synergism for greater efficacy.

The absorption of enzymes

The pharmacological principle of systemic enzyme therapy depends on the absorption of enzymes as intact molecules after oral administration. Thus their biological effects are fully preserved. The tablets or coated tablets must resist gastric secretion, to prevent destruction by the acid milieu of the stomach. Once in the small bowel, the large enzyme molecules, like all macromolecules, may be absorbed in two ways:

1. They may bind to specific receptors in a particular area of the intestinal mucosa, and be transported through the gut's epithelium (pinocytosis).

2. They may be taken up by lymphocytes "roaming" in the lumen of the bowel, and be released again after passage through the gut wall.

In this way about 25% of the administered dose may find its way into the circulation and the lymph system still in an active form.

As already stated, it is important that the structure responsible for enzymatic activity remain largely intact so that the enzyme retains its activity.

In the blood, enzymes do not exist in a free form but are bound to a carrier, e.g., the antiproteinase, a[2]-macroglobulin. This protects the enzyme from interactions with other molecules and "neutralizes" potentially allergenic properties of these proteases. In spite of this carrier binding, the enzyme remains active.

The fact that, after absorption from the gastrointestinal tract, these enzymes reach their site of action via the blood and lymph systems, is referred to as "systemic action."

Enzymes promote the body's own regeneration processes.

Certain proteolytic enzymes possess pronounced anti-inflammatory and anti-oedematous properties. They promote the breakdown of toxic metabolites and inflammatory products and thus contribute substantially to the detoxification of the human body. Simultaneously, the additional fibrinolytic activity of the enzymes and the "vessel-sealing" effect of rutin accelerates the blood flow. Together with the dissolution of fresh blood clots (microthrombi), this allows normalization of the microcirculation.

Therefore, the inflammatory products that mediate pain are eliminated more quickly, the improved blood supply enhances local oxygenation, and tissue tension decreases in parallel with the reduction in oedema. All of this provides some analgesic effect.

In sharp contrast to the mechanisms of action of conventional non-steroidal and steroidal anti-inflammatory drugs, systemic enzyme therapy thus does not block the natural healing processes of inflammation.

It is also characteristic for some enzymes, that they activate or stimulate macrophages and natural killer cells (NKcells). These cells have a well-recognized essential role in the body's own immunological defense. They are part of a larger system, the reticulo-endothelial system.

Therefore, enzymes also affect the whole of the body's immune system as a "biological response modifier." Macrophages stimulated by the enzymes secrete tumour necrosis factor (TNF) and other cytokines. For these two reasons, enzymes are predestined to become a future chemotherapeutic agent, they do not lead to the destruction of all cells with high mitotic activity, but only of those that are actually malignant.

A further characteristic feature of enzymes is their carrier function. Enzymes are able to transport antibiotics and cytostatic drugs to sites which would be nearly impossible for them to reach otherwise. Enzymes can therefore be used as "transportmedia," e.g., in the therapy of sinusitis, prostatisis, bronchitis or specific tumours.

Enzymes destroy immune complexes

Immune complexes arise from the combination of an antigen with an antibody. If the antigen is formed by the body itself, as, for instance, in rheumatism, or if very large complexes form through the conglomeration of several antigen and antibody molecules, pathogenic immune complexes may result. This may subsequently lead to autoimmune disease, especially if these complexes activate the complement system. In conventional medicine, pathogenic immune complexes are eliminated via plasmapheresis, lymphopheresis and cryoprecipitation. It is much easier, however, to remove the pathogenic immune complexes using enzymes that activate the "phagocytic macrophage system," or by breaking down the large complexes into smaller ones which can be eliminated far more efficiently.

These mechanisms of action justify the large number of indications for systemic enzyme therapy; it is, therefore, the basis of treatment in acute and chronic inflammatory conditions, autoimmune diseases such as polyarthritis, states of impaired resistance (viral and neoplastic diseases), and also for vascular conditions, in which the additional improvement in blood flow is of great importance. There is also increasing evidence for their prophylactic efficacy (prevention of tumour metastases.)

CONCLUSION
(Instructions for side effects during use)

Orally administered enzymes should not be taken with food. They should be taken at least one hour before or 1-1/2 hours after meals. Otherwise, there is a risk that some of the dose will merely help to digest the food.

From the start, relatively high doses must be used in systemic enzyme therapy, since enzymes are large molecules and their absorption, transport and distribution are different from those of small molecules.

It is worth emphasizing, that even with large doses taken over prolonged periods of time, no immunological dysregulation will occur.

Concommitant oral administration of vitamin preparations represents an ideal adjunct to systemic enzyme therapy. For this purpose, emulsions are particularly suitable, especially in higher dosages.

'Healing' Enzymes for Arthritis and Sports Injuries

In their August/September 1993 issue, Townsend Letter for Doctors and Patients *[911 Tyler St., Port Townsend, WA 98368-6541; p. 878] published our article "Bees: The Perfect Food." Based on now deceased Royden Brown's work,* How to Live the Millennium, *[C.C. Pollen Company, 3627 E. Indian School Rd., Suite 209, Phoenix, AZ 85018-5126], this article was important because virtually all essential human nutrients are available in the properly chosen and prepared bee pollen. Among those nutrients were literally tens of thousands of important enzymes. [See "Bees: The Perfect Food," http://www.arthritistrust.org.]*

In our 1995 newsletter we published two excellent articles by Hector E. Solorzano del Rio, M.D., Ph.D., D.Sc., "How do Enzymes Work?," and also "Enzymes, Great Healers."

Dr. Solorzano introduced us to Wobenzyme N, a German developed product that, perhaps, has been greatly underrated by the alternative medical profession, and especially by arthritics.

The following article explains why. It was provided to us by NutriHealth International, a publisher, through one of its representatives, Shailesh Patel. We hereby print the article with some changes with their permission.

We do not have a financial interest in Wobenzym N.

Proteolytic Enzymes as an Arthritic Breakthrough

Wobenzym N is actually not a single substance but rather a unique, synergistic combination of various proteolytic (protein-destroying) enzymes, or proteases. Wobenzym N was developed over 30 years ago by world-renowned immunologist and biochemist Dr. Kari Ransberger and Dr. Max Wolf of Germany. Wobenzym N is in fact endorsed by leading European scientists and is backed by over 30 years of scientific research and clinical studies confirming its benefits. Although individual proteolytic enzymes are useful, the extraordinary combination of these enzymes yields a combination greater than the sum of its parts. Systemic multi-enzyme therapy has proved helpful in cases of arthritis and related diseases, offering a wide range of benefits from anti-inflammatory to

vascular system protection, and regulating the immune system. The precise formulation of Wobenzym N has evolved over the years, but its basic ingredients remain the same. The ingredients include the enzymes, bromelain, papain, pancreatin, trypsin, and chymotrypsin and the flavonoid rutin.

One of the most important potential benefits of systemic multi-enzyme therapy is in the treatment of arthritis. Proteolytic enzymes are essential regulators and modulators of the inflammatory response.

They help to hinder pain and inflammatory reactions in a number of ways.

The Wobenzym N formulation has been shown to help :

* Break down proteins in the blood that cause inflammation by facilitating their removal via the blood stream and lymphatic system. (See "Lymph Drainage Therapy," and "Lymphatic Detoxification," http://www.arthritistrust.org also at kindle..)

* Remove "fibrin," the clotting material that prolongs inflammation.

* Clear up edema (excess water) in the areas of inflammation.

* Counteract chronic, recurrent inflammation, a primary cause of chronic degenerative joint disease.

Conventional treatment of inflammatory diseases such as arthritis involves powerful drugs like steroidal and non-steroidal anti-inflammatory drugs (NSAIDs), as well as more exotic treatments, such as methotrexate and D-penicillamine. [This foundation, of course, does not recommend the traditional approach. See *Arthritis: Osteoarthritis and Rheumatoid Disease Including Rheumatoid Arthritis* at www.arthritistrust.org, book stores and at Amazon.com also on Kindle.] Although NSAIDs reduce inflammation and pain, they are toxic and do very little to start the healing process. In this sense, enzymes may be superior as they have a profound influence on the immune system.

Proteolytic enzymes degrade circulatory immune complexes (CIC's) that can inhibit normal immune function. These immune complexes, which consist of an antigen bound to an antibody, are a normal part of the immune response. But when immune complexes occur in excess, they are a principal cause of a number of [symptoms of] rheumatologic diseases, including [those observed in] rheumatoid arthritis. Evidence suggests that trypsin, papain, and other proteolytic enzymes can break up existing circulatory immune complexes and possibly even prevent their formation in the first place. The bottom line of these actions is a regulatory or stimulatory effect on the immune system.

Numerous studies in animals and people with rheumatoid arthritis indicate that Wobenzym not only manages symptoms of pain and inflammation but provides immense healing benefits as well. Most recently, researchers from the Ukrainian Rheumatology Centre, in Kiev, tested Wobenzym N on 78 patients with severe, crippling rheumatoid arthritis and who were using other prime treatment drugs. All of the patients in the study showed a decrease in circulatory immune complexes (CIC) concentrations, averaging between 28%

and 42%, and decrease in rheumatoid factors. Of all the patients 20% reduced their NSAID doses and one patient stopped taking methotrexate and experienced a clinical remission.

A number of sufferers of arthritis have indeed applauded Wobenzym. Hedy Mink from Oviedo, Florida boasts "my whole family has been using Wobenzym since 10 years when I lived in Germany. It has helped me keep my arthritis under control and we take Wobenzym for all possible inflammations in our body".

A Case History

Elizabeth Bapes, Illinois has said, "There are no words to describe what Wobenzym N has done for me. My homeopath started me on this about 4 months ago, and the change in me is miraculous. I haven't felt this good in a very, very, very long time. I used to dread getting up in the morning — now I look forward to starting the day with enthusiasm. My energy is remarkable.

Before taking these wonderful enzymes I felt like an old, old, lady, because even though I am now 75 years YOUNG, no one believes that I have arthritis and lupus. I have a handicapped husband that I take care of without help …… praise to the makers and developers of Wobenzym."

Proteolytic Enzymes Bring Relief to Sufferers of Lupus

One of our former referral physicians and Board Member, Ron Davis, M.D. of Seabrook, TX has had excellent success bringing about complete remisssions in patients with Systemic Lupus Erythematosus and Progressive Systemic Sclerosis. Dr. Davis' method is available on our website, http://www.arthritistrust.org, under the same title, "Systemic Lupus Erythematosus and Progressive Systemic Sclerosis." or at Kindle. Wobenzym N, he felt, was an additional nutrient that will help to speed up the day of wellness.

Systemic Lupus Erythematosus (SLE or lupus) is a chronic inflammatory disease [said to be] of unknown cause. Lupus is [classified as] an autoimmune disease. [There are several theories as to] why the immune system, normally designed to fight infections and tumors, turns on its own human host. Many components, particularly certain white blood cells, are involved in the development of Lupus. Lupus can be a life-threatening disease and may affect every organ in the body. It strikes women far more often than men, and is most common among women of childbearing age.

Enzymes help to dissolve circulating immune complexes and antibodies that cause the severe inflammation of Lupus. A 1996 study of Lupus patients demonstrated how clinical and laboratory immuno-inflammatory activity decreased more quickly when medical drugs were used in combination with Wobenzym. Some patients were able to reduce their dose of the medical drugs Voltaren [a non-steroidal anti-inflammatory drug] and prenisolone [a form of cortisone, not recommended by this foundation]. This is important as these drugs often pose serious complications.

Enzymes may be particularly important for Lupus sufferers for another reason: they've been strongly shown to help prevent kidney disease and failure, both of which are commonly associated with Lupus.

The Wider Benefits of Multi-Enzyme Therapy

The body's inflammatory response to sinusitis, chronic bronchitis, and cystitis is benefited by multi-enzyme therapy. For bronchitis, enzymes lead to a reduction of mucosal swelling and an improvement in expectoration and ventilation. In cases of chronic sinusitis, improvements were seen in the normal inflammatory process and the natural clearance functions while stimulating the immune system. In cases of cystitis and UTI (urinary tract infections), Wobenzym N was an ideal partner with antibiotics and chemotherapeutic drugs, as it helped to deliver increased serum concentrations of these conventional medical treatments. A complete cure without recurrence was achieved only by this combination therapy.

Enzymes interrupt the causative pathogenic sequence of chronic inflammation. They cause dissipation of inflammatory edema and counteract the pathogenicity of inflammatory products and antigen-antibody complexes by causing their breakdown and elimination.

Systemic multi-enzyme therapy has practical uses for anyone suffering from acute bronchitis, sinusitis, prostatitis, cystitis and pelvic inflammatory disease (PID). They can help reduce heart disease and circulatory disorders, as well as providing relief for some of the most painful cases of ulcerative colitis, Crohn's disease, and multiple sclerosis. Women will be happy to know that they will also be able to get relief from the painful disorder of fibrocystic breast disease with the aid of enzymes.

Enzymes for Sports Injuries

Just ask Boris Becker and Steffi Graf, two of Germany's leading internationally recognised tennis stars. Both use Wobenzym to help battle the aches and pains of sports injuries. Meanwhile, the German and Austrian Olympic teams ordered one million Wobenzym tablets for the 1998 Olympics. Why? Because they wanted to win and combination oral enzymes offer them a super competitive edge.

It was the German National Hockey Team (in the early 1990's) who began experimenting with Wobenzym N in an attempt to shorten the recovery time for common hockey injuries. All of the injuries suffered by the hockey players were well documented. The convalescence process was carefully and systematically monitored with regard to multiple criteria. Hockey players suffered bruises, contusions, torn muscles, and ruptured ligaments. The swelling, pain, and immobility left the players feeling uncomfortable, and diminished their performance, or kept them off the ice altogether.

Both the physicians and the players of the Hockey Team were pleased with the results of taking Wobenzym N. Bruises and hematomas shrank in size faster, swelling was less severe and resolved faster, spontaneous pain, pain on mobility, and pain on pressure were all lower than expected, and full mobility returned quicker. Moreover, they found that taking Wobenzym N as a preventative measure worked better than taking it right after an injury.

Recommended Nutrient Quantity

Wobenzym N is available in quantities of 100 capsules. The recommended dosage is 3 capsules per day at least 45 minutes before meals or as recommended by your health care professional.

Wobenzym N should be avoided during pregnancy and lactation and a physician should be consulted before use if you are currently on blood-thinning medication.

Wobenzym N can be purchased through a number of sources that can be found on the internet via search engine.

RESOURCES

In Mexico, for further information, including clinics, organizations or referral to practitioners, you can contact:

Dr. Hector E. Solorazano del Rio, M.D., D.Sc.
Programa de Estudios de Medicinas Alternativas
Universidad de Guadalajara
Calle Escuela Militar de Aviacion No. 16
Guadalajara, Jal. MEXICO
Tels. (3) 637/7237, 6515476
Fax (3) 637/0030, 619/3722

REFERENCES

1. Systemische Enzymtherapie in der Rheumatologie. 15 Abeitstagung in Munchen am 15 Juni 1991.

2. Systemic Enzyme Therapy, Medizinische Woche, 27th October to 4th November, 1990 Baden Baden, Germany.

3. Adjuvant therapy with hydrolytic enzymes in oncology — a hopeful effort to avoid bleomycinum induced pneumotoxicity? by M. Schedler. 432 J. Cancer Res Clin Oncol 1990.

4. Absorption of Intact orally ingested protein molecules from the Gut. Cichoke Anthony. Nutritional Perspectives. 1992.

5. Seminario de Terapia Enzimatica Sistemica. Universidad de Guadalajara. Programa de Estudios de Medicinas Alternativas, 1992.

6. Segundo Congreso Nacional de Enzimoterapia. Mexico City, March 1993.

Explanation of Alternative Medicine
by
Dr. Hector Solorzano del Rio, M.D., , Ph.D., D.Sc.

To facilitate comprehension for the patients who come to me on their first visit, I always explain to them through a leaflet, and when I see them, the following:

1. We claim that there is no cure-all medicine. All the different treatments may be good, but the secret is to find which ones to use and how to combine them. Most of the physicians are fanatic about the medicine they particularly practice. This is an error. There are cases in which surgery is unavoidable. We never put in danger the life of our patients. I still practice surgery when necessary. Now you can understand how I can combine many therapies. I take the good part of them all.

2. There are no sicknesses but sick ones. In (conventional) allopathic medicine, we try to find the diagnosis and consider everyone the same. It is like putting a label on each patient. In alternative medicine, everyone is different, so, although many patients can have the same allopathic diagnosis, we can treat them in a different way, because of the distinct imbalance found in each of them. The same thing happens within nutritional therapy. I can have many patients suffering from arthritis but maybe one has a subclinical deficiency of boron. Another can have a subclinical deficiency of magnesium and so on.

3. When we treat a patient, we treat the whole body. In alternative medicine, we do not divide the patients into parts, that is, there are no specialties. You know, in allopathic medicine a specialist can give you a medication that will disturb another organ. Then, you have to see another specialist, who will give you another medicine, which, in turn, will disturb another organ and so on. All medications, in allopathic medicine, have side effects; most of them are adverse.

4. To find out the micro-bioelectronic imbalance of the patients, I use different machines, such as the Dermatron invented by Dr. Voll to measure the electrical potential of the cells. We do this in certain points, so called measurement points. The normal reading is 50 in a scale of 100. Readings below indicate a degenerative process and readings above, mean an inflammatory process.

5. According to the imbalance, I choose the treatment "individually." There are 216 alternative medicines and I recommend to patients the treatments that I think are best for their case in particular.

6. As patients look for good doctors, doctors look for good patients, that is, we need our patients to indeed want to help themselves. We, the doctors, are only the instrument by which God will heal them.

7. Every patient receives a diet in quality, not in quantity, based on the principle by Hippocrates, "let your food be your medicine and your medicine, be your food." We design the diet according to the microbiolectronic readings of each person.

8. We also keep the premise from Hippocrates "first, do not harm."

Sometimes, the allopathic treatments are more aggressive than the clinical condition itself.

9. I follow the Hippocratic philosophy that says *Natura Vix Medicatrix*, that is, Nature Heals. What I do, then, is only to stimulate the homeostasis (natural force to keep our body in order) of the patients. This way, I can say that they heal themselves. I am giving them a little push to help them.

Also see "Thyroid Hormone Therapy: Cutting the Gordian Knot," http://www.arthritistrust.org.)

Brief Curriculum Vitae

Hector E. Solorzano del Rio, M.D., Ph.D., D.Sc.

Medical Doctor (Surgeon) from Universidad de Guadalajara

Master of Acupuncture Degree from Chinese Culture University, Taiwan

Doctor of Science from Open International University for Complementary Medicines

Professor of Pharmacology at Universidad de Guadalajara

Professor of Traditional Practices at the Specialty on Public Health Course at Universidad Guadalajara

Coordinator of the Program for Studies of Alternative Medicines at Universidad de Guadalajara

Organizer of more than 150 seminars on Alternative Medicines at Universidad de Guadalajara

Lecturer in several congresses domestic, as well as national and international ones

Author of many articles for different magazines for laymen and for doctors

President of la Sociedad de Investigacion de Acupuntura y Medicina Oriental, A.C.

President of La Sociedad Medica de Investigaciones Enzymiaticas, A.C.

Co-author of the book *Enzyme Therapy* published by Universidad de Guadlajara

Co-author of the book *Tunia* (Infantile Massage)

Breve Curriculum Vitae

Medico Cirujano y Partero egresado de la Universidad de Guadalajara

Maestria en Acupuntura en la Chinese Culture University de Taipei

Doctorado en Ciencias en la Open International University for Complementary Medicines.

Profesor de Farmacologia de la Universidad de Guadalajara

Profesor de Practicas Tradicionales en la Especialidad de Enfermeria en Salud Publica en la Universidad de Guadalajara

Coordinator del Programa de Estudios de Medicinias Alternativas de la Universidad de Guadalajara, donde se han hecho muchas investigaciones sobre varias diferentes medicinas alternativas.

Organizador de mas de 150 seminarios sobre medicinas alternativas.

Ponente en varios congresos tanto locales, como nacionales e internacionales.

Autor de mas de 100 articulos para varias revistas tanto legas como medicas.

Presidente de la Sociedad de Investigacion de Acupuntura y Medicina Oriental, A.C.

Presidente de la Sociedad Medica de Investigaciones Enzimaticas, A.C.

250

Treatment and Prevention of Osteoporosis
by
Anthony di Fabio and Alan R.Gaby and Jonathan V. Wright

"There are three things you can count on,
if you live long enough.
They are death, taxes, and osteoporosis."
William Campbell Douglass[1], M.D.,

Since we are all going to suffer from Osteoporosis, it might be well to learn how to prevent the condition, if possible, and also to learn how to repair the damage.

More than likely your idea of bone is that it is a dead stick, an item that can be seen in the carcass of dead animals and is used to make up skeletons that hang in doctors' offices. Not so!

Bone is live tissue, and like all cells it has some that die and some that are born anew — bone is a growing tissue that sheds dead cells and grows new cells daily. Bone absorbing cells called osteoclasts dig microscopic cavities in the inner surface of bones. Bone-building cells called osteoblasts fill in these cavities with new bone cells. These cells begin rebuilding bone materials by first producing the collagen matrix, and then calcium and phosphorus crystals are laid down in the matrix in a process called bone mineralization. Would you believe that somewhere between 10 and 30 percent of our entire skeleton is remodeled in this manner each year?

There are two types of bone: cortical and trabecular. Cortical bone is very dense and solid, as in the long, hard bones of your arms and legs, and usually the outside layer of bone everywhere. Trabecular bone is much more porous, honeycombed with minute spaces. Inside of the bones, and especially inside the spinal vertebrae is trabecular. All bones have both a hard layer and an inner soft layer in differing proportions.

Osteoporosis literally means "porous bone." Bone is made up of calcium and phosphorus compounds that are laid in a matrix of protein fibers. It gains its strength and rigidity from calcium. The protein — mostly collagen tissue — makes the bone flexible. Other materials that can be found in bone are flouride, sodium, potassium, magnesium, boron, molybdenum, cobalt, strontium and citrate. Mostly these latter elements help hold the calcium and phosphorus compounds together.

Osteoporosis affects first the trabecular areas, which means those bones, like the spine, that have the greatest percentage of trabecular cells show osteoporosis first.

During childhood and early adulthood we grow bone faster than we lose it. By the mid-thirties, we begin to experience a slight and gradual bone loss. But, after menopause, women lose bone mass more rapidly — six times more rapidly than men do. Since men start usually with greater bone mass, they can also afford to lose more than women can.

The rate of bone loss then begins to slow about 65 years of age.

If you are fair-skinned, female, with ancestors from Europe, Japan, or China, you have one chance in four of being genetically predisposed to osteoporosis.

Loss of estrogen[21] after menopause increases the rate at which calcium is lost from your body. If you've had your ovaries removed, your chances of getting osteoporosis increases to one out of two[22]. Unlike the rapid decline of estrogen in women, men have a gradual decline of testosterone, except for those who are chronic alcoholics, a condition that increases the chance of osteoporosis.

One million three hundred thousand women suffer annually from spontaneous fractures because of osteoporosis. As men and especially women age, they become shorter, stooped and often suffer from hip or wrist fractures. When osteoporosis is advanced to the place where thirty to forty percent of bone mass has been lost, the vertebrae start collapsing, and in women this is called the "dowager's hump." As much as five to eight inches in height is lost. Clothing no longer fit, and the proportional features of the body are lost.

Osteoporotics suffer ceaselessly from bone fractures and broken hips — 1.3 million each year. Those who have hip fractures — about 80% in the U.S. (about 200,000 per year) — have Osteoporosis. About twenty percent of those die within three months. According to Rex E. Newnham, Ph.D., D.O., N.D.[27], "magnesium and boron levels in the diet are of utmost importance" for prevention and healing of bone fractures caused by Osteoporosis.

The fear of falling and breaking one's hip keeps osteoporotics from doing many routine errands, thus placing needless restrictions reflecting a dwindling life style.

Most of these cases can be prevented!

Bone loss is not visible, and the problem begins in middle age, or earlier, somewhere around thirty-five to forty-five. There are no diagnostic tests that will warn you when you are beginning to lose more bone than you are building up bone tissue, until the problem has become overlarge.

According to William Campbell Douglass, M.D.[1] originally from Georgia but now from Panama: "There are two types of osteoporosis and you need to understand the difference.

"The first type, a gradual thinning of the bones over the years, all women will get if they live long enough. A study in the *American Journal of Medicine*[20] reported that '. . . by age 75 years, virtually the entire population of aging women will be subject to fractures . . .' You don't have to panic, but be careful.'

In this study, Dr. Riggs found that there was no difference in the sex hormone levels of women with or without osteoporosis. I emphasize that because if this is so then why are millions of women taking synthetic, cancer-causing estrogen (Premarin, Ogen, etc.) 'to prevent osteoporosis'?

Do you suppose somebody has been putting us on? [Natural hormonal replacement is safe. Ed.]

According to Rex E. Newnham, Ph.D., D.O., N.D.[27], "Animal studies have shown that the boron status of the animal affected the response to low dietary calcium. This apparently is seen because boron is active in the parathyroid of the rat. Magnesium is also most important, possibly more important than dietary calcium."

William Campbell Douglass[1] continues with, "As you get older your parathyroid gland starts over-working. . . . It does this because as you get older you don't absorb as much calcium from your food. If your blood calcium falls below a certain level you get spasm of the muscles called tetany. Your heart stops beating. You're finished, dead, kaput.

"The parathyroid gland comes to the rescue by raising your blood calcium level. But you pay a price. <u>That calcium is pulled out of your bones — osteoporosis</u>. So that hydrochloric acid . . . is very important in the prevention of osteoporosis — no hydrochloric acid, no calcium absorption. (That's the punch line.)

"The other type of osteoporosis comes earlier and progresses faster. If you fit in that category you'd better have a doctor who understands nutrition or you are going to be in big trouble."

What Causes Osteoporosis?

<u>**Hype from pharmaceutical companies interested in selling a lot of calcium in over-expensive packaging leads most of the American public to believe that taking calcium supplements will prevent or reverse the problem.**</u>

Not so!

Most of the calcium preparations that are touted through news media do not work on many women, mainly because for the most part they are calcium carbonate or some calcium compound of equal difficulty to absorb.

According to Pizzarno and Murray's *Textbook of Natural Medicine*[2], "Recently there has been an incredible push for supplementing calcium in an effort to halt bone loss. While this appears to be sound medical advice, osteoporosis is much more than a lack of dietary calcium. It is a complex condition involving hormonal, lifestyle, nutritional, and environmental factors."

According to William Campbell Douglass[1], M.D., as reported in "Death, Taxes and Osteoporosis", over forty percent of women over [the age of] fifty produce less stomach acid than normal. Without stomach acid, calcium carbonate, and like compounds, cannot be utilized. Therefore they do not solve the osteoporotic problem.

If you are achlorhydric (no stomach acid) or hypochlorhydric (reduced stomach acid), then you need to take calcium citrate or calcium lactate, as this form can be absorbed better. Some physicians use Calcium/ Magnesium Aspartate. Calcium/Magnesium Orotate is excellent. Newnham[27] says that "Calcium and magnesium ascorbate are two compounds of which both the acid radical and the metal are needed by the body. These should be the ultimate compounds of choice. These are both in the ultimate of the many boron tablets available."

Douglass[1] also suggests that you can get your doctor to furnish you with hydrochloric acid drops, which will solve digestion problems. Some physicians feel that use of hydrochloric acid is cumbersome and out-of-date and prefer to recommend use of Betaine Hydrochloride with or without Pepsin or Glutamic Hydrochloride with or without Pepsin. The FDA has recently denied use of Betaine Hydrochloride for this purpose, but it is still available without being labeled for digestive purposes.

According to a pamphlet published by Physicians Committee for Responsible Medicine[6], entitled *Osteoporosis*, "Some have suggested that osteoporosis is caused by lack of calcium. But studies show that increasing calcium intake after bones are formed does not prevent or reverse osteoporosis. It now appears that the amount of calcium women consume has nothing to do with the rate at which they lose bone mass with age."

Science magazine[5] noted "the large body of evidence indicating no relationship between calcium intake and bone density." Lawrence Riggs[5] of the Mayo Clinic measured bone densities and calcium intake in women for several years. He reported: "We found no correlation at all between calcium intake and bone loss, not even a trend."

From the same source: "Studies now show that high levels of protein — particularly animal protein — in the American diet drain calcium from the body. Observations of various populations worldwide show that societies with high protein consumption have a high incidence of osteoporosis. Eskimos, for example, eat large amounts of protein due to their heavy consumption of fish. Their diet is also extemely high in calcium, yet they suffer from high rates of osteoporosis. The amino acids released by protein in the body tend to deplete calcium from the bones. The calcium is then excreted in the urine.

"Those who consume smaller amounts of protein and avoid animal protein require far less calcium in order to stay in calcium balance. Vegetarians have a lower incidence of osteoporosis than those on a meat-based diet. This is probably due to two factors: they eat more reasonable amounts of protein and they avoid animal proteins. It is important not to overindulge in protein.

Again, according to Dr. Douglass[1] : "One of the best preventives is diet. You don't have to avoid animal protein as long as you get adequate folic acid, B[6] and other nutrients. Refined sugar, cigarette smoking and birth control pills should be avoided. All food should be cooked below the critical temperature of that particular food. Excess cooking of food at a high temperature is one of the major causes of degenerative diseases including osteoporosis."

Homocysteine

William Campbell Douglass, M.D.[1] further adds that, ". . . Methionine, an essential amino acid, is converted into homocysteine. The homocysteine, if not converted to something else, . . . will build up in the blood and tissues causing hardening of the arteries and probably osteoporosis.

"You've got to get rid of the homocysteine in your blood. Dr. Brattstrom[19] from the University Hospital in Lund, Sweden, has shown that women after menopause have significantly higher levels of homocysteine than younger women. He also found that 5 mg. of folic acid daily will dramatically reduce homocysteine blood levels.

Dr. Douglass says that "Your doctor can test you to determine if your blood contains excessive homocysteine. Tell him you're worried about your homocysteine level and you want an MDS (mixed disulfide) test."

Other physicians, including Dr. Jonathan Wright[4], feel that testing for excessive homocysteine is easier said than done, that the tests are expensive, and not especially easy to do. They agree that the idea is good, but feel that laboratory testing procedures are not "patient oriented."

Quoting Douglass[1] again: "Dr. Kilmer McCulley of Harvard . . . found that vitamin B6 is also essential to convert homocysteine to the form that can be excreted in the urine. It's not necessary to get a B6 test. Just take 50 mg of B6 twice a day. It's perfectly safe." [Sometimes Pyridoxal HCl (B6) is not as easily absorbed as its metabolite, Pyridoxal-5-Phosphate: Ed.]

Nutritional Supplementation

Many minerals, besides calcium, are important for the treatment and prevention of osteoporosis, including manganese, molybdenum, selenium and vanadium.

Boron

Boron is another mineral that has been shown to be extremely important for retaining calcium. In a study conducted by the U.S. Department of Agriculture[31], within 8 days of supplementing 3 mg. of boron, a test group of postmenopausal women lost 40 percent less calcium, one third less magnesium, and slightly less phosphorus through their urine.

The first scientific paper showing beneficial effects of boron on various forms of arthritis, and osteopororsis, was in 1979 entitled "Boron Beats Arthritis" to the Congress of the Australian and New Zealand Association for the Advancement of Science, Auckland, New Zeland, by Rex E. Newnham, Ph.D., D.O., N.D.[3]

Dr. Newnham had conducted many studies, both retrospective and clinical to show that boron is essential and helpful and if it is lacking, various problems will occur, including osteoporosis[3].

While Boron may not rebuild lost bones, it does seem to prevent the bone loss. Newnham[27] says, "It has been shown with a number of patients that boron will help broken bones to mend in about half the normal time, in men, dogs and horses. No clinical trials have been completed, but the indication is that when boron is added to the diet at the rate of 3 mg. 3 times daily the rate and quality of bone repair is enhanced.

"It is well known that the parathyroid helps control bone mineralization, and work done by Dr. Nielsen[29,30,31] and others has shown that boron is probably essential for the proper parathyroid function in the animal. More research is needed. But this would explain why boron is so effective in the healing of many kinds of arthritis, osteoporosis and broken bones."

Several companies now produce and sell special products containing boron. Tablets made to Dr. Newnham's specification are available in the USA.

According to Alan R.Gaby & Jonathan V. Wright

(*References to Gaby/Wright Article are given immediuately after their nutritional summary.*)

According to Alan R. Gaby, M.D. of Maryland and Jonathan V. Wright, M.D.[5] of Washington, a wide range of additional supplements may aid the osteoporosis problem.

The following summary has been taken from their article *Nutrients and Bone Health*.[12] Supplements for osteoporosis should include more than calcium, but also Vitamin K, Vitamin D, Magnesium, Manganese, Folic Acid, Boron, Strontium, Silicon, Pyridoxine (Vitamin B6), Zinc, Copper, and Ascorbic Acid (Vitamin C).

"Vitamin K

"Vitamin K is known primarily for its effect on blood clotting. However, this vitamin is also required to synthesize osteocalcin, a protein found uniquely and in large amounts in bone.[12] Osteocalcin is the protein matrix upon which calcium crystalizes. The component of osteocalcin that attracts calcium ions is a modified amino acid, gamma-carboxyglutamic acid, formed by the vitamin K-dependent carboxylation of glutamic acid. Because of its role in osteocalcin production, vitamin K is essential for bone formation, remodeling, and repair.

"It is generally assumed that vitamin K deficiency is rare. However, assessment of vitamin K status is based on relatively insensitive tests, such as prothrombin time. Recent advances have made it possible to measure vitamin K levels in blood. In a series of 16 patients with osteoporosis, mean serum vitamin K concentration was only 35% that of age-matched controls.[13] If osteocalcin synthesis is sensitive to changes in serum vitamin K levels, then the low levels in osteoporotic patients may have clinical significance. That possibility was supported by a recent study in which vitamin K supplementation of a typical Western diet increased urinary excretion of gamma-carboxyglutamic acid by 23%.[14]

"Vitamin K deficiency is probably more common than previously believed. Deficiency may occur in individuals whose vegetable consumption is low. Another factor that could promote deficiency is frequent use of antibiotics which can destroy naturally occurring vitamin K-producing bacteria in the intestines.

"Rats fed a vitamin K deficient diet had significantly increased urinary calcium excretion.[15] Furthermore, vitamin K supplementation accelerated the healing of experimental fractures in rabbits, even though they were already receiving 'adequate' levels in their diet.[16] In a preliminary study of osteoporotic patients, treatment with vitamin K reduced urinary calcium loss by 18-50%.[17] The evidence suggests that, when accelerated bone formation is desirable, as in osteoporosis or after a fracture, a greater amount of vitamin K is required.

"Vitamin D

"Vitamin D is required for intestinal calcium absorption. Reduced plasma vitamin D levels are common in elderly individuals, especially women.[18] Factors that lower vitamin D levels in the elderly include reduced exposure to sunlight, decreased dietary intake, and malabsorption.

"Impaired conversion of vitamin D to its biologically active form, 1,25-dihydroxyvitamin D3, may in some cases exacerbate a marginal deficiency. Indeed, abnormal metabolism of vitamin D precursors may sometimes be a more significant problem than dietary deficiency.

"Treatment of osteoporotic patients with 1,25-dihydroxyvitamin D3 increased calcium absorption, improved calcium balance,[19] and reduced bone loss[20] in some studies. However, in other trials, this treatment was without benefit.[21] Routine use of 1,25-dihydroxyvitamin D3 has been limited by its high cost and by the risk of hypercalcemia associated with long-term therapy.

"Vitamin D should be supplemented in cases where dietary intake and sunlight exposure are inadequate. Measures should also be taken to enhance the conversion of vitamin D precursors to the biologically active 1,25-dihydroxyvitamin D3. This conversion may be facilitated by treatment with magnesium and boron (see below).

"Magnesium

"Magnesium participates in a number of biochemical reactions that take place in bone. Alkaline phosphatase, an enzyme involved in forming new calcium crystals, is activated by magnesium.[22] The conversion of vitamin D to its biologically active form, 1,25-dihydroxyvitamin D3, also appears to require magnesium.[23] Deficiency of magnesium can produce a syndrome of "vitamin D resistance."[24]

"Whole-body content and bone concentrations of magnesium were below normal in 16 of 19 osteoporotic women.[25] All sixteen women with low magnesium levels also had abnormal crystal formation in their bones, a factor which might increase the risk of fractures. The three women with normal magnesium status had normal crystal formation.

"The typical American diet is often low in magnesium. Dietary surveys have shown that 80-85% of American women consume less than the RDA for this mineral.[26] Daily magnesium intake in two other studies was only about two-thirds of the RDA.[27,28] These studies suggest that magnesium deficiency is common in the United States.

"Manganese

"Manganese is required for bone mineralization,[29] and for synthesis of connective tissue in cartilage and bone.[30] Rats fed a manganese deficient diet had smaller, less dense bones with less resistance to fractures than those fed adequate amounts of manganese.[29] The optimal intake of manganese is not known, but at least half of the manganese in a typical diet is lost when whole grains are replaced in refined flour.[31] Genetic factors influence the susceptibility of animals to manganese deficiency.[32] It is therefore likely that certain subsets of the human population are unusually sensitive to the effects of marginal manganese intake.

"Interest in the relationship between manganese and osteoporosis was stimulated by observations on a famous professional basketball player, who had repeatedly suffered poorly healing fractures and who was found to have unexplained osteoporosis. Examination of his blood revealed no detectable manganese, as well as deficiencies of other minerals. Within six weeks of supplementing his diet with these minerals, he was back to playing basketball. These observations led to a study of osteoporotic women, in whom blood manganese levels were found to be only 25% that of controls.[33]

"Folic acid

"The importance of folic acid for bone health seems to be related to its role in homocysteine metabolism. Methionine, one of the eight essential amino acids present in food, is converted in part to homocysteine, a potentially toxic compound. The danger of homocysteine has been discovered by studying individuals with a genetic disorder in which abnormally large amounts of homocysteine accumulate. These individuals develop severe osteoporosis at an early age, possibly due to an adverse effect of homocysteine on bone.[34]

"Prior to menopause, women are especially efficient at converting homocysteine to less toxic compounds. This unique metabolic efficiency may account in part for the resistance of premenopausal women to bone loss.[35]

"The following study suggests that, at the time of menopause, a breakdown of homocysteine metabolism occurs, which can be partly corrected by folic acid supplementation. Serum homocysteine levels were measured in female volunteers after administration of methionine. These levels were substantially greater in postmenopausal than in pre-menopausal women, with no overlap between the two groups. Treatment with folic acid partially prevented the methionine-induced rise in serum homocysteine, even though none of the women were deficient in folic acid by standard laboratory criteria.[36] Thus, it appears that menopause is associated with an increased requirement for folic acid which, if unmet, may result in an elevation of serum homocysteine.

"Folic acid deficiency is relatively common, occurring in as many as 22% of individuals 65 years of age.[37] Typical American diets often contain only half of the RDA for folic acid.[38] Tobacco smoking, drinking alcohol, and using oral contraceptives also tend to promote folic acid

258

deficiency.

"Boron

"Previously thought to be essential only for plants, boron now appears to play a role in human nutrition, particularly in relation to bone health. Postmenopausal women were fed a standard diet for 119 days, supplying about 0.25 mg of boron/day. Supplementation of this diet with boron (3 mg/day) reduced urinary calcium excretion by 44% and markedly increased serum concentrations of the estrogenic hormone, 17 beta-estradiol.[39,50] In fact, the levels of 17-beta estradiol in boron-supplemented women were the same as in women receiving estrogen therapy. This increase in hormone concentration may be important, since 17-beta estradiol is the most biologically active form of naturally occurring human estrogen.

The way in which boron acts in the body is not known. However, it seems to be required for the formation of activated (hydroxylated) forms of certain steroid hormones. Boron is known to complex with organic compounds containing hydroxyl groups. It may therefore participate in hydroxylation steps necessary for the synthesis of 17 beta-estradiol and 1,25-dihydroxyvitamin D3. Boron deficiency exacerbated signs of vitamin D deficiency in chicks, including abnormal bone formation and elevation of alkaline phosphatase.[41]

Based on animal studies, Nielsen has estimated the human boron requirement to be approximately 1-2 mg/day. Fruits, vegetables and nuts are the main dietary sources of boron. Diets containing inadequate amounts of these foods may be deficient in boron.

Toxicity studies in animals have shown a comfortable margin of safety for 'nutritional' doses of boron (1-3 mg/day). No adverse effects were seen in dogs and rats fed chronically with 350 ppm of boron,[42] which corresponds to approximately 117 mg/day in humans. In certain parts of the world where the diet contains as much as 41 mg of boron/day,[43] no problems have been reported.

The fact that boron raised endogenous estrogen levels does not suggest that this mineral poses the same risks as estrogen therapy. The cancer-causing effect of estrogen is dose-related. Because orally administered 17-beta estradiol (conjugated estrogens) is mostly converted to estrone by the gastrointestinal tract, large amounts of estrogen must be given by mouth to achieve a clinically useful serum level of 17-beta estradiol. In contrast, the amount of endogenously produced 17-beta estradiol required to maintain beneficial serum levels may be as little as 5% of the oral dose.[44] Thus, boron appears capable of producing an estrogenic effect without exposing the body to dangerous amounts of estrogen.

Another factor that argues against a cancer risk is the apparent participation of boron in hydroxylation reactions. Synthesis of estriol, a weak estrogen with documented anti-cancer activity, involves a hydroxylation step, which would presumably be catalyzed by boron.

Increasing estriol levels (as a proportion of total estrogens) may reduce the incidence of certain types of cancer.[45] If boron does indeed increase estriol production then it might actually help prevent cancer.

"Strontium

"Strontium occurs in relatively large concentrations in bones and teeth, where it is thought to replace a small fraction of the calcium in hydroxyapatite crystals.[46] Awareness of the nutritional significance of strontium has been overshadowed by the fear of radioactive strontium, a component of nuclear fallout. Because strontium tends to accumulate in bone tissue, radioactive strontium may be particularly hazardous to vertebrates. On the other hand, non-radioactive strontium occurs naturally in food. This mineral is apparently quite safe, even with long-term administraiton at doses hundreds of times greater than the usual dietary intake.[57]

"Several studies suggest a beneficial effect of strontium on calcified tissues. The incidence of dental caries was reduced in geographical regions with high levels of strontium in drinking water. Furthermore, addition of 0.27% strontium to the drinking water of mice reduced bone-resorbing activity by 11.3%.[48]

"The effect of strontium in human osteoporosis has also been investigated. Thirty-two patients were given pharmacologic doses of strontium (1.7 g/day) for periods ranging from 3 months to 3 years (10 also received estrogen and testosterone). Twenty-seven (84%) experienced marked reduction in bone pain. Radiologic examination showed possible improvement in 78% of the strontium-treated patients.[47]

"The effect of physiologic doses of strontium (several milligrams/day) has not been studied. However, chronic consumption of strontium-depleted, refined foods[49] may adversely affect bone strength.

"Silicon

"High concentrations of silicon are found at calcification sites in growing bone.[50] This mineral appears to strengthen the connective tissue matrix by crosslinking collagen strands.[51] Chicks fed a silicon deficient diet developed gross abnormalities of the skull and had unusually thin leg bones. The number of trabeculae was reduced and there was evidence of impaired calcification.[51,52]

"It is not known whether the typical American diet provides adequate amounts of silicon. As with other nutrients, subclinical deficiencies could result from overconsumption of refined foods. In patients with osteoporosis, where accelerated bone regeneration is desirable, silicon requirements may be increased.

"Pyridoxine (Vitamin B6)

"Vitamin B6 deficient diets produced osteoporosis in rats.[53] The effect of B6 on bone health may involve several different mechanisms. this vitamin is a cofactor in the enzymatic crosslinking of collagen strands,[54] which increases the strength of connective tissue. Vitamin B6 also helps break down homocysteine,[55 a methionine metabolite which is believed to promote osteoporosis (see section on folic acid).

"Dietary surveys indicate that B6 intake by American women is frequently less than the RDA.[56,57] Biochemical evidence of B6 deficiency was found in more than half of a group of presumably healthy volunteers.[58]

"Zinc

"Zinc is essential for normal bone formation.[59] This mineral also enhances the biochemical actions of vitamin D.[60] Zinc levels were low in serum and bone of elderly patients with osteoporosis.[61] Low serum zinc levels were also found in individuals with accelerated bone loss of the alveolar ridge of the mandible.[62]

"The typical American diet is low in zinc. In one dietary survey, 68% of adults consumed less than two-thirds of the RDA for zinc.[63] Widespread dietary zinc deficiency has been reported in other studies.[64,65]

"At present, the picolinic acid salt of zinc (zinc picolinate) appears to have a greater degree of bioavailability than other zinc supplements.[66] Picolinate is a naturally occurring metabolite of tryptophane which is believed to enhance zinc absorption and transport in humans.

"Copper

"Rats fed a copper deficient diet had reduced bone mineral content and reduced bone strength.[67,68] Copper supplementation also inhibited bone resorption in vitro.[69] The mechanism of action of copper is not known. However, this mineral is a cofactor for the enzyme lysyl oxidase,[70] which strengthens connective tissue by crosslinking collagen strands.

"Since a typical American diet contains only about 50% of the RDA (2 mg/day) for copper,[71] deficiency of this trace mineral may be quite common.

"Ascorbic acid (Vitamin C)

"Osteoporosis can result from vitamin C deficiency.[72] Although frank scurvy is rare in the United States, subclinical ascorbic acid deficiency may be common. Biochemical evidence of vitamin C deficiency was found in 20% of elderly women, even though they were consuming more than the RDA of 60 mg/day.[73]"

These twelve nutrients, and ten more, (in appropriate quantities) are supplied in OsteoPrime™ and Osteo Prime™ forte distributed by Bio-Therapeutics, Post Office Box 1348, Green Bay, Wisconsin 54305 [1-800-553-2370].

The above twenty-two combined nutrients were formulated by two physicians, Jonathan Wright, M.D. and Alan Gaby, M.D. as a supplement. OsteoPrime forte is designed for high risk individuals. **They are both available only through health care practitioners**. (Since they both contain Vitamin K, individuals taking the prescription drugs Coumadin or Warfarin should not take these supplements.)

"References to "According to Gaby & Wright

[Editorial Note: The first eleven and the last nine of the original Gaby/ Wright references are in their original article but not in this slight condensation.]

1. Riggs BL, Melton LJ III. Involutional osteoporosis. *N Engl J Med* 1986;314:1676-1686.

2. Avioli LV *The Osteoporotic Syndrome*, Harcourt Brace Javonovich, New York, 1983.

3. Recker RR, Saville PD,Heaney RP. Effect of estrogens and calcium carbonate on bone loss in postmenopausal women. *Ann Intern Med* 1977;87:649-655.

4. Burnell JM, Baylink DJ, Chesnut CH III, Teubner EJ. The role of skeletal calcium deficiency in postmenopausal osteoporosis. *Calcif Tissue Int* 1986;38:187-192.

5. Albanese AA. Calcium in the prevention and management of osteoporosis. *J Nutr Elderly* 1984;3(3):57-65.

6. Lee CJ, Lawler GS, Johnson GH. Effects of supplementation of the diets with calcium and calcium-rich foods on bone density of elderly females with osteoporosis. *Am J Clin Nutr* 1981;34:819-823.

7. Nordin BEC, Horsman A, Crilly RG, Marshall DH, Simpson M. Treatment of spinal osteoporosis in postmenopausal women. *Br Med J* 1980;280:541-454.

8. Horsman A, Gallagher JC, Simpson M, Nordin BEC. Prospective trial of oestrogen and calcium in postmenopausal women. *Br Med J* 1977;2:789-792.

9. Health and Public Policy Committee, American College of Physicians. Radiologic methods to evaluate bone mineral content. *Ann Intern Med* 1984;100:908-911.

10. Riis B, Thomsen K, Christiansen C. Does calcium supplementation prevent postmenopausal bone loss? *N Engl J Med* 1987;316:173-177.

11. Albanese AA, Lorenze EJ Jr, Wein EH, Carroll L. Effects of calcium and micronutrients on bone loss of pre- and postmenopausal women. Scientific Exhibit presented to the American Medical Association in Atlanta, Georgia, January 24-26, 1981.

12. Gallop PM, Lian JB, Hauschka PV. Carboxylated calcium-binding proteins and vitamin K. *N Engl J Med* 1980;302:1460-1466.

13. Hart JP, Shearer MJ, Kelnerman L, Shearer MJ, Caterall A, et al. Electrochemical detection of depressed circulating levels of vitamin K_1 in osteoporosis. *J Clin Endocrinol Metab* 1985;60:1268-1269.

14. Suttie JW, Mummah-Schendel LL, Shah DV, Lyle BJ, Greger JL. Vitamin K deficiency from dietary vitamin K restriction in humans. *Am J Clin Nutr* 1988;47:475-480. (The 23% increase noted in the text was not statistically significant.)

15. Robert D, Jorgetti V, Lacour B, Leclerq M, Cournot-Witmer G.

Hypercalciuria during experimental vitamin K deficiency in the rat. *Calcif Tissue Int* 1985;37:143-147.

16. Bouckaert JH, Said AH. Fracture healing by vitamin K. *Nature* 1960;185:849.

17.Tomita A. Post menopausal osteoporosis [47]Ca study with vitamin K_2. *Clin Endocrinol* (Jpn) 1971;19:731-736.

18. Anonymous. Vitamin D supplementation in the elderly. *Lancet* 1987;1:306-307.

19. Gallagher JC, Riggs BL, DeLuca HF. Effect of treatment with synthetic 1,25-dihydroxyvitamin D in postmenopausal osteoporosis. *Clin Res* 1979;27:366A.

20. Anonymous. Two studies indicate vitamin D metabolite curbs osteoporosis. *Family Pract News* 1984(March15):2.

21. Brautbar N. Osteoporosis: Is 1,25-(OH)D$_3$ of value in treatment? *Nephron* 1986;44:161-166.

22. Iseri LT, French JH. Magnesium: nature's physiologic calcium blocker. *Am Heart J* 1984;108:188-193.

23. Rude RK, Adams JS, Ryzen E, Endres DB, Niimi H, et al. Low serum concentrations of 1,25dihydroxyvitamin D in human magnesium deficiency. *J Clin Endocrinol Metab* 1985;61:933-940.

24. Medalle R, Waterhouse C, Hahn TJ. Vitamin D resistance in magnesium deficiency. *Am J Clin Nutr* 1976;29:854-858.

25. Cohen L, Kitzes R. Infrared spectroscopy and magnesium content of bone mineral in osteoporotic women, Isr *J Med Sci* 1981;17:1123-1125.

26. Morgan KJ, Stampley GL, Zabik ME, Fischer DR. Magnesium and calcium dietary intakes of the U.S. population. *J Am Coll Nutr* 1985;4:195-206.

27. Lakshmanan FL, Rao RB, Kim WW, Kelsay JL. Magnesium intakes, balances, and blood levels of adults consuming self-selected diets. *Am J Clin Nutr* 1984;40:1380-1389.

28. Srivastava US, Nadeau MH, Gueneau L. Mineral intakes of university students: magnesium content. *Nutr Rep Int* 1978;18:235-242.

29. Amdur MO, Norris LC, Heuser, GF. The need for manganese in bone development by the rat. *Proc Soc Exp Biol Med* 1945;59:254-255.

30. Leach RM Jr, Muenster AM. Studies on the role of manganese in bone formation. I. Effect upon the mucopolysaccharide content of chick bone. *J Nutr* 1962;78:51-56.

31. Wenlock RW, Buss DH, Dixon EJ. Trace nutrients. 2. Manganese in british food. Br *J Nutr* 1979;41:253-261.

32. Hurley LS, Bell LT. Genetic influence on response to dietary manganese deficiency in mice. *J Nutr* 1974;104:133-137.

33. Raloff J. Reasons for boning up on manganese. *Science News* 1986(Sept.27):199.

34. Grieco AJ. Homocystinuria: pathogenetic mechanisms. *Am J Med Sci* 1977;273:120-132.

35. Boers GH, Smals AG, Trijbels FJ, Leermakers AI, Kloppenborg PW. Unique efficiency of methionine metabolism in premenopausal women may protect against vascular disease in the reproductive years. *J Clin Invest* 1983;72:1971-1976.

36. Battstrom LE, Hultberg BL, Hardebo JE. Folic acid responsive postmenopausal homocysteinemia. *Metabolism* 1985;34:1073-1077.

37. Infant-Rivard C, et al. Folate deficiency among institutionalized elderly. *J Am Geriatr Soc* 1986;34:211-214.

38. Clark AJ, Gates R. Folacin status of adolescent females. *Fed Proc* 1983;42:830.

39. Nielsen FH. Boron - an overlooked element of potential nutritional importance. *Nutr Today* 1988(Jan/Feb):4-7.

40. Nielsen FH, Hunt CD, Mullen LM, Hunt JR. Effect of dietary boron on mineral, estrogen, and testosterone metabolism in postmenopausal women. *FASEBJ* 1987;1:394-397.

41. Hunt CD, Nielsen FH. Interaction between boron and cholecalciferol in the chick. In Gawthorne JM, Howell JM, White CL (eds). *Trace Element Metabolism in Man and Animals*, Springer-Verlag, Berlin, 1982, pp. 597-600.

42. Weir RJ Jr, Fisher RS. Toxicologic stuides on borox and boric acid. *Toxicol Appl Pharmacol* 1972;23:351-364.

43. Schlettwein-Gsell D, Mommsen-Straub S. Ubersicht spurenelemente in lebensmitteln. *IX. Bor. Int Z Vitaminforsch* 1973;43:93-109.

44. Barnhart ER (Publisher). *Physician's Desk Reference*, Medical Economics Company, Inc., Oradell, N.J., 1988, p. 867.

45. Lemon HM, Wotiz HH, Parsons L, Mozden PJ. Reduced estriol excretion in patients with breast cancer prior to endocrine therapy. *JAMA* 1966;196:1128-1136.

46. Anonymous. Strontium and dental caries. *Nutr Rev* 1983;41-342-344.

47. McCaslin FE Jr, Janes JM. The effect of strontium lactate in the treatment of osteoporosis. *Proc Staff Meetings Mayo Clin* 1959;34:329-334.

48. Marie PJ, Hott M. Short-term effects of fluoride and strontium on bone forming and bone resorbing cells in the mouse. *Calcif Tissue Int* 1985;38(Suppl):S17.

49. Schroeder HA, Tipton IH, Nason AP. Trace metals in man: strontium and barium. *J Chronic Dis* 1972;25:491-517.

50. Carlisle EM. Silicon localization and calcification in developing bone. *Fed Proc* 1969;28:374.

51. Anonymous. Silicon and bone formation. *Nutr Rev* 1980;38:194-195.

52 Carlisle EM. Silicon an essential element for the chick. Fed Proc 1972;31:700.

53. Benke PJ, Fleshood HL, Pitot HC. Osteoporotic bone disease in the pyridoxine-deficient rat. *Biochem Med* 1972;6:526-535.

54. Anonymous. Vitamin B$_6$ deficiency affects lung elastin crosslinking. *Nutr Rev* 1986;44:24-25.

55. Seashore MR, Durant JL, Rosenberg LE. Studies on the mechanism of pyridoxine-responsive homocystinuria. *Pediatr Res* 1972;6:187-196.

56.Kirksey A, Keaton K, Abernathy RP, Greger JL. Vitamin B6 nutritional status of a group of female adolescents. *Am J Clin Nutr* 1978;31:946-954.

57. Hampton DJ, Chrisley BM, Driskell JA Vitamin B$_6$ status of the elderly in Montgomery Country, Va. *Nutr Rep Int* 1977;16:743-750.

58. Azuma J, Kishi T, Williams RH, Folkers, K. Apparent deficiency of vitamin B$_6$ in typical individuals who commonly serve as normal controls. *Res Commun Chem Pathol Pharmacol* 1976;14:343-348.

59. Calhoun NR, Smith JC Jr, Becker KL. The effects of zinc on ectopic bone formation. *Oral Surg* 1975;39-698-706.

60. Yamaguchi M, Sakashita T. Enhancement of vitamin D$_3$ effect on bone metabolism in weanling rats orally administered zinc sulphate. *Acta Endocrinol* 1986;111:285-288.

61. Atik OS. Zinc and senile osteoporosis. J *Am Geriatr Soc* 1983;31:790-791.

62. Frithiof L, Lavstedt S, Eklund G, Soderberg U, Skarberg KO, et al. The relationship between marginal bone loss and serum zinc levels. *Acta Med Scand* 1980;207:67-70.

63. Holden JM, Wolf WR, Mertz. Zinc and copper in self-selected diets. *J Am Diet Assoc* 1979;75:23-28.

64. Patterson KY, Holbrook JT, Bodner JE, Kelsay JL, Smith JC Jr, et. al. Zinc, copper, and manganese intake and balance for adults consuming self-selected diets. *Am J Clin Nutr* 1984;40:1397-1403.

65. Greger JL, Higgins MM, Abernathy RP, Kirksey A, DeCorso MB, et. al. Nutritional status of adolescent girls in regard to zinc, copper, and iron, *Am J Clin Nutr* 1978;31:269-275.

66. Barrie SA, Wright JV, Pizzorno JE, Kutter E, Barron PC. Comparative absorption of zinc picolinate, zinc citrate and zinc gluconate in humans. *Agents Actions* 1987;21:223-228.

67. Smith RT, Smith JC, Fields M, Reiser S. Mechanical properties of bone from copper deficient rats fed starch or fructose. *Fed Proc* 1985;44:541.

68. Follis RH Jr, Bush JA, Cartwright GE, Wintrobe MM. Studies on copper metabolism. XVIII. Skeletal changes associated with copper deficiency in swine. *Johns Hopkins Hosp Bull* 1955;97:405-409.

69. Wilson T, Katz JM, Gray DH. Inhibition of active bone resorption by copper. *Calcif Tissue Int* 1981;33:35-39.

70.Anonymous. Activation of lysyl oxidase by copper. *Nutr Rev* 1979;37:330-331.

71. Wolf WR, Holden J, Greene FE. Daily intake of zinc and copper from self selected diets. *Fed Proc* 1977;37:1175.

72. Hyams DE, Ross EJ. Scurvy, megaloblastic anaemia and osteoporosis. *Br J Clin Pract* 1963;17:332-340.

73. Morgan AF, Gillum HL, Williams RI. Nutritional status of aging. III. Serum ascorbic acid and intake. *J Nutr* 1955;55:431-448.

74. Spencer H, Menczel J, Lewin I, Samachson J. Absorption of calcium in osteoporosis. *Am J Med* 1964;37:223-234.

75. Brechner J, Armstrong WD. Relation of gastric acidity to alveolar bone resorption. *Proc Soc Exp Biol Med* 1941;48:98.

76. Sharp GS, Fister HW. The diagnosis and treatment of achlorhydria: ten year study. J Am Geriatr Soc 1967;15:786-791.

79. Ivanovich P, Fellows H, Rich C. The absorption of calcium carbonate. Ann Intern Med 1967;66:917-923.

79. Mahoney AW, Hendricks DG. Role of gastric acid in the utilization of dietary calcium by the rat. Nutr Metabol 1974;16:375-382.

80. Hunt JN, Johnson C. Relation between gastric secretion of acid and urinary excretion of calcium after oral supplements of calcium. Dig Dis Sci 1983;28:417-421.

81. Nicar MJ, Pak CYC. Calcium bioavailability from calcium carbonate and calcium citrate. J Clin Endocrinol Metab 1985;61:391-393."

Additional Suggestions
Environmental Toxins

The *Textbook of Natural Medicine* (Pizzorno and Murray)[13] disagrees with the presumption that Flouride strengthens bone structure, as "its validity has not survived the scrutiny of controlled studies."

Newnhan[27], says"People who have been ingesting fluoride for years can develop dental fluorosis which can be seen easily, and they also develop skeletal fluorosis which cannot be seen. Because doctors were never taught about this few of them recognize it and simply call the problem arthritis. Boron is the natural antagonist to fluoride and will overcome its effects. Too much fluoride in the diet tends to osteosclerosis and this uneveness in bone density will show as more marked areas of poor bone structure when osteoporosis starts to occur. A worthwhile study would be to examine X-rays of cases of osteoporotic fracture in areas of high fluoride and areas of low fluoride in the water. See the work of Mark Diesendorf, Ph.D.[28]." (See : "Fluoride: Governmentally Approved Poison," http://www.arthritistrust.org.)

Also Aluminum over-exposure, Pizzorno and Murray[13] feel, "may be an important [negative] factor in some patients."

David Watta[14], Ph.D. says that "Lead is known to interfere with collagen synthesis, and Cadmium has been shown to decrease the mineral content of bone, thereby contributing to osteoporosis."

Hormonal Therapy
Estrogen

Estrogen has long been used in treatment of osteoporosis, especially for those women who no longer produce a sufficient quantity. Estrogen as normally used and available in the United States, however, has some serious side effects, such as cancer of the uterus, gall bladder disease, high blood pressure, blood clots and abnormal vaginal bleeding. Furthermore, estrogen may not be doing the job it is thought to do. The problem has to do with the kind of estrogen available in the United States, according to Jonathan Wright, M.D. There is a form of estrogen available on prescription that, taken along with Vitamin E and Omega 6 and Omega 3 fatty acids will do the job. It is called *Triest*, and contains a small amount of Estradiol and Estrone and a major amount of Estriol. I understand that this combination can also be used for prevention of Osteoporosis by cancer patients under medical supervision. The Vitamin E and Omega 6 and Omega 3 fatty acids assist in preventing thrombolic diseases[4].

Edward Thorpe, Ph.D., suggests caution in the use of Triest, because females of certain families have a genetic sensitivity to estriol. This sensitivity can be determined by appropriate urine screening during mid-teens. Apparently, after the mid-teens, there is no further danger in the application of estriol[23].

Progesterone

According to John R. Lee, M.D., "Conventional treatment with vitamin D, calcium, and estrogen will delay but not reverse osteoporosis. The addition of fluoride may increase bone mass but fails to increase bone strength; fracture incidence is actually increased in non-vertrebral bone by fluoride. . . . The hypothesis that progesterone and not estrogen is the missing factor was tested in a clinical setting and was found to be extraordinarily effective in reversing osteoporosis[24]."

Dr. Lee followed 100 post-menopausal white woman average age of 65.2 years. The majority had already noted height loss, and many had already observed one or more bone fractures. He said, "The benefits from the treatment program were so obvious to these patients that no problems with patient compliance arose. . . . Height loss was stabilized, previous musculoskeltal aches and pains disappeared and no osteoporotic fractures occurred. . . .the average 3-year change in density, instead of losing an expected 4.5% actually increased 15.4%. Patient age was found not to be a factor; the increase in bone density for those 70 years older was identical with that of those less than 70. The most important factor in relative gain in bone density was found to be the initial lumbar bone density; i.e., those with the lowest bone densities experienced the greatest relative improvement.[24]"

Additional studies by Jerilynn C. Prior, M.D., Yvette Vigna, R.N. and Nenita Alojado, R.N.[25] seem to support John Lee's use of progesterone. They concluded in their studies that "Cyclic medroxyprogesterone (Provera) treatment replaces the hormone progesterone that is missing during anovulatory cycles. This treatment may prevent spinal bone loss and promote gains in bone density. Cyclic Provera also produces a predictable flow and prevents a potentially increased endometrial cancer risk. Cyclic progesterone replacment is a rational treatment for amenorrhea and ovulation disorders, which must be suspected, documented and treated. Recent studies suggest that this treatment may be important in the prevention of osteoporosis."

John R. Lee, M.D. and other physicians have learned to apply a progesterone cream directly to the skin, and have found relief for PMS, Pre- and Post-menopausal conditions and Osteoporosis.

Nandrolone Decanoate

Nandrolone decanoate, under the name of Decadurabolin[R], has been reported to be used for reversal of Osteoporosis in parts of Africa and Europe[26]. It is injected intra-muscularly, 100 mg. once each month.This was Dr. Paul Pybus, deceased Chief Medical Advisor for The Rheumatoid Disease Foundation and also by our former Research Director, John Simoons, PhD formerly employed by Organon pharmaceuticals, the company that owns and produces Decadurabolin[R]. As this substance is not widely used for Osteoporosis in the United States, caution is advised. It may be perfectly safe, but, on the other hand, since hormone stimulation must be involved in its use, one should take care that your physician knows its safety and efficacy for this particular use.

According to Newnham[27], "Work done by the Human Nutrition Research Center in North Dakota[29,30] has shown that a boron supplement would restore the hormone levels to normal in elderly women after they had been eating a low boron diet. Many elderly people eat a low boron diet these days. Boron supplements are safer and better than using synthetic hormones."

Exercise

"Exercise is another important feature of an osteoporosis prevention program. At about age 35, human bones begin to lose mass. To prevent osteoporosis, one must build bone mass early in life in order to withstand bone loss in later years. This is accomplished by weight-bearing exercises such as walking, dancing and playing tennis."

Notice emphasis on "weight-bearing exercises."

Until relatively recently it was felt that exercise alone would help to prevent or reverse osteoporosis. After all, the body and its parts, respond as a demand system: i.e. the more one uses the muscles, the stronger one becomes, the more one uses one's brain, the better one can use the brain and so on. It therefore follows that the more one uses your muscles and bones in exercise, the less osteoporosis.

Relatively recent studies of the effects of weightlessness on the human body by American, English, Russian, and French scientists demonstrate that exercise alone is not enough to prevent bone loss. The exercise must be "weight-bearing;" i.e **against gravity**.

These same studies also show that there is no apparent difference between bone loss suffered by astronauts, bone loss suffered by those immobilized in bed (disuse Osteoporosis), and those of us conducting our everyday activities and who have Osteoporosis. It's quite predictable, therefore, that space

268

research funds are being expended to find a way for astronauts to travel for long durations in space without bone loss, and that such discoveries, when found, will help us here on earth. If a positive means is not discovered, we will not be able to explore or even to colonize moons or planets a long distance from earth.

According to L. Schultheis[6] "Mechanical forces appear to coordinate the fundamental bone shaping processes by a negative feedback control system."

In "Can The Adult Skeleton Recover Lost Bone?" A. LeBlanc and V. Schneider[7] say: "We conclude that recovery [from bone loss] can be expected, but the rate and extent will be individual and bone site dependent."

In P. Minaire's[8] article "Immobilization Osteoporosis; A Review," he says that "The prevention is based on exercise if the load is applied intermittently for a daily period. It seems also that muscle weight is an important determinant of bone mass. There is a potential for recovery during subsequent late (about six months) inactive phase. Permanent losses [from immobilization] could be prevented by appropriate measures, pharmacology or exercises applied during the first months of immobilization. No recovery has been demonstrated after the inactive phase has been reached, whatever the treatment."

And finally, Schoutens, Laurent and Poortmans[9] say:" Bone mass and muscular mass show a parallel evolution during growth, and parallel involution with age. However, the bone loss related to the withdrawal of oestrogens is independent of muscular waste. The extensive study of disuse osteoporosis shows that exercise without weight-bearing cannot counteract the loss of bone mass provoked by bed rest or weightlessness. Physical training, even at low frequency (30 to 60 min/day, 2 or 3 days/week), can increase bone mass or reduce bone loss associated with age. This effect is even present when exercise is practised by very old people at a seemingly low level of muscular tension on bone . . . . Equal distribution of tension on all parts of the skeleton is probably not mandatory to obtain a general effect of exercise on bone mass. It is assumed that muscular exercise acts through tension exerted on bone, but the exact mechanism is unknown, as are the specifications of effective exercise in terms of site of application, intensity, frequency and duration. Moreover, little is known about the expected synergy between exercise and occupational activity."

In the *JAMA* section, State of the Art/Review[10] "'Senile' Osteoporosis Reconsidered" by Neil M. Resnick et. al. The summary is quoted: "Osteoporosis is a devastating, morbid, and costly condition whose ravages are felt most profoundly by women over age 70 years. Yet most research on its prevention and treatment has focused on perimenopausal women [women just before, during, or just after menopause], although there are significant differences between perimenopausal and older women in factors related to bone mineral metabolism, rates of bone loss, the structural integrity of remaining bone, risk factors for fractures, and the types of fractures sustained.

Currently recommended therapies, which slow bone loss in perimenopausal women, may be of less benefit for older women whose loss of bone has already slowed or ceased and whose remaining bone may be of inadequate quantity and quality to prevent fracture. Thus, the application of currently available modalities is unlikely to mitigate significantly the consequences of osteoporosis in this population. Further research is urgently needed, and some directions for future investigation are suggested."

Chelation Therapy

Ethylene diamine tetracetic acid, known as EDTA, is successfully used for treating many diseases, because repeated infusions make it easier for the body to more fully and properly nourish each cell. Better nourished cells produce healthier organs, which, in turn, provide for greater reserve potentials and improved functioning. (See : "Chelation Therapy," http://www.arthritistrust.org also at Kindle on Amazon.com.)

But, Chelation Therapy also reverses Osteoporosis! This was verified by a one percent sampling using a densitometer on bones of 20,000 patients who had Chelation Therapy. This retrospective study covered 15 years in many clinics and was privately funded by John M. Baron, D.O.[11] of Cleveland, Ohio, along with other physicians and PhDs.

What happens is this: As EDTA is dripped into the veins over a three and one half hour period, it picks up calcium from the circulatory system, thus lowering the calcium present in the blood serum. The body senses this lowered amount of calcium and turns on the parathyroid gland. That gland produces parathormone, a substance that activates calcium from other places in the body, and stuffs the calcium where it belongs, in the teeth and bones, thus helping to reverse Osteoporosis.

Herbal Medicine

The *Textbook of Natural Medicine*[15] recommends, in addition to most of the above supplements, Pranthocyanidins and Anthocyanidins from many berries, including hawthorn berries, blackberries, blueberries, cherries and raspberries. "Supplementation with concentrated extracts of high intake of those berries rich in these flavonoids may offer significant benefit in preventing osteoporosis."

Phytooestrogens are "components of many medicinal herbs. . . that may be suitable alternatives to estrogens in the prevention of osteoporosis in menopausal women.

"Herbs which possess both proven estrogenic activity and a long historical use in treating various female complaints include: *Angelica sinensis* (Dong quai), *Glycyrrhiza glabra* (licorice), *Aletris farinosa* (unicorn root), *Cimicifuga racemosa* (black cohosh), *Foeniculum vulgare* (fennel), and *Helonias opulus* (false unicorn root)[15]."

A physician versed in naturopathic medicine will be able to individually define necessary supplements and supporting or reinforcing supplements.

Rules of Prevention

Although physicians may differ on details of treatment, there are some rather constant agreements on the specifics of prevention and treatment of Osteoporosis:

1. One should consume a diet consisting mainly of vegetables. Or at least minimization of protein consumption is recommended, along with the other elements of a healthy diet, including fresh vegetables and fruits, whole grains and nuts, proper essential fatty acids (which implies avoiding the wrong kinds of fatty acids), cold water fish,and avoidance of birth control pills, tobacco, alcohol, sugars and processed grains, such as white flour. Increasing folic acid consumption may permit increased protein consumption

According to Newnham[27], "It is important that the fruits and vegetables consumed should be organically grown. That is, no chemical fertilizer should be used to force them to grow faster or bigger than is normal. Whenever plants are forced with soluble chemical fertilizers the trace elements suffer. A native corn plant grown in unfertilized soil will absorb say 1000 mg of trace elements which enters into two corn cobs weighing one kilogram, but a similar hybrid corn plant grown in a well fertilized soil will absorb no more than 1000 mg of trace elements, and often less, but this is then spread over 20 corn cobs weighing 15 kilograms. So each kilogram of corn from the commercial plant has one fifteenth of the trace elements of the native corn. Then in the processing of the corn more minerals are lost as these help to cause rotting of the corn. White flour lasts indefinitely but whole flour lasts only a few months, because white flour lacks the minerals that are needed for the spoiling process. Packet foods lack these essential minerals. It is important to never discard the water used for cooking vegetables as most of the valuable minerals are in that water.

"Fruits grown on a backyard tree contain more trace minerals for the same reason. A good, small well-grown apple can contain 5-10 mg. of boron, but a commercially grown apple may have as low as 1 mg of boron. We need at least 3 mg a day and if we have osteoporosis or arthritis to overcome it is wise to take up to 9 or 10 mg boron a day."

2. One should insure — lacking proper soils (not polluted with herbicides, et. al. and holding appropriate minerals) and fresh vegetables from good soils — that vitamin and mineral supplements include Vitamin K, Vitamin D, Magnesium, Molybdenum, Vanadium, Manganese, Folic Acid, Boron, Strontium, Silicon, Pyridoxine (Vitamin B6), Zinc, Copper (to be taken at a different time than the Zinc), and Ascorbic Acid (Vitamin C), and Vitamin E, this latter in a non-esterfied, mixed tocopherols form. Prior to indiscriminate use of various vitamins and minerals, it may be useful to use any of several clinical tests for their deficiencies or over-abundances. If done correctly, blood sera, hair analysis and tissue analysis may be in order.

3. As one ages, to insure that stomach acids (HCl) are of sufficient strength and, if not, to supplement HCl or its equivalent.

4. To exercise via any mode that allows the muscles (and bones) to work against gravity: running, dancing, walking, tennis, other ball games, "pumping iron" and so forth.

5. However possible, stay away from Aluminum, Floride, Cadmium and Lead excesses[13].

It's interesting to note that for almost all disease conditions, recommended preventive measures follow the same roadway: proper nutrition, exercise and appropriate vitamin and mineral supplements!

Rules of Treatment

Since we are all of us bound to suffer from some degree of Osteoporosis, the question occurs as to what should we do when this happens?

According to "Osteoporosis Prevention May be Achieved by Early Intervention," *Townsend Letter for Doctors*[16], in a study "which involved more than 800 women, Jeffrey Bland, Ph.D., and his colleagues at the Bionutritional Research Foundation confirmed the importance of premenopausal assessment of bone density in the prevention of postmenopausal bone fractures. . . Screening and intervention are particularly critical for women with a family history of bone loss and easy fracture.

"In the study, one group of women identified as high risk were given hormonal therapy and placed on a program of diet modification and regular exercise. When they were compared to a control group of women at high risk who did not receive intervention therapy, the treatment group showed increased bone density. Methods of screening and monitoring included CT scanning, duophoton absorptiometry and radiographic photodensitometry.

"An aggressive program of therapy to maintain bone density, according to the authors, includes diet modification, hormonal support after menopause, increased physical activity and life style modification, including cessation of cigarette smoking.

"'If the bad news is that bone loss in older women is a growing and serious problem,' Dr. Bland stated, 'the good news is that preventive techniques and dietary modification can help most women affected by bone loss. Screening, as our study shows, can match the problem with the solution."

1. It should be understood without saying it, therefore, that all of the above recommendations for prevention, should also be followed for treatment, and in addition we can do the following:

2. Following Newnham's advice[27], "When treating osteoporosis it is wise to make sure that one is consuming at least 3 mg of supplementary boron with each meal. This gives the parathyroid every opportunity to improve the bone mineralization. We don't want chelated boron as so many are trying to sell. The boron must be readily available to every part of the body that needs it. Only one boron tablet has ever passed any hospital trial, and these have been improved by" Dr. Newnham.

3. As one ages and/or if one has circulatory problems, to have treatments with EDTA Chelation Therapy.

4. Ask your physician for the MDS (mixed disulfide) test to determine homocysteine level and supplement with folic acid, if warranted.

5. If estrogen replacement is indicated, get *Triest* instead, and a physician who knows how to use it along with the proper kind of Vitamin E, and the correct forms of Omega 6 and Omega 3 fatty acids; or, find a physician

who understands the usage of herbs for Osteoporosis, as described earlier.

6. If indicated try progesterone ointment. John R. Lee, M.D., found that nightly application of a topical ointment of 3% natural progesterone for two weeks per month resulted in a significant increase in bone mass, in an uncontrolled study of 100 postmenopausal women. Although studies like this are not well accepted by established medicine, they are surely worthwhile looking into.

7. Whenever the body is subject to disease there are often two components that you and your doctor must separate out, and treat. The first, of course, is the basic cause of the disease itself. The second, is the damage that the disease has done to your body.

We cannot leave the subject of Osteoporosis without mentioning that there are many treatment modalities which you and your doctor must look at — to ease the load on your body — any portion of which might in some way either known or unknown be contributing to the Osteoporotic condition. Any and all treatments that will improve your overall health are important. Physicians will differ as to the "best" treatment, and perhaps they should, as each of us also differs. According to Newnham.[27], Before Dr. newham passed away, he wrote: "Far too many methods such as screening and chelation for osteoporosis and arthritis involve expensive medical procedures, and that is, I am afraid, what the medical industry wants. They don't want a simple, cheap supplement. I did have patents but too many companies have copied more or less, but I try to stay one jump ahead with a better formula. That is why I use calcium and magnesium ascorbate, so that all the molecule is used. I try to keep things cheap so that everybody can afford the tablets. I will never get rich this way but I don't want riches, it is better to know that people are being helped." That, after all, is the point of every good physician's viewpoint — to help. But even more important, is the effort that leads to your own personal insight on how to help yourself.

8. There is a treatment modalitiy of great import that is often overlooked — or at least has been greatly overlooked for more than 35 years.

It is a therapy practiced by only about 600 U.S. physicians, both MDs and DOs. It is known as Sclerotherapy by DOs and as Proliferative Therapy by DOs. Some physicians have also recently began calling this form of treatment Reconstructive Therapy, which defines what it does for the human frame.

As there is now two excellent books on the subject, *Pain, Pain Go Away*[17] by William J. Faber D.O. and Morton Walker, D.P.M. and *Prolo Your Arthritis Pain*[17] Away by Ross A. Hauser, M.D. and Marion A. Hauser, M.S., Rd. we won't dwell too much on its nature. Briefly it is based on the observation that the human skeleton in its living form is held together — maintains its natural human configuration — by tendons and ligaments. The muscles do not hold the body together — it's the tendons and ligaments. Muscles give power.

As the body ages, collagen tissue, that acts as a spacer and shock absorber throughout the skeleton, decreases. There is, indeed, a shrinking of bone tissue accompanied by a decrease in this collagen tissue with Osteoporosis. As the bones shrink and the shock absorbers decrease in size, the tendons and ligaments are no longer of the correct lengths to properly stabilize the skeleton.

Consequence is that the body — in a very unconscious and automatic manner — attempts to compensate by doing several things: growing calcium spurs in painful locations, crushing or grinding bone tissue, placing more tension on various tendons or ligaments on opposite sides of the body, thus creating additional pain, and so on. X-rays do not show where the ligments and tendons are stretched or torn.

Many pains appear in remote parts of the body; i.e., remote from the actual source of skeletal disturbance.

Physicians who use this treatment modality will find those points in the skeletal structure where tendons and ligaments need to be tightened up. At those specific points they will insert any of several substances — often a natural bodily substance called sodium morrhuate — which promotes the growth of collagen tissue and fibroblasts by normal physical mechanisms.

Your body, then, begins building fibroblasts and collagen tissue in such a way that tendons and ligaments are restored to their natural tautnesses with appropriate lengths.

It is necessary, however, to have a reasonably good metabolism; i.e. your thyroid should be functioning reasonably well. If not, then best to have thyroid supplements for a number of weeks prior to seeking this kind of therapy. If your metabolism is running low, or marginally low, your body will not build fibroblasts and collagen tissue very rapidly, and therefore you will not perceive results that are your due.

It is clear that this kind of treatment is virtually a must for anyone who begins to suffer or has suffered from Osteoporosis, Osteoarthritis, or Rheumatoid Disease — not to mention various kinds of accidents or sports problems.

Indeed, specialists in this mode of treatment state that 30% of all human pains can be solved by Reconstructive Therapy coupled with Neural Therapy, (*Instant Pain Relief*[18] by William J. Faber DO and Morton Walker, DPM) a treatment modality that has proven effective in releasing bound-up energy resulting from scars from various kinds of internal or external operations. (Also see *Intraneural Injections* on www.arthritistrust.org, book stores and at Amazon.com also on Kindle.)

Case History of Rex E. Newham, Ph.D., D.O., N.D. [27]

"I was not a medical man, but a teacher of soil science, agricultural botany and chemistry. Thirty years ago I developed arthritis and was given drugs which failed to help the condition. There is a cause for every effect and I soon realized that I should try to find the cause for my arthritis. Then I realized that most of the fruit and vegetables I was eating was mineral deficient. Even the pastures around Perth, Australia were often deficient in several minerals.

"All the common minerals were checked and none were relevant, but boron was written off as being not relevant to man or animal, yet it was very necessary for plants and it helped in their calcium metabolism. I looked into boron and 45 or more grams was a poisonous amount, so I took less than a thousandth of this amount twice daily and in 3 weeks all pain swelling and stiffness had gone. I was cured with no side effects.

"The next thing was to tell the university medical people and the public health authorities, but none of them were interested. Then I told a few people who had arthritis and they were thrilled as they were getting better. But it meant that they buy a packet of chemical that was labelled 'Poison — for killing cockroaches and ants.' Some people believed the label and stayed with their arthritis. In due course of time people persuaded me to have tablets made with a safe quantity of boron. This I did.

"I tried to enter a normal medical school but was too old to be accepted. So I quit teaching and qualified in alternative or complementary medicine, as a naturopath, homoeopath, osteopath and nutritionist. This latter was fortunate as doctors normally fail to study nutrition, yet it holds the key to nearly all of our maladies today. I later qualified for Ph.D. in nutrition.

"The first [boron] tablets took 2 years for me to sell 1000 bottles, but within 5 years they were selling at 10,000 per month; and that was without advertising, but every satisfied user told a few more so the business just grew. It was getting too much for me and I went to a drug company for help in marketing. They made most of their money from aspirin which was the main medical drug for arthritis and I thought they would be interested in finding a real cure for arthritis. I was wrong and a fool for thinking so.

"They said they were not interested, but they were most concerned; not about people with arthritis, but about losing some of their profits. This company had members on at least two government committees, and these men had boron declared poison in any concentration. It actually has about the same toxicity as common salt. But I was fined nearly $1000 for selling a poison, and they succcessfully put me out of business in Australia. So I moved overseas where boron is not poison by law. Actually there is no such thing as a poisonous substance, there are only poisonous concentrations. We don't call oxygen a poison, yet pure oxygen will soon kill a person if breathed continuously for a time.

"Following up on my early work the U.S. Human Nutrition Research Center in North Dakota[29,30,31] has shown that boron works through the parathyroid to stop or reduce calcium loss in osteoporotic women. Boron also helps to increase the natural hormones in these older women to normal. This could obviate the use of hormone replacement therapy which can be cancer forming when synthetic hormones are introduced into the body. I have tried to have formal studies done on bone density but those concerned don't seem to want to work with boron. Those patients who have used boron just don't seem to develop osteoporosis, they just remain well.

"The effect of boron on bone fractures is also interesting as these fractures just heal well in about half the normal time, in both man and animal. Horses and dogs with broken legs or even a broken pelvis have recovered fully. Yet it has been impossible to get orthopaedic surgeons to try this remedy in a proper trial.

"I did have patents in six countries for my formula, but these [for scientific proof] are not worth the paper they are written on. Other people can copy the important aspects of a formula but vary it a little and they are not infringing the patent. Even one company copied exactly and even used my patients in their advertising. Then in court they were made to apologise. This all means that I will never gain much from a monetary aspect, but there is a lot of satisfaction in knowing that people are getting better. I only wish that more knew about it and that the authorities did not just try to cover up this work.

"It seems as if the 'health authorities' just want more and bigger hospitals with more top jobs and expensive drug bills with more undertakers in business. I would rather see a healthy population and healthy people to not need hospitals."

Dr. Newnham's experiences are normal in the field of health treatment and prevention. It is consistent with every other field of medicine for every condition. There is almost always alternative or complementary paths to health.

As there are many paths to freedom of the spirit, there are many ways to seek bodily health.

In using any therapy, the important part is knowing that you are better, and that the treatment you've selected works for you!

DR. MERCOLA'S COMMENT

in www.mercola.com regarding an article *The Protein and Calcium Paradox in Osteoporosis* By Dr. Robert Heaney in *American Journal Clinical Nutrition* April 2002;75(4):609-10.

"One of the arguments vegetarians are fond of stating is that increased protein intake, especially animal protein, results in loss of calcium from the bone.

"As Dr. Heaney explains this is not entirely true. If one has inadequate protein intake it is clearly quite detrimental to bone density. There are many studies that clearly demonstrate this.

"However, if one has excess protein intake and does not adequately have sufficient calcium in the diet, the protein will cause loss of calcium from the bones into the urine to buffer the system.

"Having large amounts of raw vegetables which are high in calcium and other acidic buffering agents will clearly compensate for this.

"Additionally, sufficient quantities of vitamin D in the summer from sun and in the winter from cod liver oil will also maximize calcium absorption to more than compensate for the loss of calcium from protein intake in most people.

"So if you have osteoporosis, or osteopenia you will clearly want to have sufficient."

Information Sources, References and Supplement Suppliers

Listed in what follows are sources of information that may help you in preventing or treating Osteoporosis:

Information Sources

1. American Academy ofAdvancement in Medicine, 6151 West Century Blvd., Los Angeles, CA 90045. Source of physicians who do Chelation Therapy.

2 Candidia Research and Information Foundation, PO Box 2719, Castro Valley, CA 94546; (510) 582-2179. Non-Profit, Tax-Exempt, Charitable Foundation.

3. Douglass, William Campbell, M.D. writes and publishes a newsletter *Second Opinion,* interesting for layfolks. PO Box 888, Warwoman Road, Thurmond Building, Clayton, GA 30525.

4. Newnham Rex , PhD, DO, ND *Away With Arthritis,*, Cracoe House Cottage, Cracoe, Skipton, North Yorkshire BD23 6LB England. This pamphlet, written for layfolks, discusses Newnham's research on use of Boron.f postage and handling. (See http://www.arthritistrust.org.)

5. Price-Pottenger Nutrition Foundation, Inc. 5871 El Cajon Blvd, San Diego, CA 92115; (619) 582-4168. Their newsletter and other literature are good sources for data on proper nutrition. Non-Profit, Tax-exempt, Charitable Foundation.

6. Physicians Committee for Responsible Medicine, PO Box 6322, Washington, D.C. 20015 (202) 686-2210. Non-profit, tax-exempt charitable foundation.

7.The Arthritis Trust of America/The Rheumatoid Disease Foundation, 7111 Sweetgum Road, Fairview, TN 37062, (Also at http://www.arthritistrust.org.)

8. *Townsend Letter for Doctors* is an informal newsletter for doctors communicating to doctors — but it is also excellent for layfolks. It is published monthly, contains a large number of interesting articles on various medical conditions, is generally easy to read and to understand. ISSN 1059-5864, 911 Tyler Street, Port Townsend, WA 98368-6541 or call (206) 385-6021 regarding subscription price.

9. Wright/Gaby Nutrition Institute, PO Box 32188, Baltimore, MD 21208.

Supplement Suppliers — an Incomplete Listing

Sources for various essential fatty acids, minerals and vitamins and vitamin supplements follow. Note, some are for physicians only!

1. Bronson Pharmaceuticals 4526 Rinetti Lane, PO Box 628 La Canada, CA 91012-0628. An excellent source for powdered Vitamin C in the form of Ascorbic Acid, Sodium Ascorbate, and Calcium Ascorbate.

2. AC Grace Co. 1100 Quitman Road, Big Sandy, TX 75755 (214) 636-4368. Source of proper type of Vitamin E.

3. Advanced Medical Nutrition, Inc. 2247 National Avenue, PO Box 5012,Hay- ward, CA 94540-5012. Various vitamins and minerals.

4. Bio-Therapeutics, PO Box 1745, Green Bay, WI 54305, outside U.S. call collect (414) 435-4200, inside U.S. 1-800-553-2370. Note: Physicians only!

5. Bio-Tech, PO Box 1991, Fayetteville, AR 72702, 1-800-345-1199. Various vitamin and mineral supplements.

6. Cardiovascular Research Ltd. 1061-B Shary Circle, Concord, CA 94518; 1-800-351-9429. Various vitamin and mineral supplements.

7. Henderson Metabolic Services, Inc., 8304 Harford Road, Baltimore, MD 21334;1-800-289-4674. Various vitamin and mineral supplements.

8. Inter-Cal Corporation, 421 Miller Valley Road, Prescott, AZ 86301; (602) 445-8063. Source of Ester C[R].

9. Klabin Marketing, 115 Central Park West, 5A, New York, NY 10023; (212) 877-3632. Among other products, distributes a new form of Vitamin C, called Ester C[R].

10. Klaire Laboratories, Inc., 1573 W. Seminole, San Marcos, CA 92069 1-800-533-7255 or (619) 744-9680. Various vitamin and mineral supplements.

11. Miller Pharmacal Group, Inc. 245 W. Roosevelt Rd., PO Box 279, West Chicago, IL 60185; 1-800-323-2935 or 1-708-231-3632. Various vitamin and mineral supplements.

12. New Dimensions Distributors, Inc. 16458 East Laser Drive, Suite A-7, Fountain Hills, AZ 85268; 1-800-624-7114; (602) 837-8322. Source for good Flaxseed Oil (Fatty Acid).

13. Thorne Research, Inc. 901 Triangle Drive, PO Box 3200, Sandpoint, ID 83864; (208) 263-1337. Note Physicians only! Various vitamin and mineral supplements.

14. Vitaline Formulas 722 Jefferson Ave., Ashland, Or 97520; 1-800-648-4755. Various vitamin and mineral supplements.

15. For Your Health Pharmacy, Kent Washington for supplies of Triest. Write to Edward Thorpe, Ph.D., Box 5198, 349 West Georgia, Vancouver, Canada V6B 4B3.

16. Professional and Technical Services, Inc., 3331 N.E. Sandy Blvd., Portland Oregon 97232 for supplies of Progesterone creams and oils for topical treatment.

17. Dr. Don Breen, Osteo-Trace tablets, 1535 North Limestone Street, Springfield, OH 45503. These are tablets made to Rex E. Newnham's specifications.

18. Mumme Enterprises, Osteo-Trace, 1321 Meridican Ave., South Pasadena, CA 91030. These are tablets made to Rex E. Newnham's specifications.

References

1. *Cutting Edge*, April 1987, p. 19, 22. Name of Douglass' publication is now *Second Opinion*.

2. *Textbook of Natural Medicine*, Pizzorno & Murray, 1989, VI: Osteop-3.

3. Rex Newnham, Personal Communication from; also see *Away With Arthritis*, Rex E. Newnham, Cracoe House Cottage, Cracoe, Skipton, North Yorkshire BD23 6LB, England.

4. Jonathan Wright, M.D., Alan R. Gaby, M.D., Personal Communication.

5. *Science News*, August 1, 1986.

6. Schultheis, L. *Exp-Gerontol.* "The Mechanical Control System of Bone in Weightless Spaceflight and In Aging," 1991; 26(2-3): 302-14

7. LeBlanc A., Schneider, V., *Exp-Gerontol.* 1991; 26 (2-3): 189-201.

Reversing Type II Diabetes Naturally
by
Jaime E. Dy-Liacco and Anthony di Fabio

In America when you sit down before your TV, reach for your remote and snap on your TV to a news channel, what's the odds that you'll first see an advertisement?

1 to 10? Even up? 10 to 1?

I'm willing to bet the odds are even up that you'll see an ad before you see your program.

Believe it or not the odds in the Philippines are 0 to any number you care to name!

In the United States the airways belong to the people and that's interpreted to mean advertisers, those with the big bucks to pay for the time.

In the Philippines the airways also belong to the people, and that's interpreted to mean zero advertising, the airways do not belong to the big bucks corporations.

Another interesting difference between the United States and the Philippines is that in the United States the odds are quite high that the ad you see before you see your program is that of a patent medicine company selling a patent medicine that has deceptively been declared safe and effective in relieving a symptom of your medical problem. The odds are pretty high that along with the expensive glossy advertising there will be listed — almost too fast to read or comprehend — a long list of bad things that will happen to you if your doctor chooses to provide you with this chemical.

One more question: What's the odds that the patented drug advertising that you tune in on is about Diabetes I?

I've not measured the odds but it's pretty darned high.

The FDA, American Congress and the American President should be as ashamed of themselves as possible for permitting this kind of scam to be played on the American Citizens but then scamming regarding patented drugs to treat this or that symptom is what the American medical system is all about.

Roselyn S. Yalow in 1977, shared one-half of the Nobel prize with two others, Roger C.L. Guillemin and Andrew V. Shally. They were able to show that in Type II Diabetes the pancreas' beta cells swelled up and refused to permit insulin to be released in the blood stream!

It takes neither a rocket scientist or a patented medicine director of research to immediately guess that the reason the beta cells swell up is because the patient has a food allergy that causes the swelling!

Can the cause of Diabetes II be so simple?

Diabetes is a very common disease, which, if not treated, can be very dangerous. There are two types of diabetes. They were once called juvenile-onset diabetes and adult diabetes. However, today we know that all ages can get both types so they are simply called type 1 and type 2 diabetes.

Type 1, which occurs in approximately 10 percent of all cases, is thought to be an autoimmune disease in which the immune system, by mistake, attacks its own insulin-producing cells so that insufficient amounts of insulin are produced — or no insulin at all. Type 1 affects predominantly young people and usually makes its debut before the age of 30, and most frequently between the ages of 10 and 14.

Type 2, which makes up the remaining 90 percent of diabetes cases, commonly affects patients during the second half of their lives. The cells of the body no longer react to insulin as they should. This is called insulin resistance.

In the early 1920s, Frederick Banting, John Macleod, George Best and Bertram Collip isolated the hormone insulin and purified it so that it could be administered to humans. This was a major breakthrough in the treatment of diabetes type 1. But at the same time this was the beginning of the scam for treating Diabete II.

The primary treatment for Diabetes II is a daily race between supplying too much or too little insulin while eating too much or too little sugar (or easily converted carbohydrates). Other portions of the accepted treatment specializes in how to measure insulin or sugar and how to deliver insulin.

Millions upon millions of dollars are wasted treating these symptoms when Diabetes, since 1977, is known to be simply a food allergy problem.

Several medical doctors have written books advising everyone of this simple solution. One such is referenced in William Philpott's *The Magic of Magnetic Healing* which is found on www.arthritistrust.org, book stores and at Amazon.com also on Kindle.

This is where we blend in our important story of the Philippines and Diabetes II.

One of us (Anthony di Fabio) was very much aware of the relationship between Diabetes II and food allergy. During a long a year and a half sojourn there he met a young Filipina who became his wife. Her mother had Diabetes II. The doctor was recommending that her toe be cut off. Although di Fabio strongly objected, it seems that the family has priority over what one of their own will have done medically. The vote was against di Fabio.

The wound healed slowly.

On the next visit to the hospital the mother was told she'd need to have her leg amputated. Again the vote, and this time di Fabio won. The doctor, like so many American doctors, got very angry and told the mother "Don't ever come back to my hospital!"

Unlike the United States, where alternative/complementary doctors are persecuted by the controllers of medicine, the Philippines has a law requiring allopathic doctors to cooperate with alternative/complementary doctors. Di Fabio easily found a doctor, Fe Merced, M. D., in the middle of Manila who fully understood the allergenic component to Diabetes II.

Shortly thereafter di Fabio's future mother-in-law was off of insulin completely and thriving on a new diet, one that excluded her most likely allergenic diet of rice, rice, rice.

The rules for identifying allergenic foods is well known. Go to "Allergies and Biodetoxification" at www.arthritistrust.org, bookstores or to Amazon.com at Kindle.

Also because of the Philippines' legal liberality between alternative/ complementary doctors and allopathic physicians one can easily locate an annual alternative medical conference. Di Fabio and his wife attended one such where a remarkable healer described his variation of applied kinesiology when diagnosing and treating patients. He also was happy to share without cost his method of treating Diabetes. You will immediately recognize it as being designed for those without a lot of wealth. Here, then, is Jaime E. Dy-Liacco standard treatment of Diabetes.

Jaime Dy-Liacco teaches:

This protocol works every single time, even curing diabetic gangrene in one week and saving legs from getting amputated. Look at the bottom half of the last page which lists what to do in case of diabetic gangrene.

If the patient has been taking the diabetic drugs for less than 6 months, they can be stopped abruptly without harm, so long as she starts immediately with the natural remedies. But if she has been taking them for more than 6 months, she cannot stop them abruptly. Instead overlap them with the natural remedies, and monitor her fasting blood sugar every week or at least every 10 days with laboratory blood tests. After the fasting blood sugar has stabilized within the normal range for 3 months, phase out the drugs gradually.

The 6 food supplements listed are readily available in health food stores, the green leafy vegetables in supermarkets and produce stores. If she lives in the U.S., she probably will not be able to find raw pork pancreas, but try China town. The raw pork pancreas are very rich in natural insulin. It brings down blood sugar from 500 to 84 in 5 minutes with just 2 tablespoons. It doesn't have the side effects of synthetic insulin injections.

The protocol does not yet mention the use of red siling labuyo (red cayenne peppers) which I will add to the protocol after having seen how well it works. If it's the big red ones (about 1.5-2" long) which is what is available in Metro Manila, take 9 silis 3x a day. If it's the small ones (less than 1" long) which is what is abundant in the provinces, take 12 silis 3x a day. Be sure there is food in the stomach, because sili gives a stomach ache if taken on an empty stomach.

I always give the sili together with 1/2 teaspoon of rock (sea) salt, 2 bananas, 3 glasses of water, and if available 3 tablespoons of dark chocolate ice cream. The ice cream helps to digest the food just taken because it makes the stomach acidic within 5 minutes of eating it. I have found dark chocolate ice cream does not raise blood sugar, especially if it's taken together with the red silis.

Please keep me posted. Am happy to help.

REVERSING TYPE II DIABETES NATURALLY

Jaime E. Dy-Liacco, trustee, Philippine College for the Advancement in

Medicine; Former Director General, Philippine Institute of Traditional & Alternative Health Care, DOH; Tel. #632-924-2487, Fax #632-929-9173, email: mito@pacific.net.ph

Diabetes is due to a deficiency of 5 minerals, and to eating habits that load the body with too much simple sugars, wearing down the insulin-producing beta cells of the pancreas and weakening the potency of the insulin they produce. (A different interpretation than the Nobel Prize winners, but still effective in results.) So to reverse Type II or adult-onset diabetes naturally, correct the mineral deficiency with 5 food supplements, regenerate the beta cells in the pancreas producing insulin with a 6th supplement, correct eating habits, and do regular exercise. Here's how:

CORRECTING THE MINERAL DEFICIENCY with these 5 food supplements:

1. Vanadyl Sulfate, 50 mg capsules. Take 50 mg or 1 capsule after every meal. So, it's totally 3 capsules or 150 mg daily.

2. Copper, 2 mg capsules. Take 2 capsules after every meal. So, it's 6 capsules or 12 mg daily.

3. Zinc Picolinate, 22 mg capsules. Take 2 capsules after every meal. So it's 6 capsules or 132 mg of zinc daily.

4. Manganese, 30 mg capsules. Take 30 mg or 1 capsule after every meal. So it's 90 mg or 3 capsules daily.

5. Chromium Picolinate, 500 mcg capsules. Take 1000 mcg or 2 capsules after every meal. So it's 3000 mcg or 6 capsules daily.

IMPORTANT: Items 2-5 must be taken together. If one is missing, the others won't work.

REGENERATING INSULIN-PRODUCING BETA CELLS with this 6th supplement:

6. Gymnema Sylvestre, 300 mg capsules. Take 300 mg or 1 capsule 15 minutes before each meal. So totally it's 900 mg or 3 capsules daily.

FIRST AID FOR VERY HIGH BLOOD SUGAR

Eat 2 tablespoons of raw pork pancreas. It is very rich in natural insulin, and has brought down in 2 minutes blood sugar from as high as 240-502 down to 84-85. Have the pancreas on standby in your freezer, for use in emergency situations, or eat it daily if you wish. Eaten with every meal keeps blood sugar normal every day, like having insulin shots. Always eat it with a clove of crushed raw garlic, to kill bacteria and viruses.

Because raw pork pancreas are also very rich in the animal-protein digesting enzymes that digest cancer cells, 2 tablespoons with every meal will also prevent cancer.

Here's how to prepare: buy the pancreas early in the morning from the market, to be sure it is freshly slaughtered. Do not buy more than a week's supply. Wash it well of soil and dirt. Soak for 10 minutes in a basin of water with half a cup of rock salt. After soaking, rub well on both sides with rock salt until the sliminess is gone. Cut into small cubes so you can measure it by the tablespoonful. Put 2 tablespoons each into a small plastic bag. Put the bags in the freezer, and take as needed.

You can season it any way you want to make it palatable, so long as you don't cook it or use vetsin (MSG). Some use wasabi and toyo. Others eat it with chopped onions, ginger, green sili, garlic, salt, kalansi. Others like it as is from the freezer. It has a nice, cool clean taste and melts in the mouth.

Please note, the raw pancreas are not a permanent cure, just like insulin shots are not. To cure diabetes permanently, you need to correct the mineral deficiencies and regenerate the beta cells in your own pancreas that produce your own insulin, but this time with the mineral deficiencies corrected, your own insulin production will now be potent.

So you can use the raw pancreas to keep your blood sugar down while you are correcting your mineral deficiencies and regenerating your pancreatic cells.

CORRECTING EATING HABITS

1. Fresh vegetables. Eat 3x a day 1 cup of raw saluyot leaves, or camote leaf tops (talbos ng kamote) either dark green or purple in color, or kangkong (swamp cabbage), or spinach leaves, or sea grapes (lato) as a salad to start every meal.

These raw dark green vegetables are rich in vanadium, copper, zinc, manganese, chromium and will lower your blood sugar. You may blanch these vegetables, or juice them, but do not cook them. Anything cooked beyond 40 degrees centigrade loses all enzymes, vitamins, and the organic minerals become inorganic which the body cannot absorb.

2. Garlic. Eat 3 large cloves of crushed raw garlic with every meal. It has to be crushed or chewed thoroughly to release the active ingredients, allicin and alliin. Besides being anti-viral and anti-bacterial, garlic lowers blood sugar levels. If you cannot take raw garlic, take garlic pills: either 1 pill of Garlinase 4000 (from Healthy Options), or 2 tablets of Kyolic Garlic (from GNC, get the one that's all garlic, no mixtures) after every meal.

3. Water. Take 15 8-oz glasses of non-chlorinated, mineral water every day to keep your body's water level at the 75% that the body needs to metabolize properly. If you let it drop below 75%, you are dehydrated. All your vital organs, your cells, your tissues, your blood (75% water), your brain (85% water) will be dehydrated. Your immune system drops when your water level drops below 75%, and you become vulnerable to infections. No medication that you take will work if your body is dehydrated.

One simple way to check if your water level is at 75% is to look at the color of your urine every time you urinate. If it is yellow, you are dehydrated. Drink a glass of water right away. Your objective must be to make the color of your urine as clear as water.

To be free of dehydration, you need salt. Without salt the body cannot retain water and you will still be dehydrated even with the 15 glasses of water a day, because water is a natural diuretic. So take 2½ teaspoons of salt a day. Sprinkle 1/2 teaspoon of salt on each meal, eat 1/2 teaspoon with your merienda with a glass of water, and eat 1/2 at bedtime with a glass of water which will help keep you from urinating frequently during the night. Use natural salt from the sea (rock salt), not refined table salt which is synthetic.

If you cannot avoid using tap water, which is chlorinated, let the water sit for half an hour, without a cover, to evaporate the chlorine. Do not take distilled water. It strips the body of minerals, and aggravates your diabetes. Take mineral water.

4. Foods and drinks to avoid. All processed foods (canned goods, foods made with white refined flour such as pan de sal, white bread, noodles, etc., white refined sugar, confectionery, margarine, any food that comes in a box or package made by a manufacturer and sold in stores, junk food), dairy products (milk, cheese except cottage cheese), red meats, soft drinks, coffee, alcoholic drinks.

For frying, use only extra virgin, cold-pressed olive oil or coconut oil. All other oils are not heart-healthy (the polyunsaturated oils) and some, like Canola and soybean oil, are even conducive to cancer. Fresh fruits in moderation are OK, they are complex sugars.

Fish, chicken, and turkey without the skin are OK. Proteins from plants, like beans, are incomplete and not usable by the body. To make them complete, eat them with grains, like brown rice. It's delicious mixed with sticky red rice (red malagkit). Mix 1 cup brown with 1 tablespoon red. Avoid white rice. It's a simple sugar.

5. Sweeteners. Use raw honey, or muscovado sugar. To sweeten cereal, use fruits like sliced raw bananas. Do not use synthetic sweeteners like aspertame (Equal or NutraSweet). They aggravate diabetes and can cause brain tumors. Avoid diet softdrinks with NutraSweet. NutraSweet is converted in the body into formaldehyde (it's embalming you while you are still alive). A natural sweetener that's acceptable is Stevia. If health food stores don't have it, order it from the U.S.

6. Flax seed. Eat ¼ cup of ground raw flax seed daily. Sprinkle it on food or mix it with fruit juice or water. Raw flax seed is available at Healthy Options, either ground or as whole seeds. Do not buy the ground seed. It oxidizes once the package is opened. Get the whole seeds. Grind 1/4 cup in a small electric coffee grinder for 10 seconds, only when you are about to eat it, because it oxidizes in 15 minutes after grinding. You can eat kesong puti with it. The two make a healthy combination.

DO REGULAR EXERCISE

Three hours a week. This can be mild like walking or rebounding 30 minutes 6x a week, or vigorous like 1 hour of tennis, squash, badminton, basketball, swimming, or gym workouts 3x a week. The key is to do it regularly.

Rebounding is going up and down on a circular mini-trampoline which is available for about P1,500 (Pesos) from sporting goods stores like Toby's. Rebounding is actually the best exercise because it exercises all the cells, not just certain muscles. It is the exercise prescribed for astronauts.

12-HOUR FASTING BLOOD SUGAR TESTS

Take this at least every 2 weeks or more frequently to help guide possible adjustments in dosages.

WHAT TO DO WITH DRUGS

If you have been taking pharmaceutical drugs for diabetes, do not drop them abruptly, because that might cause an adverse reaction, since the body has become addicted to their use. Overlap them with the natural remedies. With your diabetes doctor's help, phase the drugs out gradually after your fasting blood sugar has normalized or fallen below normal. Normal is 70-105.

MAINTENANCE PROTOCOL

1. Nutritional Supplements. After the blood sugar level normalizes, and after you have phased out the drugs, cut back on the 6 food supplements until finally you are taking only one 10 mg Vanadyl Sulfate a day, not the 50 mg capsule you started with. Keep using fasting blood sugar level tests (at least every 2 weeks) to guide you in how much to cut back. If the blood sugar rises again after the last cut back, put back the last dosage that was cut out. If it has remained stable or within normal limits or has dropped, you can make another dosage reduction.

2. Other measures. Continue the eating habits changes and other measures. These alone, even without the one Vanadyl Sulfate a day, may already be enough to keep the blood sugar level within normal limits.

BASIC OPTIMUM HEALTH

1. Constipation. The healthy bowel movement frequency is 3x a day or as often as you eat a major meal. The healthy texture is soft, like soft peanut butter or even loose, like sawdust with a little water. So it's all over in one minute, no need to strain, and no need to read a newspaper or magazine.

Blood circulates every 3.5 miinutes, and if you keep fecal waste inside you for 24 hours (only 1 BM a day) or longer, the blood will pick up the toxins and parasites and distribute them every where, to your pancreas, all the vital organs, all your cells.

If you are already moving 3x a day, do not take diatabs or immodium or lomotil to bring it down to 1. LBM is not bad. What is bad is diarrhea, which is all liquid, no substance. If you get diarrhea, take 3 cloves of crushed raw garlic with every meal; that will kill the bacteria causing the diarrhea. Or use the Mayco Bio-Zapper, which will kill the bacteria by zapping it with low voltage electricity (12-18 volts, not enough to kill a cockroach, but enough to kill all bacteria, viruses, worms, other parasites).

The Mayco Bio-Zapper was invented by Fr. Howard May, an American missionary living in Quezon City who supplies his missionaries in Mindanao with the zapper to heal their parishioners, who are too poor to afford pharmaceutical drugs, of all kinds of ailments caused by bacteria, viruses, and parasites.

How do you get 3 BM's a day? (1) Avoid dehydration; that makes you constipated. (2) Eat a cup of raw saluyot leaves as a salad 3x a day to start your every meal. (3) Take 3 tablespoons of Extra Virgin cold-pressed Coconut Oil after every dinner. (4) If all this fails, take Dr. Richard Schulze's Intestinal Formula #1. Take 1 capsule with a glass of water after dinner. If 3 BM's do not result the next day, keep adding 1 capsule to every dinner until 3 BM's result. Then maintain that dosage.

Keep your blood clean, not filthy. Do not be a walking septic tank. Have 3 BM's a day.

2. Detoxification. Follow Dr. Schulze's Incurables Program to detoxify the body thoroughly. It will unclog and cleanse the intestinal tract, the liver, gall bladder, the kidneys, and the bladder, removing old dried up fecal matter, heavy metals like mercury, lead, drug residues, parasites, the rotting food and fecal waste trapped in loops of the colon (diverticulosis), polyps in the colon, and gallstones and kidney stones. The 3 BM's a day is the start of the program.

The first thorough detoxification process takes 3 months. Month 1 — get 3 BM's a day. Month 2 — remove the old dried up fecal wastes, remove the heavy metals, polyps, diverticulosis. Month 3 — Clean up the liver, gall bladder, kidneys, and bladder.

3. A basic high potency multi-vitamin/mineral food supplement. Do not take Centrum. It is synthetic. Get a natural multi-vitamin/mineral complex from health food stores. What is best is Dr. Schulze's Superfood nutritional drink. All the ingredients are food, not chemicals. It gives you 2-5 times the vitamins and minerals you get from regular food. As a liquid, it is in your blood stream and already nourishing all your cells within 15 minutes of drinking it.

4. Clear the arteries of blockages. Super Phos 30 will dissolve the calcified plaques with 90 drops a day mixed with fruit juice, or with the SuperFood drink. Rinse the mouth well or brush teeth immediately after taking Superphos 30, because it can strip the calcium from teeth if allowed to stay too long in the mouth.

Pancreatic lipase enzymes will dissolve the fat blockages. Natural Vitamin E will remove inflammation of arterial walls that narrow the channels. Your blood will be free-flowing, delivering oxygen and nourishment to all cells.

For pancreatic enzymes, take the raw pancreas or Dan Raber's CardioClean lipase enzymes, 2 capsules with every meal and 1 with every snack. This will dissolve fat blockages and help digest the fats you eat, lightening the burden on your own pancreas.

For natural Vitamin E, take 1,000 to 1,200 IU's after breakfast daily. The bottle label will say "d-alpha tocopherol..." without an l after the d. If it says "dl-alpha...," it is synthetic. Avoid synthetic Vitamin E.

5. Prevent future blockages. High cholesterol and/or high homocysteine cause the calcified plaques, high triglycerides the fatty deposits, and a Vitamin E deficiency the inflammation. Have blood tests taken for cholesterol, triglycerides, homocysteine, and C-Reactive Protein (CRP). If the CRP is positive, there is inflammation of the arteries, if negative, none.

Normalize high cholesterol with Flush-Free Niacin (Vitamin B-3, the non-flush type), 1,000 mg after every meal, high homocysteine with 2 capsules a day (1-0-1 after meals) of the Homocysteine Formula (which corrects the Vitamin B-6, B-12, folate, and trimethyl glycine deficiencies that cause homocysteine to rise), high triglycerides with 2 capsules a day (1-0-1 after meals) of 20 mg Policosanol (a food supplement extract from sugarcane), and inflammation with 1,000 or 1,200 iu's of Vitamin E daily after breakfast

Ed Wendlocher, founder and president of the former Arthritis Help Centers, Inc., suffered from arthritis for many years until he discovered his sensitivity to various foods. He promoted clinical studies that resulted in several booklets, the latest being Pain Foods! *which was available at his address listed below, a landscape service, his primary business address.*

After careful studies over many years it was learned that many taste enhancers, such as capsaicinoids, were exempted by the food labelling act and were also found in small quantities in many ordinary foods. These, it was discovered, caused many people, including Ed Wendlocher himself, to suffer from the classical phenomena of "arthritis."

Now the mechanism is revealed through further academic research that capsaicinoids do, indeed, play a serious role in creating inflammation, tissue damage and "arthritis!"

We highly recommend obtaining the Arthritis Help Center booklet describing foods that may be causing arthritic problems.

Chemicals in 'hot' Chili Peppers Confirmed to be a Cause of Arthritis!
by
Professor Jack Abel, Ph D

"Harvard Medical School researchers have now found that the receptor activated by chemicals in 'hot' chili peppers is also responsible for the ongoing, burning pain associated with inflammation, tissue damage and arthritis!"
The chemicals in the 'hot' chili peppers that cause them to be 'hot' are the capsaicinoids. Capsaicinoids are strong irritants that act directly on the pain receptors in your skin and mucous membranes. The strongest capsaicinoids are capsaicin and dihydrocapsaicin. Capsaicin is so strong that a single drop diluted in one million drops of water will still warm your tongue. Like dihydrocapsaicm, it delivers a sting all over your mouth. A third capsaicinoid, nordihydrocapsaicin, produces a warmer, mellower sensation in the front of your mouth and palate. A fourth, homodihydrocapsaicin, packs a delayed punch, delivering a stinging, numbing burn to the back of your throat.

Until now, capsaicin has been reported to primarily have beneficial effects on the body. It is best known as an effective 'pain relief' substance when applied topically to the skin where it destroys certain nerve cells and prevents pain signals from reaching the brain. However, increased research of capsaicin is now uncovering that it also has significant detrimental effects on the body.

Capsaicin is now confirmed to be a primary cause of the on-going, burning pain associated with inflammation, tissue damage and arthritis!
Capsaicin is a strong irritant. Applied to the skin, it causes the small blood vessels under the skin to dilate; increasing the flow of blood to the area and making the skin feel warm. It stimulates nerve endings in your mouth normally

stimulated by a rising body temperature, sending impulses to your brain that release endorphins giving you a false sense of well-being. Eating 'hot' chili peppers may upset your stomach, irritate the lining of your stomach, irritate your bladder so that you have to urinate more frequently or even make your urination painful.

The 'hot' chili pepper plants are 'cousins' of tobacco [and tomatoes] being in the same Solanaceae plant family. The 'hot' chili peppers contain many of the same natural toxins as tobacco. By comparing the established LD-50 values (measures of toxicity), we see that the capsaicin in 'hot' chili peppers is in the same league as a dangerous toxin as is nicotine in cigarette smoke.

Capsaicin is now used commercially as a pesticide on fruits and vegetables as it both kills insects and repels animals from crops. Again, based on LD-50 values, it is one of the more dangerous toxic pesticides in use today!

'Hot' chili pepper, also known as cayenne pepper, is made from the seeds and pods of Capsicum peppers, a species completely different from *Piper nigrum*, the plant whose fruit is used as black pepper (the one in the shaker on your table). The Capsicum peppers are native to Mexico, Central America, the West Indies and much of South America, but similar varieties are also native to the Far East. They may be long and thin like the cayenne pepper, large and firm like the Anaheim, cone shaped like the jalapeno or small and cherry shaped. Tabasco peppers, used to make a popular hot sauce, are a variety of 'hot' peppers known as *Capsicum frutescens*. Ground red pepper labeled cayenne pepper or simply red pepper is made by grinding the smaller, more pungent Capsicums. The term "red pepper" may also be used to describe ground red pepper milder than, cayenne. Crushed red pepper, the spice you find in pizza parlors, is made from the seeds of the 'hot' varieties of *Capsicum annuum* and *Capsicum frutescens*. Chili powder is a blend of red pepper with other herbs and spices.

Recent studies completed in association with scientists at a major university show that persons with arthritis can significantly reduce their pain, swelling and stiffness by conscientiously avoiding the foods containing the 'hot' chili peppers and certain other food ingredients!

The problem: 'hot' chili ingredients are not easy to avoid as they are rarely shown on the food label by that name. They are usually shown on the label as spices, spice extracts, flavorings, natural flavorings or seasonings; or added as colorings or preservatives and not shown at all!

For complete information on the foods to avoid, contact

Arthritis Help Centers is located in the city of Wharton, New Jersey, county — Morris — at the address 394 Berkshire Valley Rd. The main activity of company is Agricultural Services (Services), Standard Industrial Classification — Ornamental Shrub And Tree Services (SIC code is 0783). You can contact (with President, Edwin Wendlocher) by the phone number (973) 361-1867 (ZIP code is 07885-1008). "FOOD PAIN!" $11.95 + $3.00 S&H. We highly recommend this book to those suffering from any kind of arthritis.

What Harvard Medical School researchers seem to have concluded is as follows:

1. When chili peppers activate certain nerve receptors, this activation is also responsible for a burning sensation associated with inflammation, tissue damage and "arthritis."

2. When inflammation occurs, a "p38" molecule switches on. This is an intracellular signaling molecule which causes a "cascade" of enzymes to increase the amount of heat that passes through a protein known as "TRPV 1," sometimes called the "ion-channel protein." It is also sometimes called the "chili pepper receptor."

3. The "chili pepper receptor" is very sensitive to capsaicin. Capsaicin causes chili peppers to feel "hot."

4. Regulation of the chili pepper receptor was not expected, according to Harvard anesthesia researcher professor Clifford Woolf as large increases in the amount of receptor from increasing inflammation does not change production of mRNA. However, "The gene itself is not being changed, the mRNA that is being translated is."

5. Dr. Woolf may perform further research in using p38 inhibitors for treatment of inflammation and accompanying pain. Footnote from: "Hot research, burning pain: the protein TRPV1 is sensitive to capsaicin, found in chili peppers."

[(Frontlines), Hal Cohen. *The Scientist*, copyright Scientist, Inc., Oct. 14, 2002, v16 i20 p8(1); from Lehigh University Library; http://www.web m a s t e r @ t h e - s c i e n t i s t . c o m; h t t p ://web1.infortrac.galegroup.com/ itw/infomark/147/680/30131280w1/purl=rcl_EAIM_ (Article A93348351)]

Potassium Deficiency as a Cause of Rheumatoid Disease
 by
Charles Weber — weber@brinet.com
(A more complete discussion of the role of potassium in arthritis may be found at Weber's homepage http://members.tripod.com/~charles_W/ arthritis.html.)

This discussion of potassium is presented in the hope that one of its readers will consider performing an experiment establishing the effect of potassium on rheumatoid arthritis. There is no report in the literature going back to 1914 of such an experiment.

Every essential nutrient should have been explored before this. In view of the way hormones which are regulated by or regulate potassium, such as cortisol and deoxycorticosterone (DOC) are involved with rheumatoid arthritis (RA), and the low whole body potassium content in Rheumatoid Arthritis (RA), potassium especially should have been investigated before now.

INTRODUCTION

Since the most serious aspect of the diarrheas is wasting potassium, cortisol has acquired the attribute of conserving potassium by moving it into the cells when cortisol declines. Cortisol (but not corticosterone) is reduced during a potassium deficiency, and this reduction accounts for many of the symptoms of RA.

Cortisol shuts down most of the copper enzymes when it declines so that excretion of copper is increased and Lysil oxidase inhibited. These last two attributes are proposed to account for most of the mortality from aneurysms and infections during rheumatoid arthritis (RA).

Thus the urgent necessity to survive during virulent diarrheas has set people up in the course of evolution for some of the worst symptoms of rheumatoid arthritis.

DISCUSSION

Judging by the drastic decline of mortality in babies suffering from a virulent strain of diarrhea by potassium supplements,[1] potassium loss in those diseases which force cyclic AMP to excrete water into the intestines[2] must be the most serious effect of the diarrheas. I suggest that this is the reason why cortisol has acquired the attribute of moving potassium out of cells[3] and therefore into the cells upon declining. It is also undoubtedly the reason why the adrenal's cortisol secretion is inhibited by low serum potassium in vitro (in the test tube) but not corticosterone.[4] The body thus has a way of signaling for a decrease in cortisol secretion during a serious intestinal disease independently of ACTH. Thus the body inversely mobilizes defenses.

Endotoxin bacterial diseases force the body to secrete cortisol by increasing ACTH[5] probably an adaptation by the bacteria to force the body to inhibit the immune system. Glucosteroid response modifying factor (GRMF) secreted by T- cells then prevents the cortisol from having full effect on white cells other than suppresser cells[6] and thus raises the set point, as does interleukin-1.[6] Interleukin-1 also stimulates cortisol secretion,[7] as does cachectin (tumor necrosis factor).[8] I suspect that this is an adaptation to provide some cortisol maintenance[9] when normal ACTH production is later cut off during endotoxin attack.[10]

In other words, the immune system takes over its own regulation but at a higher set point. The role of GRMF has not yet been demonstrated for physiological processes. GRMF will probably prove to inhibit cortisol for most of those processes as well, surely at least for cortisol's various affects on potassium.

One of the most important of the cortisol controlled immune defenses is the mobilization of the availability of copper to the white cells, an attribute which probably arose because copper is crucial to an adequate immune defense.[11] The primary way cortisol does this is by, inversely to its concentration, shutting down production of copper-containing enzymes such as Lysil oxidase and superoxide dismutase.[12] Lysil oxidase catalyzes the formation of cross links in all connecting tissue including elastin.[13] Since elastin makes up the main strength of normal blood vessels[12] and has a rapid turnover, this is the most serious problem in arthritis. Ruptured aneurysms along with poor resistance to infection and heart disease are the chief terminal events in arthritis.[14]

The body uses ceruloplasmin to carry copper to the immune system during infection.[12] Probably the main reason for this development is that the copper is not in equilibrium with the serum and so is not available to pathogens. However, ceruloplasmin is also used to carry copper to the bile for excretion.[15] Therefore I submit that the rise in serum ceruloplasmin in RA[16] causes an increased excretion in members of a society who, even before this, were receiving less than the minimum daily requirement.

CONCLUSIONS

Evidence can be provided for this proposal in several ways. Arthritic people should have a lower whole body potassium content than normal people. This has been proved.[17] Red blood cells have a higher potassium content than normal during RA.[18] This should not be taken as counter evidence because I suspect that this is an adaptation to help avoid circulatory collapse when dehydration reduces the blood volume during diarrhea. There should be a lower incidence of RA among people on potassium supplementation or who eat Morton's Lite Salt (TM) or Stirling's Half and Half (TM). I know of no epidemiologic study showing this. However, people who work in potash mines have a 25% lower incidence of heart disease than the surrounding population[19] and heart disease is prevalent in RA. There should be a healing of RA upon starting potassium supplements. No controlled experiment has been reported which would indicate this. However there is a case history of a single arthritic brought up to 3.5 grams per day in order to explore the effects of various steroid hormones on the body's mineral balance.[20] A total of 3.5 grams is about the amount an adult would obtain from unprocessed food. The subject showed consistent improvement throughout the experiment even though potassium was the only consistent change. His total body potassium consistently rose. There should be a negative correlation between potassium-caused muscle spasms and RA, but I have no supporting data. Neither do I know of a positive correlation with eating licorice or potassium losing diuretics, both of which increase potassium loss. There should be a negative correlation between eating acids which have an indigestible anion and RA since the hydrogen ion interferes with potassium excretion.[21] I know of no good experiment or epidemiologic study.

However, it has been suggested from folk custom that eating vinegar[22] or cherries is efficacious. The vinegar seems doubtful since it is my understanding that acetate can be metabolized by the body. However, it is conceivable that people on a diet high in calories do not utilize all the acetate. RA should not be present in people who eat predominantly vegetables instead of grains.

An experiment has been performed in which RA was healed in a group of people by switching to a vegetable diet.[23a]

I suspect that people with rheumatoid arthritis tend to have a poorer ability to conserve potassium than other people because of damage to their kidneys by a poison such as bromine gas or long term poisons in plant foods (such as solenaceous vegetables) or by poisons excreted by pathogenic bacteria. Screening some common poisons currently in use in food might be enlightening. Since GRMFs inhibit cortisol, it is possible that a discordance in the immune response or some infection types may accentuate RA. (See **"Chemicals in 'hot' Chili Peppers Confirmed to be a Cause of Arthritis!"** prior article, this book.)

If animals are used for experiments, it is futile to use rats or mice because they rely primarily on corticosterone to regulate the immune response, not cortisol. I suspect that this developed because they have a factor in their intestinal fluid which counteracts cholera toxin.[23] They also have the ability to absorb water under cyclic AMP stimulation in part of their colon[24] instead of excretion, unlike other animals.

Since the disturbance in copper metabolism is proposed as the most serious aspect of RA, evidence for copper's effect should be possible. Supplementing with copper should remove some of the symptoms of RA. I know of no such experiment. (See "The Use of Ionic Copper in the Treatment of Arthritis," http://www.arthritistrust.org.)

However, it is known that Finnish men who work in copper mines have little arthritis or susceptibility to infection.[25] The high milk diet along with frequent saunas may be two reasons why other Finns have one of the highest rates of arthritis in the world,[26] since milk is the poorest source of copper[27,p92] and perspiration loses potassium.[28] Milk has been shown to have a high statistical correlation with cardiovascular disease, said to be as great a risk as smoking.[29] which disease in turn is correlated with RA. Laplanders on a meat diet have a lower rate of RA not much further north.[26] The Massai of Africa have a higher rate of RA than the surrounding tribes.[30,p268].

The Masai also use a lot of milk as well as very few vegetables, which vegetables would have increased potassium intake. Men who work in copper mines must have stronger tissues than other miners because the percentage of injuries which result in lost time is significantly lower[31] even though injuries like eye damage and burns which are not affected by strength are part of the data. Eating a lot of shellfish or liver should reduce those symptoms related to copper deficiency since they are the richest sources, but I know of no study. The same is true of drinking acid water out of copper plumbing.

I believe that it is unwise to give cortisol to any class of people whose immune system is weak, such as arthritic people. If it is felt that cortisol should be raised in the body, why not use something relatively safe, like potassium supplements? If potassium supplements are used, be certain that vitamin B1 is adequate because the "wet" heart disease of Beri-Beri can not materialize when potassium is deficient.[32] Obviously the reverse is also true for vitamin B1 supplementation. For this reason, If the patient has heart trouble, it is very important to determine whether it is caused by vitamin B1 or potassium. If potassium chloride is dissolved in fruit juice it tastes good and avoids the danger to the intestines that even slow release enteric tablets may present.

The chloride is the most efficacious form.[33] It would be better and safer yet to provide potassium from food high in potassium such as celery or bamboo shoots as Effinger proposed.[34] Unboiled, unfrozen, uncanned vegetables low in starch are the richest sources.[35] However, removing a deficiency will be slower since the potassium is not associated with chloride and would take a few months longer.

A deficiency can arise from diarrhea, processed food, reliance on grain or fatty foods,[35] psychic stress stimulation of aldosterone[36,p209] (which is the main regulator of potassium)[37], stress stimulation of cortisol (as in an operation, for instance.[38]) diuretics, licorice[39] as well as probably grapefruit,[39a] profuse perspiration,[28] excessive vomiting,[40] eating sodium bicarbonate,[41] hyperventilating,[41] laxatives,[43] enemas,[44] shock from burns or injury,[45] hostile or fearful emotions,[36] and very high or very low sodium intake.[46] All of these increase excretion or decrease intake of potassium.

A chronic potassium deficiency must surely cause a degenerative disease. I believe it materializes in some people as RA. If not, then what is the name of the degenerative disease which attends a potassium deficiency ? It is not hypokalemia. This is only a word which describes low serum potassium, a marker.

BIBLIOGRAPHY

1. Darrow, D.C. 1946 "Retention of Electrolyte during recovery from severe dehydration due to diarrhea," Journal of Pediat. 28; 515.

2. Mekalanos, J.J.; Swartz, D.J.; Pearson, GDN.; Harford, N.; Groyne, F.; Wilde, M. 1983. "Cholera Toxin Genes: Nucleotide Sequence, Deletion

Analysis and Vaccine Developement," Nature 306; 551.

3. Bronner, F.; Comar, C.L. 1961 Mineral Metabolism Vol I, Academic Press.

4. Mikosha, A.S.; Pushkarov, I.S.; Chelnakova, I.S.; Remennikov, G.Ya. 1991 "Potassium Aided Regulation of Hormone Biosynthesis in Adrenals of Guinea Pigs under Action of Dihydropyridines: Possible Mechanisms of Changes in Steroidogenesis Induced by 1,4-Dihydropyridines in Dispersed Adrenocorticytes." Fiziol. ZH (Kiev) 37:60.

5. Melby J.C.; Egdahl, R.H.; Spink, W.W. 1960 "Secretion and Metabolism of Cortisol after Injection of Endotoxin." Journal of Lab. Clin. Med. 56;50.

6. Fairchild, S.S.; Shannon, K.; Kwan, E.; Mishell, R.I. 1984 "T-cell Derived Glucocorticosteroid Response Modifying Factor (GRMFt): A Unique Lymphokine Made by Normal T Lymphocytes and a T-cell Hybridoma." Journal of Immunology 132; 821.

7. Besedovsky, H.O.; Del Rey, A.; Sorkin, E. 1984 "Integration of Activated Immune Cell Products in Immune Endocrine Feedback Circuits." p. 200, Leukocytes and Host Defense Vol. 5 (Oppenheim, J.J.; Jacobs, D.M., eds) Alan R. Liss, NY.

8. Milenkovic, L.; Rettori, V.; Snyder, G.D.; Beutler, B.; McCann, S.M. 1989 "Cachectin Alters Anterior Pituitary Hormone Release by a Direct Action in Vitro." Nat. Acad. Sci. 86; 2418.

9. Finlay, G.J.; Booth, R.J.; Marbrook, J. 1979 "Antibody Responses of Human Lymphocytes in Vitro; Enhancing Effects of Hydrocortisone." Austr. Journal of Exp. Biol Med. Sci. 57; 597.

10. Jones, R.S.; Howell, E.V.; Eik-Nesk. 1959 "Inactivation by Plasma of ACTH Releasing Property of C-14 Labeled Bacterial Polysacharride." Proc. Soc. of Exper. Biol. Med. 100; 328.

11. Prohaska, J.R.; Lukaseqycz, O.A. 1981 "Copper Deficiency Suppresses the Immune Response in Mice." Science 213; 559.

12. Weber, C.E. 1984 "Copper Response to Rheumatoid Arthritis." Medical Hypotheses 15; 333.

13. Harris, E.D.; Rayton, J.K.; Baltriop, J.E.; Di Silvestro, R.A.; Garcia de Quevedo. "Copper in the Synthesis of Elastin and Collagen," p. 163, Biological Roles of Copper, Ciba Foundation Symposium No 79, Exerpta Medica NY.

14. Matsuoka, Y.; Obana, M.; Mita, S.; Kohno, M.; Irimajiri, S.; Fujimori, I.; Fukuda, J. "Studies of Death in Autopsied Cases with Rheumatoid Arthritis," p. 27, New Horizons in Rheumatoid Arthritis. (Shiokawa, Y.; Abe, T.; Yamauchi, Y., eds.) Excerpta Medica Internat. Cong. Series #535.

15. Frieden, E. 1981 "Ceruloplasmin: A Multifunctional Metalloprotein of Vertebrate Plasma." Metal Ions and Biological Systems, Vol. 13, p. 117 (Sigel, H.; Sigel, B., eds.) Marcel Dekker, NY & Basel.

16. Aiginger, P.; Kolarz, G.; Wilvonseder, R. 1978 "Copper in

Ankylosing Spondylitis and Rheumatoid Arthritis." Scand. Journal of Rheumatol. 7; 75.

17. LaCelle, P.L., et al. 1964 "An Investigation of Total Body Potassium in Patients with Rheumatoid Arthritis." Proc. Ann. Meeting of the Am. Rheumatism Assoc. Arth. Rheum. 7; 321.

18. Knudsen, E.T.; Thomas, M.J. 1957 "Erythrocyte Potassium Level in Rheumatoid Arthritis." Lancet 272; 251.

19. Waxweiler, R.J., et al. 1973 "Mortality of Potash Workers." J. Occup. Med. 15; 486.

20. Clark, W.S, et al. 1956 "The Relationship of Alterations in Mineral and Nitrogen Metabolism to Disease Activity in a Patient with Rheumatoid Arthritis." Acta Rheum. Scand. 2; 193.

21. Berliner, R.W, et al. 1951 "Relationship between Acidification of the Urine and Potassium Metabolism." Amer. Journal Med. 11; 274.

21a. Mills, J.H.; Stanbury, S.W. 1954 "A Riciprocal Relationship between K+ and H+ Excretion in the Diurnal Excretory Rhythm in Man." Clin. Sci. 13; 177.

22. Jarvis, D.C. 1960 "Arthritis and Folk Medicine." Pan Books Ltd. London.

23a. Kjeldsen-Kraw, J. 1991 Lancet Oct. 12; 899.

23. Donowitz, M.; Binder, H.J. 1976 "Effect of Enterotoxins of Vibrio Cholerae, Escherichi coli, & Shigelladienteriae Type 1 on Fluid and Electrolyte Transport in Colon." Journal of Infect. Dis. 134; 135.

24. Hornyck, A.; Meyer, P.; Milliez, P. 1973 "Angiotensin, Vasopressin, and Cyclic AMP: Effects of Sodium & Water Fluxes in Rat Colon." Am Journal of Physiol. 224; 1223.

25. Sorrenson, JRJ;. Hangarter, W. 1977 "Treatment of Rheumatoid and Degenerative Diseases with Copper Complexes." Inflammation 2; 217.

26. Kellgren, J.H. 1966 "Epidemiology of RA" Arh. Rheum. 9; 658.

27. Underwood, E.J. 1972 "Trace Elements in Human and Animal Nutrition." Academic Press NY.

28. Consolazio, C.F., et al. 1963 "Excretion of Sodium, Potassium, Magnesium, and Iron in Human Sweat and the
Relation of Each to Balance and Requirements." Journal of Nutr. 79; 407.

29. Seely, S. 1981 "Diet and Coronary Disease: A Survey of Mortality Rates and Food Consumption Statistics of 24 Countries." Med. Hypotheses. 7; 907.

30. Best, C.H.; Taylor, N.B. 1950 The Physiological Basis of Medical Practice, 5th ed. Williams and Wilkins Co., Baltimore (p. 768).

31. U.S. Dept. of Labor, Mine Safety and Health Administration. 1981 "Injury Experience in Metallic Mineral Mining, IR 1142 Table # 6. pp. 24 & 58.

32. Folis, R.H. 1942 "Myocardial Necrosis in Rats on a Potassium Low Diet Prevented by Thiamine Deficiency." Bull. Johns-Hopkins Hospital

71; 235.

33. DeLand, E.C., et al. 1979 "A Theoretical and Experimental Study of Ionic Shifts Induced by K Depletion and Replacement." Journal of Theor. Biol. 76; 31.

34. Eppinger, H. 1939 "Einiges Uber Dietetische Therapie." Ztschr. F. Artzl. Fortbild. 36; 672 & 709.

35. Weber, C.E. 1974 "Potassium in the Etiology of Rheumatoid Arthritis and Heart Infarction." Journal of Applied Nutrition. 26; 41 (Bibliography published separately).

36. Glaz, E.; Vecsei, P. 1971 "Aldosterone." Pergamon Press NY (p 209).

37. Weber, C.E 1983 "Corticosteroid Regulation of Electrolytes." Journal of Theor. Biol. 104; 443.

38. Elman, R., et al. 1952 "Intracellular and Extracellular Potassium Deficits in Surgical Patients." Ann. Surgery 136; 111.

39. Stormer, FC, Reistad, R, Alexander, J 1993 Glycyrrizic acid in licorice - evaluation of health hazard. Food Chem. Toxicol 31; 303-312.

39a. Lee YS, Lorenzo, BJ, Koufis, T, Reidenberg, MN 1996 Grapefruit juice and its flavenoids inhibit 11 beta -hydroxy steroid dehydrogenase. Clin. Pharmacol. Ther. 59; 62-71.

40. Barter, F.C. 1980 "Clinical Problems of Potassium Metabolism, Contributions to Nephrology." p. 21, Disturbances of Water and Electrolyte Metabolism. Bahlmann, J.; Brod, J., eds. S. Karger, Basel.

41. Berliner, R.W, et al. 1951 "Relationship between Acidification of the Urine and Potassium Metabolism." Amer. Journal of Med. 11; 274.

42. Kilburn, K.H. 1966 "Movements of Potassium during Acute Respiratory Acidosus and Recovery." Journal of Applied Physiol. 21; 679.

43. Schwartz, W.B.; Relman, M.B. 1953 "Metabolic and Renal Studies in Chronic Potassium Depletion Resulting from Overuse of Laxatives." Journal of Clin. Invest. 32; 58.

44. Dunning, M.F.; Plum, F. 1956 "Potassium Depletion by Enemas." Amer. Journal of Med. 20; 789.

45. Fox, C.L.; Baer, H. 1947 "Redistribution of Potassium, Sodium, and Water in Burns and Trauma and Its Relation to Phenomena of Shock." Am. Journal of Physiol. 151.

46. Williams, G.H.; Dluhy, R.G. 1972 "Aldosterone Biosynthesis: Interrelationship of Regulatory Factors." Am. Journal of Med. 53; 595.

Root Canal Cover-Up
Conceals Numerous Dangerous Side Effects
book by
George Meinig, D.D.S.
Report by Anthony di Fabio

Since the discovery of penicillin and antibiotics, root canal specialists and some physicians have come to believe infections resulting from tooth extractions, root canal work, tonsillectomies, and adenoidectomies no longer cause diseases in other parts of the body. They incorrectly claim that long-standing focal infections are a thing of the past. Most disturbing is their failure to accept the existence of the bacteria that become trapped inside the dentin tubules which make up 90 percent of the structure of teeth. Added to that fact is the inability of antibiotics and other medicaments to be able to get at and kill these organisms.

Extensive research studies in which 5000 animals took part, clearly demonstrate how these bacteria, or their toxins, escape into the circulation of the tooth's surrounding bony socket, and how these organisms are responsible for a high percentage of the chronic and degenerative disease conditions that are so epidemic in America today.

Confusing the issue is the fact that twenty-five percent of individuals who have root canal fillings (or tooth extractions) are free from trouble for extended periods of time. These are individuals who have <u>excellent</u> health and exceptionally good immune systems.

This group's freedom from side effects unfortunately has led many root canal specialists to believe their treatment of infected teeth is always successful and can cause no harm.

On the other side are the 75 percent whose immune systems have been compromised by illnesses, accidents, poor nutrition, stress, etc. This group develop a variety of conditions which end up in their going from doctor to doctor, in desperate attempts to find the cause of their problems. A high percentage of these cases are due to the bacteria coming from their root canal filled teeth, or from tooth extractions, or other foci of infection.

Once confronted with root canals, or teeth extractions, being a possible source of their illnesses, these patients often recall their health problems seemed to start right after the root canal treatment was undertaken or teeth extracted. When these infected gums are removed, many find their illnesses disappear.

To visualize what happens, picture the bacteria trapped in the dentin tubules; see them mutate and become more virulent and their toxins more toxic. In their escape into the blood circulation of the tooth's socket, these bacteria, like cancer cells, metastasize to other parts of the body. As they migrate, they infect the heart, kidneys, joints, nervous system, brain, eyes — and can endanger pregnant women and in fact may infect any organ, gland or other tissue.

The Root Canal Cover-up book was compiled and written by George E. Meinig, D.D.S., F.A.C.D., one of the 19 founding members that organized the American Association of Endodontists and a former Twentieth Century Fox Studio dentist.

His book provides the public and health professionals with their first real look at the serious illnesses that can arise as a result of root canal therapy. This 7 X 10, soft cover 237 page third edition (the first and second edition (sold out in record time) should be read by all patients and all health specialists!

The World's Greatest Medical Discovery

If you heard there was a source of disease which caused literally hundreds of different illnesses, wouldn't you think that would be one of the world's greatest medical discoveries?

What will be your reaction when you learn this phenomenal work has been covered up and buried for over 80 years? Be prepared for a series of shocks. Just such a wide assortment of diseases were found and proven to come from focal infections present in infected teeth, jaws and tonsils. While these degenerative diseases could come from almost any oral infection, a high percentage come from bacteria that remain locked in root canal filled teeth. No doubt your first reaction to these words will be — what kind of crazy man is this Dr. George to make such statements?

Stay with me for a few moments. It will be to your advantage to learn what this unfortunate cover-up is all about. It will be helpful for you to know that I was one of the 19 dentists who started the Root Canal Association now known as the American Association of Endodontists (AAE). My love affair with trying to save teeth led to graduate studies about root canal therapy from Professor Edgar Coolidge, foremost root canal researcher and teacher of the subject in the world. He was my first mentor in the field of dentistry.

It was also my good fortune to be one of the six members of his study and teaching group. Keep in mind at that time, very few dentists did root canal therapy. In fact some dental schools didn't even teach the subject.

To spread the word, Dr. Coolidge arranged for our study group to be guest speakers at numerous dental meetings. Those efforts, and those of the AAE, has resulted in some 20 million root canals now being treated each year. In my general, holistic practice of 47 years — I did several thousand.

Four years ago I learned there had been a 25 year research program which covered all phases of root canal treatment. This was no small program; 5,000 animals were used and it was directed by Dental Research Specialist, Weston A. Price, D.D.S., M.S. The last ten years was conducted under the auspices of the American Dental Association and its Research Institute. That Research Institute was governed by 60 of the nation's leading medical and dental scientists.

All of those thousands of studies and experiments were documented in two large volumes containing 1,174 pages and in more than 25 articles which can be found in the dental and medical literature.

A vast array of discoveries were forthcoming from that extensive and meticulous research which found many root canal therapy common beliefs of dentists and endodontists to be false. The most startling one clearly and emphatically demonstrated with 5,000 animal studies, that root canal filled teeth always remain infected no matter how good they look or how good they feel.

You can readily see after 47 years of practice, upon learning about all of the conclusive evidence of this discovery why I was in more of a shock than you. How in the world could it be that these vital and important revelations have been kept from the entire dental profession for over 70 years? During the last four years I have probably talked to two or three thousand dentists and have found only one who knew about Dr. Price's great discoveries.

While I knew from Dr. Coolidge's teaching that infections could be present in the lateral canals of teeth even if they appeared normal on x-ray pictures, I had no knowledge that the infection problem was so immense.

Let me get right to the heart of the problem. To do so requires that you have a little knowledge about the anatomy of a tooth. The crown of a tooth, I am sure you know, is covered by a little less than 1/4 inch of enamel. The root with

1/8 of an inch of cementum. All of the rest of the tooth (over 90 percent of it) is composed of what is called dentin.

Though the dentin is almost as hard as enamel, it is composed of tiny tubules measuring 1.5 microns, which is smaller in size than the thickness of a sheet of paper. In the normal, healthy tooth, these tubules are filled with a liquid which contains nutrients.

Running through the center of the tooth is the root canal. Everyone knows it contains a nerve. Many are not aware that it also contains an artery, vein, and other tissue. As the blood flows through the artery every day and night, it drops nutrients into the fluid in each of those dentin tubules — the same way blood vessels drop nutrients into each cell of the body. The nutrients present in those tubules travel to all parts of the tooth. That is the real hidden secret about what keeps teeth alive and healthy.

When we get a small cavity in a tooth which is just breaking through the enamel into the dentin, the bacteria that are part of the decay process get into the tubules in the vicinity of the decay area. Dentists in cleaning out the decay quite readily stop the process.

The problem arises when the person doesn't go to their dentist regularly and that tiny cavity becomes a deep one. Once the decay gets so deep that it penetrates into the root canal itself, the bacteria present in the decayed tooth substance enter the canal and quickly travel it down to the end and then out of the apex of the root into the surrounding bone. Along the way, they spy those dentin tubules and their nutrient food content.

They find those tubules are excellent new home sites. Herein lies the problem. Dentists, in doing root canal treatment, feel they adequately kill the bacteria that are present, but are unaware that the medications they use cannot penetrate into those tiny tubules far enough to kill them. Most dentists are entirely unaware of the bacteria in the tubules, and the fact that hundreds of experiments showed not a single one of over 100 commonly used disinfectants could penetrate those tubules.

When we confront dentists with these facts they often will say, "So what? When we place the root canal filling, the organisms will die off." Here again their opinion is incorrect as they are unaware that these bacteria are polymorphic, which means they can mutate and change form and are able to actually live under the most severe, adverse conditions. [See *Cell-Wall Deficient Forms*, by Lida Mattmann, Ph.D.]

Undaunted, your dentist will now say, "What difference does it make? The germs can't escape because the root canal filling blocks them out" That too is untrue, as the bacteria can readily escape from the lateral, accessory root canals present in all teeth. Not only that, the toxins formed by bacteria can escape right through the cementum of the tooth. In another series of intelligent experiments, Dr. Price showed that the hard cementum outer covering of the roots was actually a semi-permeable membrane. That means liquid substances like bacteria toxins could travel right through the cementum and escape into the periodontal membrane which holds the tooth in its bony socket. It is that membrane which attaches the tooth to the jaw bone and keeps teeth from falling out.

The peridontal membrane is a hard fibrous tissue but it has a blood supply and the bacteria and their toxins now infect it. From there, the organisms and their toxins have easy access into the surrounding jaw bone and its blood supply. It is similar to cells breaking away from a cancer lesion and metastasizing and setting up a new cancer some other place in the body. These bacteria from teeth and their toxins also metastasize via the blood stream. In their travels when they find a gland, organ or body tissue that appears attractive, they make it their new home and promptly set up a new infection. This eventually results in a degenerative disease.

Now that you know the source of the problem, let me tell you about how a rabbit revealed the actual devastation that occurs.

Dr. Price had treated a root canal infection for a patient who subsequently developed a severe case of arthritis in her hands and legs. He was well aware that physicians in trying to discover the cause of a disease would isolate the bacteria, grow them in culture, and then inject the organism into animals to see if they could reproduce the disease and subsequently find a cure.

At that particular moment, Dr. Price did not know just where the infection was in the tooth, but in thinking how doctors were discovering the causes of diseases, he thought of a similar way that might lead to an answer. After a little trouble he convinced the patient to let him remove the tooth. He washed and bathed it in a disinfectant. He then made a small buttonhole incision in the skin of the back of a rabbit, inserted the extracted root canal tooth, placed a couple of stitches so it wouldn't fall out, and returned the animal to its spacious cage and waited developments.

It didn't take long. In just two days the rabbit's limbs had developed the same arthritic swelling as that of the patient and in ten days it died from the infection coming from that tooth.

Now, Dr. Price immediately thought of all those patients he had who were suffering from heart, kidney, liver, joint disease, eye problems, etc., etc., and he wondered if their root canals were the source of their degenerative health problems. Those who had root canals he suggested their removal and he implanted them under the skin of an animal.

What happened was surprising and unexpected. In the vast majority of cases the animal developed the same disease as the patient and most passed away in from two or three days to a week or two from the infections present in the root canal treated teeth. Different kinds of animals were used: Rats, Guinea pigs, dogs and monkeys, but it didn't matter, the same results occurred. They usually used rabbits as they seemed to react a bit more promptly and proved the better choice for such studies.

Early on in his studies Dr. Price made some reports of his research in articles which appeared in medical and dental journals. A number of dentists came to him voicing the opinion that any animal would likely get sick and die with an extracted tooth in its body. Dr. Price admitted he didn't know the answer to that question but he said let's find out. What he did was to have a group of dentists secure 100 healthy teeth. These were removed for orthodontic purposes, or impacted teeth, none of them had any tooth decay or gum trouble. He placed each single tooth under the skin of a different animal.

Well, not a single one of those 100 animals got sick or died. All lived their normal life span with the tooth under its skin. In a few, their immune systems were strong enough to expel the tooth out through the skin and in a few the tooth dissolved away. They even did bacteriologic studies of the tissue around the imbedded teeth and always found them to be sterile.

It is always a surprise to learn that Dr. Price's work was buried for over 80 years. Of course, there is the obvious objection of dentists not wanting to lose this part of their income. Actually there were a half dozen or more reasons why his work was covered up and buried. That will have to wait for another time because of space limitations.

I can assure you, hardly a dentist in the country has ever heard about this 25 year extensive and meticulous research program. The Endodontic Association says they teach about Dr. Price in dental schools, but it is strange I never find any dentists who have ever heard about it.

The AAE isn't very happy with me exposing this cover-up and they claim the focal infection theory was proven false years ago, but so many investigators have proven the accuracy of the theory, that it is unbelievable they stick to that old claim that helped bury Dr. Price's work. That story too will need to wait for another day.

I had hoped by now they would set up research to investigate the bacteria in the dentin tubules as these infections prove to be so devastating. The AAE has numbers of research projects but they have not as yet faced this critical issue.

Editor's Comments

If you have a root canal or been told you need one, your best approach is to learn all you can about this subject. See *Root Canal Cover-Up*, search online. It is written in lay language and covers the major issues covered in Dr. Price's two volumes of 1,174 pages of documentation. Even if you don't have a root canal treated or extracted tooth it is worthwhile to learn about what is taking place in so many people and how these degenerative diseases can be prevented.

An extracted tooth can cause the same problems as do the infected root canal. The executive director of this foundation found that he had sustained a 50 year long, hidden, unknown infection in upper and lower gums from having had teeth extracted 50 years ago via the Veteran's Administration.

Also a word of caution: as with the problems of mercury poisoning from mercury amalgam fillings in teeth (another sad story to be told), it's not easy to find a "biological dentist" trained in its safe removal. Removing mercury amalgams in the wrong manner can result in more harm than the mercury fillings to be replaced.

A specially trained and knowledgeable dentist (biological dentist) can use non-invasive means to determine the source of root canal or tooth extraction infection, after which surgery may be required accompanied by proper sterilization techniques. Even then, follow-up checks may be required. The Price-Pottenger Nutrition Foundation, PO Box 2614, La Mesa, CA 91943-2614; (619) 462-7600 may help you find your nearest biological dentist.

Sad to say, as critical and important as a biological dentist is to achieving wellness, it's been the editor's experience that they are usually few and far from our home stations.

CranioSacral Therapy

by
JohnPage
listed in Craniosacral Therapy
originally published in issue 13 - July/Aug 1996
http://www.positivehealth.com/articles.asp?i=486
Permission granted for reprint

Why are such a variety of healthcare practitioners excited about the tadpole-shaped bag that lines our skulls and spinal columns? The excited healthcare practitioners include massage therapists, doctors, nurses, osteopaths, dentists, physiotherapists, chiropractors, psychotherapists and – yes – vets. The tadpole-shaped bag is the dural membrane whose three layers surround, protect and connect our central nervous system, bathed and nourished in its own special liquid environment, cerebrospinal fluid.

The answer is that the insights, skill and determination of an American osteopathic physician led to a specialised and somewhat mysterious manipulative system that had been strictly reserved for osteopaths being developed and taught in ways that brought it safely within the scope of any healthcare professional with good intention and sensitivity of touch.

A new direction emerges.

In the early 1970s Dr John E. Upledger discovered for himself, in a most tangible way, the cranio-sacral rhythm or cranial rhythmic impulse. This impulse was evident in causing a section of cervical dural tube, which he was attempting to stabilise during a delicate surgical procedure, to move with a frequency that was neither cardiac nor respiratory. Furthermore the rhythmic movement was so persistent as to prevent Dr Upledger from being able to keep the dural tube still. His curiosity aroused he went on to learn about the pioneering work of Dr W.G. Sutherland who formulated Cranial Osteopathy. Impressed by the effectiveness of Cranial Osteopathy, and following his 1975 appointment as a clinician researcher and Professor of Biomechanics at Michigan State University, Dr Upledger employed extensive research facilities to help understand how the phenomena that Dr Sutherland had discovered actually worked. This research began the formulation of CranioSacral Therapy. 21 years on, it has placed profoundly effective light-touch techniques in the hands of tens of thousands of practitioners.

Dr Sutherland had been a pupil of A.T. Still, father of Osteopathy. Sutherland's cranial work was not only effective with various cases of pain that had failed to respond to osteopathic treatment, but was also helpful in restoring good metabolic function and assisting recovery from endogenous depression and respiratory disorders.

Despite Dr Sutherland's experiments including work with the human energy field and the use of very light touch, sometimes working off the body, Cranial Osteopathy was to develop very much as an extension of osteopathy, albeit with light contact, where the bones are seen as all important and the practitioner focuses on restoring to proper mobility the joints or sutures between the bones that make up the cranium. However, Dr Upledger's research and his consideration of how cranial suture restrictions tend to be maintained by structures outside the head caused him to deduce that it is within the body's membranes or fascia that the astonishing effects of Cranial Osteopathy are explained. It is interesting that A.T. Still also regarded the fascia as being of primary importance.

So now back to that tadpole-shaped envelope that contains the brain and spinal cord. Why is it so important? Apart from the obvious (that it contains and protects some rather vital equipment) it is from within this dural membrane that the cranio-sacral rhythm is generated. Also the dural membrane is centrally placed within the whole of the fascial system in such a way that it can influence, and be affected by, the condition of any and every other part of the body.

All-important membranes

The term fascia is the collective name for the membrane material that would remain were our hair, blood vessels, viscera, bones, nerves, muscle fibres and fluids to be removed. It includes our ligaments and all the membranous sheaths that surround and connect all our organs, bones and muscles. The tendency of restriction in one part of the body to transmit dysfunction to other parts is accounted for by the characteristics of fascial material and the construction of the whole fascial system. So fundamental are these aspects to a proper understanding of CranioSacral Therapy that they are worth going into in some detail.

First let's take a simplified look at the components of fascia. There are three basic components. Variations in their proportions account for the huge range of qualities and functions that fascia exhibit. They are collagen, a fibrous material that provides tensile strength, elastin which when tension is removed causes fascia to return to its original dimensions, thereby providing 'elastic memory', and ground substance which, as it were, fills in the spaces. Ground substance is wet and proteinous, and provides passage for dissolved nutrients and waste compounds. Fascia also contains sensory and motor nerves and has blood supply. It is capable of contraction. From the electrical perspective relaxed fascia carries negative electrical potential that supports healthy tissue metabolism. When under stretch the potential changes to positive. Fascia that is under continual tension will therefore suffer local metabolic deterioration and begin to lose some of its qualities.

Second we should consider the all-pervasive design of the fascial system. In the embryo, fascia forms from a single fold at a very early stage of development. Rather than being lots of different structures that have grown together, fascia is a single structure, holding together in functional relationship every part of the body. We can travel from any point on or in the body to any other without leaving fascia. In fact, it is so pervasive that it not only connects every cell but actually penetrates right into the nuclei, providing a framework for the chromosomes.

To summarise, fascia holds, connects, allows movement, helps the body remember what shape it's meant to be, contracts, feels, contains the body's fluids (blood, lymph and csf) and transmits load and strain throughout the body.

Weird connections

Now we can begin to understand the extraordinary effects of Dr Sutherland's work, how, for instance, the freeing up of the membranes inside the head by applying gentle pressure and/or traction to the cranial bones could lead to improved pituitary (and therefore endocrine) function, resolving many problems including hormone-related and metabolic illnesses. However, Dr Upledger found that many restrictions in the cranium often have causes outside the head. CranioSacral Therapy practitioners are used to the emergence of bizarre cause-and-effect connections: the appendicectomy scar that leads to chronic migraines, the compressed lumbo-sacral joint to endogenous depression, the restricted upper neck to digestive disorders or to hyperactivity, the unbalanced pelvis that may lead to eyesight problems.

Often the question is asked "What is CranioSacral Therapy useful for?" The straight, and perhaps rather unhelpful answer is "just about any health problem." But we want clear answers. "I have such-and-such a problem. What will fix it?" It is at this point that it helps to think clearly about how pain and illness really tend to occur. I find the most helpful starting point is to remember that we have our own self-healing mechanisms.

To the core of healing

As long as we are breathing, as long as our fluids are circulating, old structure is being demolished and removed while new material is being imported and built into new body parts. Our electrical and chemical systems are constantly informing each other of, and responding to, the latest developments and needs. In addition to these routine processes of renewal and repair there are exceptional items that need taking care of from time-to-time. Some of these exceptional items we will be aware of, like a minor cut or insect bite. Others will escape our attention provided we are healthy. One of the qualities of good health is the ability of our self-healing mechanism to take care of an endless list of minor insults and repairs without the need to divert our attention. Provided we don't overload our systems we have the flexibility to accommodate a whole variety of stressors. It is only when our system loses flexibility that we start running the risk of deteriorating health when problems that should be temporary tend to hang on or become chronic, or we may become very sensitive to substances or energetic influences that would not trouble a healthy person. (We call some of these sensitivities allergies.)

What sort of things happen to us that reduce our flexibility to renew and repair routinely? This is where the qualities and functions of the fascial system really start to account for themselves. Fascia has great flexibility and is fundamentally influential in all of our body processes. If fascia in one part of the body loses its flexibility due to mechanical inhibition or a toxic or malnourished environment it may affect any other part or system. Causes of mechanical inhibition include physical injury of any kind, surgery and occupational and postural strain. Injuries that can cause retained fascial restriction will include those that happen around birth. Other causes can be old or current inflammation, whether or not infection is or was involved. Inflammation tends to cause normally free-sliding fascial layers, such as the dural layers around the spinal cord, to bind together. With all of these causes resultant dysfunctions may not appear until years, sometimes decades, later.

The body tells its story . . .

So the CranioSacral Therapy practitioner is concerned about evaluating and helping to restore the flexibility of the whole fascial system. It is here that the cranio-sacral rhythm becomes a really useful tool. For while the skilled practitioner gains a fair impression of fascial mobility through light contact with the surface with the ability to project into deep tissue, working with the cranio-sacral rhythm brings greater accuracy in locating fascial restrictions. Evaluating the cranio-sacral rhythm also helps determine the involvement of the spinal nerves.

An extraordinary phenomenon that is the very essence of CranioSacral Therapy is the responsiveness of fascia to very subtle influences. Place hands very lightly on a clothed person lying supine on your treatment table and nothing may happen. Apply one or two grammes of pressure and all sorts of movements may start, where your hands are or anywhere else. Emotion may start to surface, and held-in emotion is yet another cause of reduced fascial flexibility. Even without a single gramme of imposed pressure or traction, the mere alteration of thought or attention can facilitate fascial movement. It is as if the attitude and intention of the practitioner create an atmosphere where the fascia (at last!) feels secure enough to risk the idea of starting to let go.

. . . and reveals its solutions

This is an appropriate point to consider further the idea that the elastic nature of fascia enables it to carry the memory or intelligence of exactly how the body would like to be arranged to enjoy the greatest ease. Fascia under tension is always trying to pull the body back to this state of greatest ease. One of Dr Upledger's great insights is that the body knows in full detail and with total accuracy exactly what it needs to do, and what assistance it needs, to return to this state of ease. The good CranioSacral Therapy practitioner learns to respect this fascial wisdom in preference to anyone's ability to diagnose and intervene from the outside. By listening and feeling the fascial wisdom expressing itself we are taken to the deeper causes of pain and dysfunction instead of being distracted and delayed by symptoms and their apparent causes.

The more helpful answer to the question "What is CranioSacral Therapy useful for?" would therefore be "Any condition where the self-healing mechanism can be supported through improved fascial flexibility", and that covers the majority of conditions that involve pain, restriction, lowered energy, increased susceptibility to infection, and poor circulation or breathing. CranioSacral Therapy also helps many people with specific learning difficulties such as dyslexia, dyscalclia and clumsiness, our co-ordination and proprioceptive mechanisms being easily upset by imbalance of the cranial fascia and bones. Early evaluation and treatment of newborns is recommended, as colic, feeding difficulties and hyperactivity will often be quickly and easily reduced or eliminated. Strains introduced before, during or shortly after the birth process can also be quickly and easily eliminated that may otherwise be retained through adulthood with consequences of chronic dysfunction that would take much more time and perseverance to release from a less fluid and flexible mature person.

Qualities for practice

The adoption of cranial work by healthcare practitioners other than osteopaths came about through two pieces of exploratory work which Dr Upledger led and supervised while a Professor of Biomechanics at the University of Michigan School of Osteopathic Medicine. The first was a clinical trial involving children who had brain function problems, within the Michigan public school system. Hundreds of such children would need evaluation to check if cranio-sacral problems were present and therefore if treatment by Dr Upledger would be appropriate. Insufficient of the University medical staff were interested enough or available to train to do the evaluations but some lay helpers – special needs teachers, social workers, clinic staff, etc. were keen to get involved. So Dr Upledger evolved a format for breaking down the evaluative procedures into very simple components, without any loss of sensitivity. And in fact it was this approach to training that was to form the basis of the skills development programme that Dr Upledger has designed for training healthcare practitioners. In the event too many children were found to have cranio-sacral irregularities for Dr Upledger alone to handle, so he allowed his newly-trained colleagues to do some of the treatment. Furthermore, wishing treatment to be as continuous as possible he started teaching the more motivated parents to perform simple release techniques for daily use at home, with improved results.

Dr Upledger and some of his team then became involved with helping autistic children at a special centre. There he discovered that the prerequisites for progress in treatment were not so much medical qualifications as sensitivity of touch and good intention. Experienced CranioSacral Therapy practitioners find that more is achieved by waiting and listening than by trying to 'do' anything. However, it is also true that the more detailed understanding we have of the anatomy we are waiting with and listening to, the more productive our presence becomes. It is as if our intention becomes more informed.

Putting his work on paper for the benefit of students of cranial work resulted in the publication in 1983 of Dr Upledger's first book CranioSacral Therapy, which he co-authored with Jon Vreedevogd, one of his scientific collaborators at Michigan State University, whose speciality is the study of form in relation to function, or 'natural architecture'. CranioSacral Therapy is now recognised as required reading for serious students of the cranio-sacral system. Then followed CranioSacral Therapy II; Beyond the Dura and Somato Emotional Release and Beyond, both under Dr Upledger's sole authorship. Most recently he has written a brief and inspiring introductory paperback *Your Inner Physician and You* which tells the story of his development of CranioSacral Therapy and SomatoEmotional Release – an approach to helping uncover, resolve and release deep emotional issues and their structural and functional components.

The word spreads

In 1985 Dr Upledger founded The Upledger Institute in Palm Beach, Florida. The Institute is a research and educational undertaking which incorporates a clinic offering a variety of naturopathic therapies. It provides training programmes based around intensive workshops throughout North America, the Pacific, Japan and Australasia. The Upledger Institute Europe was established in 1990. Based in Doorn in The Netherlands it provides training in continental Europe and Scandinavia. The Upledger Institute U.K. started operations in 1993 and serves the U.K. and Ireland. So far over 25,000 students have benefited from The Upledger Institute's training programmes.

One of the joys of introducing experienced healthcare practitioners to CranioSacral Therapy is to observe how students of very diverse backgrounds come to work together so quickly and with such ease through the 'middle ground' of the fascia. Osteopath, massage therapist, physiotherapist, acupuncturist and psychotherapist blending together, to me corresponds with the fascia allowing the body's rigid structures to interrelate with its liquids and gases.

Dr Sutherland started teaching Cranial Osteopathy in 1940. Notwithstanding the distinction between Cranial Osteopathy and CranioSacral Therapy, in the reality of everyday practice the distinctions have become blurred as more and more practitioners are drawn into the fascial system in pursuit of the needs of the whole person. It really does seem as if the fascia are holding the centre ground. On the one hand the more structural practitioners who like to focus on the neuromusculo- skeletal system may care to remember, as A.T. Still did, that the fascia hold it all together. And on the other hand those who have more of an affinity for fluids and energy would I am sure agree that fluids need containers and pipes if they are to be useful. Likewise energy needs storage places and pathways. The condition of those containers, pipes and pathways has, as any plumber, electrician or acupuncturist knows, a profound influence. The fascia provide all of these.

International network

The Upledger Institute provides referral services for those seeking a CranioSacral Therapy practitioner, as well as programmes of training for practitioners. Designed to be adaptable to an individual's own learning needs, the Institute's intensive training workshops are held in a variety of locations and supported by detailed study guides and sourcing of textbooks, research articles and other learning materials. Many students pursue their Upledger training in more than one country, and all have access to the resources of the headquarters in Palm Beach, Florida. The Upledger Institute also runs clinical symposia and research conferences.

About John Page

John Page has a background in osteopathy and cranial osteopathy, practising in Perth and Edinburgh. Seeking an approach which could reach the deepest causes of dysfunction he became the first student in the U.K. to complete the Upledger Institute's training in CranioSacral Therapy and SomatoEmotional Release. Since opening The Upledger Institute's U.K. satellite he has fulfilled a long-term ambition to teach by becoming an Upledger Institute Certified Instructor. John lives with his wife Carol Houston, who is also his clinic and business partner, in a tiny village in the Perthshire countryside.

Silicone Arthritis and Related Diseases
by
Stephen B. Edelson, M.D.[2]
Portions of this article were originally published by Dr. Edelson.
Permission to publish granted from Stephen B. Edelson, M.D.

Stephen Edelson, M.D. was one of those doctors who cared deeply for his patients and tried to help everyone, even those with apparently hopeless causes. He was a very rare doctor who tried to help ladies who'd been conned into getting their mammary glands enhanced. Virtually no one else even tried to correct the diseases caused by silicon implants!

Cookbook recipes sanctioned by medical health boards and the FDA are one of the evils in the practice of medicine. One might just as well have an auto mechanic treat you, and probably it would do more good than most traditional medical practices. Along with the evil of cook book medical treatments required by medical boards and the FDA there is, of course, always those who delight in bringing a good man down. Such is the — what I call — the Quack, Quack Busters. You'll find them dishonestly pooh poohing any treatment that is not in the cook book and especially if the treatment has a chance of taking money away from pharmaceutical companies, the biggest evil of all!

Edleson gave up his license rather than continue the good fight, and a lot of folks did not get well who might have been well because of this sad event. Here's what Stephen had to say, "Because I do not practice 'standard medicine,' it is easy for the FDA, the Georgia Medical Board, and patients who do not see immediate results, or the extent of the results we had hoped for, to attack me. All of this has taken a tremendous toll on me and my family. . . . I have begun the process of closing my clinic and transitioning into retirement."

The Silicone Implant Problem

Between one and two million women have had silicone breast implants to improve their physical appearance. Within and after thirty years, thousands of women have been questioning their earlier decision, and many seem to be suffering major disabilities as a result of these implants. In 1993 the FDA placed restrictions on the use of silicone for breast implants and currently (1994) there is pending a record $4.7 billion settlement in one of the nation's largest class-action suits resulting from the implant damage.

When the U.S. patent office approved the first implant in 1966, they were not legally required to test out implants, and so long as implants were treated as a "device" rather than a drug, it did not have to pass rigorous testing to satisfy the FDA.

Until 1978 no one outside of the chemical companies had reason to know that the envelope surrounding the implant was permeable to the silicone gel inside. When three researchers reported this fact, the whole world knew why certain people, who had received the implants, were becoming ill.

Silicone had long been thought to be chemically inert. This view has changed in the past 48 years. Not only is the silicone tetramer an immune system stimulant and dysregulator, but also the envelope covering breast implants does not protect the individual from the chemical inside the "sac." Slowly and at different rates the silicone oil leaks through this semi-permeable membrane and is carried around the body by cells of our immune system. "Slow contamination of the body by this chemical and the secondary effects on the body lead to what I am calling the 'Silicone Immune Dysfunction Syndrome'," Dr. Edelson[2] says.

There are several forms of the chemical breast implants that can cause a problem. Silicon is the basic element (Si) and probably causes immune system changes. Silica, or $SiO2$ (chemical formula), is the way it is mined from the earth. Silica is 45% silicon. It's chemical structure is $O — Si — O$.

Silicone gel, used for breast implants, is a synthetic material containing 38% silicon. The usual implant material is a silicone tetramer (polydimethylsiloxane). There is slow leakage ("bleeding") of the silicone gel from the implants through the semi-permeable membrane envelope and also into and through the capsule that surrounds the implants. This is picked up by the macrophages (scavenger cells) of our immune system and is broken down inside these cells which travel all over the body. The gel breaks down into Silica (SiO_2) and Silicon (Si) which causes an immune system dysregulation. Thus there are antibodies produced against the silicon and also against the silicon and protein complex (organ systems) so that one suffers from an auto-immune illness. Polydimethylsiloxane's chemical structure is

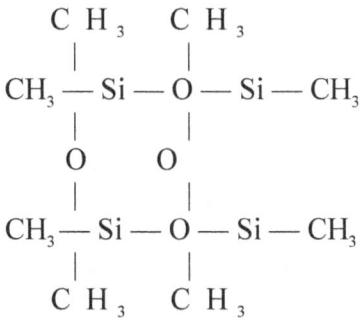

There is also damage that is not related to the immune system because the silicone gel causes oxidants (damaging molecules) to be produced that directly damage our cell walls, DNA, and enzyme systems. All of this adds up to slowly developing chronic debilitating illness affecting every organ system of the body.

As expressed by Dr. Edelson[2], and other physicians, the background burden of oxidants and toxins from our surrounding environment, and the food we eat and drink, adds hugely to the already overpowering burden from silicone leakage. Together, silicone and the oxidant burden (bacterial endotoxins, food chemicals, and chemicals in our world; i.e., xenobiotics), deplete our natural antioxidant systems. Depletion of our antioxidant systems produces respiratory damage and GI damage, the latter leading to organ damage affecting the immune, respiratory, nervous and endocrine systems, as well as other physical systems. Skin damage is also induced, leading to rapid aging of skin and cancer.

Some women whose implants have ruptured, or who suffer from continual silicone leakage, have had a difficult time finding physicians who will work with them.

According to Stephen Edelson, M.D.[2], Immune Disorder Symptoms, sometimes occurring within months of implant, but often occurring 15 to 20 years after surgical implant, include the following: Peripheral Neuropathy (weakness, tingling, numbness, etc.), Central neurotoxic Neuropathy (cognitive difficulties, memory problems, hyperactivity, attention deficits), Cervical and axillary enlarged or painful lymph nodes, fatigue, malaise, weight gain/weight loss, joint and tendon pain, hair loss, dry eyes & mouth, flu-like symptoms, burning skin, constipation, dizziness, enlarged lymph nodes, depression, thyroid problems, hair loss, night sweats, fibromyalgia (multiple tender areas), Myositis (painful inflamed muscles), abdominal pain, emotional instability, chemical sensitivity, food sensitivity, and Pulmonary Hypersensitivity (shortness of breath).

It is believed that these are only the most observable symptoms. Some patients are only moderately ill, while others suffer damage to more than one organ of the body.

Some people who have Silicone Implant illnesses have been diagnosed by their physicians with Lupus, Raynaud's SjÖgren's, Rheumatoid Arthritis, Chronic Fatigue Syndrome and Multiple Sclerosis.

Edelson [2] says that "All of these symptoms are caused by the dysregulation of the immune system and by damage occurring from the free radicals produced by our own system in response to the chemical silicone."

Before the symptoms begin, there are immune system functional abnormalities that allows physicians to pinpoint those women who may be at high risk in developing the silicone implant problem, the Silicone Immune Dysfunction Syndrome. Knowing in advance that one is at high risk, it may be possible to stop the process before it causes significant organ system damage. Edelson[2] suggests that since various studies of the immune system include natural killer cell activity, auto-antibody profile, lymphocyte subsets, silicone antibodies and many other known factors, these factors, as well as organ systems, need to be looked at to evaluate the damage, and that knowledge, in turn, can lead to suggestions on how to go about repairing the body.

Unless the implants are removed from the body, such patients will have a continuing downhill course, and, often, simple removal may not be sufficient, as the healing process may require various treatment regimens including immune modulation, nutritional therapy for sensitivities, anti-oxidant therapy, environmental controls and psycho-neuroimmunological approaches.

How the Syndrome is Evaluated

Dr. Edelson[2], and other physicians, will evaluate Silicone immune Dysfunction Syndrome by the following steps:

1. In depth history, including details of implant problems.

2. Physical examination.

3. Studies to rule out other conditions such as Lyme Disease, Multiple Sclerosis, etc.

4. Various laboratory studies

    a. immune studies (complex)

    b. T-cell silicone immune study

    c. fungal or bacteriological studies (if indicated)

    d biochemical profile

    e. skin testing (if needed)

5. Address each organ system damage individually depending on patient's complaints.

    a. brain: PET, SPECT, BEAM. EMG, etc.

    b. pulmonary: PFT

    c. rheumatological: synovial fluid

    d. breast: MRI, Xeromammography

    e. GI: Digestive studies, pancreatic malfunction

    f. immunological: chemical antibodies, silicone antibodies, T-lymphocyte subpopulation, activated lymphocytes, lymphocyte immune function, natural killer cells and activity, immune complexes, complement levels, ANA, autoantibody analysis (myelin, striated muscle, thyroid, skin antibody, collagen antibody); skin testing (chemical, foods, etc.).

6. Assessment of general damage to the immune system and direct damage from free radical oxidant molecules which has led to diffuse organ system damaging effects.

Therapy

During the course of therapy, many different, often unique, approaches are recommended, usually of one or another form of antioxidant therapy, coupled with proper diet, exercise, and other treatments.

Dr. Edelson[2] has provided the following table to demonstrate various antioxidant factors or substances that protect against oxidant molecular species. Since, apparently, during silicone breast implant leakage, most, or all of the listed oxidants occur or add to the total body burden, treatment must be based upon relieving the load, and searching for ways of eliminating harsher effects.

Free Radical/ Activated Species	Name	Antioxidants
O_2	Superoxide anion radical	Superoxide dismutases

		(SOD)
H_2O_2	Hydrogen peroxide	Glutathione peroxidase
		Catalase
HO⁻	Hydroxyl radical	Mannitol
		PUFA (red.)
		Methionine
		Guanine, cystosine, uracil (DNA bases)
		Uric Acid
		Ascorbate
		Benzoate
		Butanol, ethanol
O⁻	Singlet Oxygen	Histidine
		Beta-carotene
		Alpha-tocopherol
		PUFA (red.)
		GSH
		Uric Acid
		Bilirubin
		Cholesterol
PUFA	Polyunsaturated Fatty Acid Radical	Beta-carotene
		Alpha-tocopherol
ROOH	Organic/Fatty acid hydroperoxides	Gluthione peroxidase
		Possible other peroxidases
PR-S-SPR	Oxidized protein	GSH, sulfhydryl amino acids

Dr. Stephen Edelson[2] has also outlined the nature of the treatment protocol recommended for those with breast implant silicone leakage symptoms, as follows:

1. Diet: organic, high alkaline, semi-vegetarian, moderately high protein
2. Exercise: moderate low impact daily
3. Intravenous nutritional therapy
   a. Detoxification
   b. Antioxidant
4. Nutritional Supplementation — Oral
5. Immunotherapy
   a. Chemicals
   b. Food
   c. Silicon
   d. Inhalants
6. Environmental and Chemical Controls
   a. Transfer Factor
   b. Dehyroepiandrosterone (DHEA)
   c. Immune Stimulants: thymus, herbals, etc.

d. Intravenous gamma globulin

SBI Laboratories Antibody Tests

As reported in an abstract by Nir Kossovsky, M.D.[5], Consultant to SBI Laboratories, "Research has shown that silicone, an adjuvant, is a tacky substance that adsorbs the body's own molecules, a process that denatures the molecules[6] and may cause them to look foreign to the body's own immune system[7]. The adsorbed molecular layer then controls the biological response[8,9,10]. The body may then engage in cytokine-mediated immune and autoimmune activity[12], which, in turn, may cause a wide range of symptoms[13,14].

"Determining whether any particular set of symptoms is the result of exposure to silicone requires, in part, a test that can detect antibodies that bind to the molecules denatured by silicone[15]. Standard rheumatologic and immunologic tests for well established immune diseases may not detect the hypothesized nontraditional immune reactions caused by silicone exposure[12,16,17]. SBI laboratories offers the Detecsils™ Silicone Sensitivity Test as a research test to detect potential nontraditional antibodies. . . .

"The body's biological responses to implanted medical devices such as silicone breast implants are directed principally by the concentrated and denatured proteins bound to the implant's surface. There are five potential clinical materials and their post-surgical surface film of adsorbed proteins[5]," as follows:

1. Clinically Imperceptible

"As implied, imperceptible symptoms are below the threshold of detection. However, while the inflammatory process may not be noticeable, the consequences of chronic inflmmation may produce secondary signs and symptoms. For example, as a consequence of a local inflammatory process, the patient may perceive progressive hardening of an implant. Associated with the formation of an implant/scar mass could be such symptoms as back pain, shoulder pain, and tightness of the chest[5]."

2. Local Inflammation

"Local symptoms would mimic those above, but would be more noticeable and may be associated with a greater degree of pain as well as tenderness, swelling, and heat. The skin may be slightly reddened secondary to the increased blood flow associated with inflammation."

3. Cytokine-Mediated Systemic Inflammation

"Cytokines liberated by the inflammatory cells in the tissues surrounding the implant are designed to act locally. However, when released in large quantities, cytokines may enter the circulation where they may have an effect on both the brain and the liver. In the brain, they can reset the body's thermostat, leading to fever and chills. In the liver, they can promote the release of acute-phase reactants that increase blood sugar and cause generalized muscle and joint aches and pains. These symptoms can be 'flu-like'.[5]"

4. Systemic Immunological Activation

"With antibody production, symptoms may be identical to level 3, and although symptoms such as those in level 2 are also possible, our preliminary data suggest that local chest symptoms are less likely when there is antibody positivity shown by the Detecsil test. The biggest differences between level 3 cytokine activity and level 4 antibody activity are: first, permanent tissue damage induced when antibodies are being produced is more likely; and second, the symptoms are less likely to respond to medical therapy alone. Surgical intervention may be necessary, and even then, if silicone is still present in the body, chronic medical therapy may be required for clinical relief of the symptoms. Common symptoms associated with the anti-SSAA [anti-Silicone-Surface-Associated Antigens] study published in *The Journal of Applied Biomaterial*, December 1993, were analyzed recently. In that study, fever, sleep disturbances, and foot pain were found to be independently statistically significant symptoms (p<.05). Fever coupled with the absence of local chest pain was a statistically significant syndrome (p<.001)[5]."

5. Immunological Activation With an Autoimmune Component

"If the antibodies elicited have an autoimmune feature, the symptoms may be the same as in levels 3 and 4, but they may also include a wide range of neuromuscular and hematologic problems in organs that are distinctly separate from the breast or any region where gross amounts of silicone may have deposited. We do not have enough information to be more specific at this time[5]."

Future Research

Charles H. Farr[3], M.D., Ph.D. and other allied physicians have found that hydrogen peroxide infusions (IVs) will ease the pain, at least temporarily, of silicone symptoms. (See "Hydrogen Peroxide Therapy," http://www.arthritistrust.org also at Kindle.)

Gus Prosch, Jr.[4], M.D., through use of ELF laboratory's Light Beam Generator[1], discovered that swollen lymph glands will reduce. Whether or not a return of swollen lymph glands means that the body, under influence of the Light Beam Generator, simply recycles the tetramer and its products, or whether there is a net loss of silicone and its products has not yet been determined. (See "Lymphatic Detoxification" and "Lymph Drainage Therapy," http://www.arthritistrust.org, bookstores and also at Amazon.com's Kindle.)

An overall body detoxification process developed by Lee Cowden, M.D. of Dallas, TX has brought about complete recovery from at least one lady who suffered from a combination of breast cancer and silicone tetramer leakage, as interviewed by this writer.

References

1. Anthony di Fabio, Thomas Gervais, Courtland Reeves, *Lymphatic Detoxification*, 1994, http://www.arthritistrust.org.

2. Stephen B. Edelson, M.D., personal correspondence, lectures and

publications, Environmental and Preventive Health Center of Atlanta, 3833 Roswell Road, Suite 110, Atlanta, GA 30342-4432, received 1994.

3. Charles H. Farr, M.D., Ph.D., personal correspondence, 10101 S. Western Ave., Oklahoma City, OK 73139-2929, received 1994.

4. Gus J. Prosch, Jr., M.D. personal communication, 1994.

5. Nir Kossovsky, M.D., "A Capsule Summary of the Biological Response Triggered by Silicone Implants," SBI Laboratories, 1401 Forbes Avenue, Suite 237, Pittsburgh, PA 15219, received Janaury 1995.

The following references came from the abstract prepared by Nir Kossovsky, M.D., reference 5 above.

6. Cheng SS et al. J Colloid Interfac Sci, 1994; 1662:135-143.

7. Kossovsky N and Freiman CJ. Arch Path Lab Med, 1994; 118:686-693.

8. Kossovsky N et al. J Biomed Mater Res, 1987; 21:1125-1133.

9. Tang L and Eaton JW. J Exp Med, 1993: 178:2147-2156.

10. Bonfield TL and Anderson JM. J Biomed Mater Res, 1993; 27:1195-1199.

11. Naim JO and Lanzafame RJ. Invest Immunol, 1993; 22:151-161.

12. Kossovsky N and Stassi J. Sem Arthritis Rheum, 1994; 24 (Suppl 1):18-21.

13. Bridges AJ et al. Ann Intern Med, 1993; 118:929-936.

14. Wilhelm K. Autoimmunity, 1993; 14:341-342.

15. Bernstein RA. J Roy Coll Phys (London), 1990; 24:18-25.

16. Kossovsky N and Papasian N. J Appl Biomat, 1992; 3:239-242.

17. Kossovsky N et al. J Appl Biomat, 1993; 4:281-288.

Treating Arthritic Pain with Ginger
by
Wayne Martin, B.A.
Reprinted with permission from
Townsend Letter for Doctors & Patients,
911 Tyler St, Pt. Townsend, Wa 98368-6541, November 2000

On March 14 our local newspaper had a report on treating arthritis. I think that it may have been an Associated Press report, quoting a professor of rheumatology at a University in Michigan. It put down things such as evening primrose oil and the thrust of it was that if one had rheumatoid arthritis, one is just somewhat out of luck. I sent the following letter to the local newspaper. It was not published, I rather expect that it was shown to a local rheumatologist who said it was the bunk. If you may be so kind as to give this letter the light of day and in the process, bring a degree of pain relief to some patients with arthritis.

"I am age 88 and have been an amputee since 1929 when I lost my left leg in a motorcycle accident. From that day onward, I have been plagued with episodes of painful spasms at the severed nerve endings. These episodes are excruciatingly painful. The way out was to take about 25 aspirin in a short period of time. I would get sick from too much aspirin. When that happened, it was a good sign. The spasms were about to end. I feel fortunate that I did not kill myself with an overdose of aspirin.

"I have been almost completely free from these painful episodes now for over ten years. I read a report in the British medical journal *Medical Hypotheses,* [1989, vol. 29, pp 25 29]. Two doctors from India were at the hospital of Odense University in Denmark. The article was by R.C. Srivastava and T. Mustafa and the title of the article was "Ginger (*Zingiber officinale*) in Treating Rheumatic Disorders." Ginger is an important medication in the very old Ayurvedic and Tibb system of medicine in India dating from prehistory. They were telling how ginger is effective in treating both osteoarthritis and rheumatoid arthritis but especially, rheumatoid arthritis. They gave a few cases of success in so doing. Its effectiveness in treating these two types of arthritis was said to be due to its anti-inflammatory effect.

"I assumed that the nerve ending spasms I was having were caused by an inflammatory reaction. I began taking a heaping teaspoon per day of ground ginger bought in a food market. I mixed it in a glass of milk and in almost no time it abolished this problem that had plagued me for over 60 years. This problem has remained abolished now for over 10 years and I take my ginger almost every day.

"It is not all that easy to understand but I will try to explain the antiinflammatory action of ginger. We get a fatty acid in meat called arachidonic acid. Adult humans can make a little of it but not much. It plays a major role in arthritic pain that is caused by inflammatory action. It is acted on by two enzymes, the first one is cyclooxygenase. It converts arachidonic acid into several of what are called 2 series prostaglandins. One is a pain prostaglandin, another is involved in an inflammatory reaction. Aspirin inhibits cyclooxygenase and hence pain. Insofar as the cyclooxygenase produce prostagladins, it is both anti-inflammatory and anti pain.

"The other enzyme acting on arachidonic acid is lipoxygenase and it converts arachidonic acid to the super inflammatory 4 series leukotrienes. Aspirin will not inhibit lipoxygenase. As it tends to prevent arachidonic acid from flowing into the cyclooxygenase produced prostaglandins, more of it will tend to flow into the highly inflammatory leukotrienes. As a result aspirin is often proinflammatory and with some asthma patients, it will cause an asthma attack.

"Ginger is said to inhibit both cyclooxygenase and lipoxygenase so it may be truly anti inflammatory. The name of the game in any antiinflammatory treatment is to inhibit lipoxygenase.

"The cost of a teaspoon a day of ginger is next to nothing, and unlike aspirin it seems to have no harmful side effects. Here it is suggested that patients suffering from either osteoarthritis or rheumatoid arthritis may care to try ginger. Rheumatoid arthritis is caused by our immune cells attacking our joints, however in so doing, they cause the pain and joint destruction by an inflammatory action. It could be that patients suffering from rheumatoid arthritis may be in for a pleasant surprise if they would try ginger

"In your article an arthritic patient was quoted as saying that evening primrose oil was of no benefit. Gamma linolenic acid in evening primrose oil acts to prevent arachidonic acid from being acted on by both cyclooxygenase and lipoxygenase and as such should be antiinflammatory. It also inhibits lipooxygenase. It is likely that to have any benefit in treating arthritic pain, one would have to take about five capsules a day.

"Vegetarians get almost no arachidonic in diet. I have never heard any suggestion that vegetarians suffer less arthritic pain but if looked into, there might be something to this line of thought.

"It is my thought that ginger added to milk improves the flavor of milk. I hope that some patients suffering from arthritic pain may read this letter, try ginger and report back to me."

In a letter to this foundation dated November 3, 2000, Wayne Martin adds:

"Here is something of interest. Beginning in 1972 there have been five big expensive trials on aspirin in treating Coronary Heart Disease. The first four showed no benefit in the reduction of death from Coronary Heart Disease. It was only the last one here in the USA — The "Physician's Health Study" that showed benefit — and not all that much even so. In this last trial Bufferin™ was used and it contains aspirin and some magnesium.

"There was a letter in the *New England Journal of Medicine* about ten years ago with comment on the failure of the aspirin trials. It was said that aspirin reduces thromboxane A[2] which is good but that it also reduces prostacyclin.

"Ginger like aspirin inhibits cyclooxygenase which reduces thromboxane which is good, however ginger unlike aspirin induces rather than inhibits prostacyclin. Ginger may be far more effective in the prevention of Coronary Heart Disease than aspirin.

"The reference to this is *Medical Hypothesis* 1986 Volume 20, pp 271-278, Bockon.

Wayne Martin, born June 17, 1911 died May 13, 2006.

He was a great searcher for medical truths, and he is missed by many!

During the past twenty four years we've been fortunate to have Wayne Martin as one of our most esteemed advisors. Wayne was not just a knowledgeable advisor, but also a fine friend, one who unstiningly gave of his medical knowledge to whomever inquired.

Wayne Martin graduated from Purdue University with a BS in Chemical Engineering in 1933 with major emphasis on biochemistry and bacteriology. Depression years prevented him from obtaining a medical degree, his first love, but did not stop him from a lifetime of interesting synthesis of the world's medical literature, often resulting in discoveries of successful treatments used today by many complementary/alternative medical practitioners.

His professional work in Chemical Engineering also resulted in remarkable findings results of which are still used by people everywhere. Ninety percent of the beryllium copper alloys used worldwide contain 1.80% of beryllium instead of the more expensive form of 2.2 to 2.5% beryllium set by Germans at the Siemans and Haliske Company. Working at the Beryllium Corporation, Wayne Martin in 1935 discovered that the 1.80% beryllium to copper alloy (Berylco 180) was superior in many ways and less expensive. For more than fifty years automobiles — and you — have used Wayne Martin's beryllium alloy.

Early in World War II, at the Sperry Gyroscope Company, and also as a "dollar-a-year" consultant with The War Production Board (WPB), Wayne Martin developed two National Emergency (N.E.) aluminum casting alloys (319, 380). Ninety-five percent of today's aluminum castings are made of these two alloys. Sixty million pounds monthly of this aluminum alloy is currently used to produce the modern automobile.

At end of World War II, the Beryllium Corporation was stuck with a plant owned by the Atomic Energy Commission for which they wanted a peace-time use. Wayne suggested that it be used to make potassium titanium fluoride. The entire aluminum industry uses it to grain-refine aluminum. After it's return to the Atomic Energy Commission, Henry Kawecki, Wayne's friend, formed the Kawecki Chemical Company to manufacture potassium fluoride, becoming a multimillion dollar firm, all on Wayne's ideas.

In 1950 Wayne Martin helped to place aluminum/magnesium alloy (AL MG 35) for which there was a large market. In 1960 he developed another aluminum alloy (Precedent 71) which, over a period of 20 years, made his employer, U.S. Reduction Company, a great deal of money. (Think of airplanes, among other uses.)

Wayne retired in 1979, becoming a salesman with The Southern Aluminum Casting Company of Bay Minette, Alabama. Thereafter each retirement has led to further consulting jobs, so he never truly retired.

So why was a Chemical Engineer who invented important metal alloys featured as a consultant in medicine?

Although the great American depression had steered him elsewhere for survival's sake, he never lost touch with medicine. His enquiring mind synthesized many medical articles and research papers to bring to light remarkable treatments in heart, cancer, and other medical problems.

In one example from years' gone by, in 1963 Wayne organized the Nutrition Research Products Company dedicated to doing something about the 600,000 deaths each year from heart attacks. His idea was carried to The Royal College of Surgeons and The National Heart Hospital in London, England, where Nutrition Research Products Company spent $200,000, and proved that his ideas were effective in preventing heart disease.

Wayne periodically gave himself weak hydrochloric acid shots because he'd learned — long before the advent of antibiotics — that administration of these weakened solutions stimulated macrophage and leucocyte activity, thus killing and/or warding off invasive infections. (See *Three Years of Hydrochloric Acid Therapy*, http://www.arthritistrust.org, "Books and Pamphlets" tab.) His story about the Harvard medical school graduate who became wealthy by specializing in this treatment in Las Vegas, NV was very educational as well as hilarious.

Wayne had a lifetime love affair with study of problems related to the heart and circulation and also with various types of cancers.

Many years before the expenditure of billions of dollars to "find the cure for cancer," Coley's toxin was bringing about remarkable "permanent remissions." This so aggravated the medical monetary and power structure that the simple mixture was forbidden. Having seen at first hand cures brought about by this mixture in his early adulthood, Wayne could never cease telling about it. Several years ago he invested a good sum of his own money to have the product made in Brazil, thus making it available to any patient who wished to use it.

Again, alas! Tthe long arm of "forbidden medicine" reached into Brazil, and the US supply was again halted.

Nonetheless, Wayne found another way to help cancer patients by publishing the formula for Coley's toxin so that any patient or doctor can make up their own supply, if desired. (Coley's Toxin formula is now found at our website at http://arthritistrust.org, "Research and Letters" tab, under Wayne Martin's name; also see the earlier article on how to make Coley's toxin in this book.)

But even prior to his publication of Coley's toxin, certain doctor friends began manufacturing their own Coley's toxin and are having great success in bringing about "permanent remissions," among some of their patients!

Wayne Martin's thinking about medical treatment has been frequently reported in *Townsend Letter for Doctors* (911 Tyler St., Port Townsend, WA 98368-6541; http://www.towsendletter.com). It is there one should go for the articles.

Martin's recommendations for the safe easing of pain through the use of ginger can also be found in our Arthritis Trust of America Summer 2001 Newsletter at http://www.arthritistrust.org, "Newsletters" tab.

Martin was a remarkable human being, one who cared greatly for his fellow man, who gave without concern for rewards, who loved life, and who made each hour, each minute count toward bettering his fellow man.

We are so glad that he passed away peacefully — not in pain or suffering from degenerative disease — just a few months before his 95th birthday! But, we are not at all happy that he passed so early in his life — and we shall sorely miss this intelligent, generous, kind scientific advisor!

Exclusive Interview

Landmark Work on Niacinimide and Arthritis

of William Kaufman, Ph.D., M.D.

by Jonathan Wright, M.D. *Nutrition & Healing,* August 1997, p.5-6

See: http://www.wrightnewsletter.com/nah/nahindexie.shtml

Welcome Dr. Kaufman. During my years at the University of Michigan Medical School, 1965 1969, we heard scarcely a word about nutrition, vitamins, and disease treat-ment. And even though you were a 1938 graduate of that same Medical school, we heard nothing about your landmark work on niacinamide and arthritis. Any speculations about that?

In my medical school years, we were drilled in great detail about vitamin-deficiency disorders during our lectures in internal medicine, pediatrics, public health, neurology, psychiatry, and pathology. But after synthetic vitamins became available to treat florid deficiency diseases, not teaching about nutrition and vitamins became a national trend.

I'm not surprised they didn't refer to my books. The reviews of my 1943 book were dismissive, because the "experts" couldn't believe that the larger amounts of niacinamide I used in therapy improved joint mobility, muscle strength, maximal muscle-working capacity, and mental func-tioning.

Your two books concerning niacinamide treatment contain absolutely amazing detail about clinical signs and symptoms of the syndrome you called "aniacinamidosis." How did you gather all of this information?

Throughout my twenty-five years of private clinical practice, I always took two to three hours minimum with each new patient, and at least an hour and sometimes two hours on subsequent visits, according to the needs of the patient. Remember, I was always extremely interested in psychosomatic medicine, too, and taking this time was extremely help-ful in getting basic information that could ease psychosomatic difficulty as well as physical problems.

Not Many doctors spend that amount of time with each patient, especially with today's so-called managed care, HMOs, and all that. You've mentioned your direct observations of patients taking niacinimide. . . .

Yes, as I said, any patient I gave niacinamide had to sit in my office for at least an hour, so I could observe what happened. My first observations were made in the days before bread and other white-flour products were "enriched"...

A misnomer of the first order. . . .

... "enriched" with niacin, which eventually turned into niacinamide, but the "enrichment" used only a few B-vitamins, and not B[6] or folic acid or chromium or many of the other things milled out of flour. So I really got a chance to observe the difference that niacinamide could make, starting from a position of real deficiency or semi-deficiency.

Tell us about that.

There are many more details in my 1943 book, but let's cover a few. Within 2-1/2 to five minutes after taking the first 100 milligrams of niacinamide there was a degree of physical and mental relaxation which became marked in the next twenty minutes. The first objective change, apparent within the first five minutes, is the relaxation of previously tense muscles, and the replacement of a drawn facial expression by a more calm one, or even a smile. Without suggestion, patients began to sit, walk, and stand more erectly. Within the first five to ten minutes, the color of the hands and feet might change from a sallow yellow to a healthy pinkish or ruddy color, and the hands and feet frequently are subjectively and objectively warmer. There are many more changes detailed in that book.

What got you started studying niacinamide?

Actually I started with niacin. I had read an article in the *AMA Journal* which said that niacin was safe, so I took some and got very sick. After that I decided to concentrate on niacinamide, and looked around without success for a local supply. I couldn't find any at first, but ultimately I was shipped two boxes containing 100,000 tablets of niacinamide, 50 milligrams each, so I had plenty of material.

Your second book, published In 1949, contains carefully made clnical observations of 455 people treated with niacinamide over sev-eral years each, especially focusing on their joint disease.

I had noticed early on that joints were one of the most fre-quently improved areas among patients with aniacinamidosis. When compulsory "enrichment" of flour occurred in 1943, many of the more obvious symptoms of aniacinamidosis disappeared from the general population, but the same joint problems persisted. So in 1944, looking for objective data, I started precise measurement of the ranges of joint motion of every patient who had obvious arthritis, at the time of their first examina-tion.

You designed your own instrument. . . .

They're completely described in my 1949 book. In 1945, I designed an abbreviated but objec-tive measurement of twenty joints or joint groups that could be ob-served and recorded in five min-utes on a special form. I performed this measurement on all new pa-tients instead of just those with obvious arthritis, and it quickly became apparent that limitation of joint movement was exceedingly apparent in many individuals without joint complaints or clini-cally obvious arthritis. From there, I went on to design a "Joint Range Index" from a weighted numerical average of these twenty measure-ments.

Your 1949 book reports the very significant improvement in the Joint Range Index that could be achieved both in individuals with osteoarthritis and in those with rheumatoid arthritis. . . .

As well as the regression that occurs when individuals stop their niacinamide therapy. As long as niacinamide is continued, the improvement "holds," but it can't be stopped without ultimate re-gression.

Of course, joint mobility wasn't the only improvement, just the one we could precisely mea-sure. Nearly everyone got at least some pain relief and reduction of swelling. It takes one to three months for maximum effect, but nearly everyone needed less pain medication, and a significant num-ber needed none.

I've followed your lead in niacinamide therapy for 21 years, and have observed it to work just as you've said. Some joints respond better than others. . . .

Yes, although they all respond to a degree. The best are knees, shoulders, and the neck . . . and then wrists and fingers.

How does niacinamide work in helping joints?

Niacinamide has the special capacity of "wringing out" excess fluid from cartilage and connective tissue. Niacinamide is also anti-inflammatory, as demonstrated by reductions in the sedimentation index for patients with rheuma-toid arthritis.

What dosages of niacinamide do you recommend?

After I completed the study reported in the 1949 book, I found that larger amounts were actually more helpful. But timing is just as important: 250 milligrams of niaci-namide taken every three hours for six doses is about twice as effective as 500 milligrams taken three times daily. You actually did us a service, Dr. Wright, when you persuaded Winner Chemists in New York City to Manufacture an effective time-release niacinamide.

There is so much to learn in your books, and we're almost out of space . . . you write about "delayed post-traumatic articular syndrome," and its treatment with niacinamide. The depth and breadth of detail about clinical uses of niacinamide you provide is remarkable! But you also were a practitioner of "whole patient" medicine decades before it became popular — you write about psychogenic and allergic causes of joint problems and many other symptoms. Are your books still available?

[Dr. William Kaufman replies, but, unfortunately, his books are now collector's items: Ed]

You may have none left once this is published! thank you, Dr. Kaufman, for sharing with the reader of Nutrition & & Healing a very small portion of your knowledge of the clinical uses of niacinamide.

William Kaufman earned his BA. from the University of Pennsylvania in 1931, his Ph.D. in physiology and his M.D. from the University of Michigan graduate and medical schools in 1937 and 1938. Following internship and residency, he served as Clinical Assistant in Medicine at the Yale University School of Medicine.

From 1952 through 1969, Dr. Kaufman was variously Contributing Editor and American Editor-in-Chief of the *International Archives of Allergy and Applied Immunology*. He was in the private practice of internal medicine from 1940 to 1965 in Bridgeport, Connecticut, where he conducted and published the research on niacinamide and arthritis discussed in this interview.

Dr. Kaufman was a Fellow of the American College of Physicians, the American Association for the Ad-vancement of Science, the American College of Nutrition, the Geron-tological Society of America, the Royal Society of Medicine, and an Emeritus Fellow of the American College of Allergy and Immunology. He was co-founder, in 1950, of the Academy of Psychosomatic Med-icine.

Dr. Kaufman is the author or co-author of more than 60 profes-sional papers, and of the books *The Common Form of Niacin Amide Deficiency Disease, Aniacinamido-sis*, Bridgeport, Connecticut, 1943, printed by The Printing Office of Yale University Press, and *The Common Form of Joint Dysfunc-tion: Its Incidence and Treatment*, E.L. Hildreth and Company, Brat-tleboro, Vermont, 1949. He is also a playwright, artist, and poet.

Dr. Kaufman's complete bibliography is posted at http://www.doctoryourself.com/biblio_kaufman.html

Hubbardian Detoxification
by
Zane Gard and Anthony di Fabio

The Scandinavians generations ago pioneered the use of sweat saunas to induce a bright outlook on life and health.

L. Ron Hubbard, founder of the Church of Scientology and Dianetics incorporated a variation of the sauna for the purpose of ridding us of exo-toxins that are stored in the fatty parts of our cells and/or the metabolites of the exo-toxins that are stored there. Most medical doctors agree that there are few medical procedures that can eliminate these exo-toxins from the cell's fatty parts. The exo-toxins do, therefore, can cause serious medical conditions.

This article makes no claim that Hubbard's wild-eyed assertions to super human abilities is correct. In fact, experience by many from the 1950s forward demonstrate exactly the opposite is true. Expending tens of thousands of dollars to use the processes of Scientology or Dianetics has not resulted in the fantastic claims that Hubbard wrote about.

However, there is one area that Hubbard got right, and that's the use of the Sauna which he called The Purification Rundown available at every Church of Scientology outlet and also through a tiny handful of medical doctors.

Since the benefits from the sauna have been known by whole societies for hundreds of years, it's difficult to credit Hubbard with the finding that these exo-toxins can be eliminated in part or in whole through The Purification Rundown. So, we won't get into the question of who discovered these benefits from the sauna' use.

We do know from both medical case histories as well as from personal experience that saunas can have huge health benefits.

Zane Gard, M.D. ws one of our former referral physicians practicing in San Diego, CA. As he told the story, he, his wife and daughter had been exposed to agent Orange. Accordng to Wikipedia, Agent Orange— or Herbicide Orange (HO)—is one of the herbicides and defoliants used by the U.S. military as part of its herbicidal warfare program, Operation Ranch Hand, during the Vietnam War from 1961 to 1971 It was a mixture of equal parts of two herbicides, 2,4,5-T and 2,4-D.

In 1969 it was revealed to the public that the 2,4,5-T was contaminated with a dioxin, 2,3,7,8-tetrachlorodibenzodioxin (TCDD), and that the TCDD was causing many of the previously unexplained adverse health effects which were correlated with Agent Orange exposure.

Dr. Gard practiced medicine in Sturgeon, MO. The people of Sturgeon, MO, were exposed to toxic levels of dioxin when a train carrying two tankers full of Monsanto's pesticide orthochlorophenol derailed near the town's elementary school and high school December 27, 1979. Dioxin is an extremely toxic byproduct of phosphate fertilizer production. The

327

amount of dioxin contained in the spilled pesticides was only three to four ounces.

Unaware that the town had experienced the chemical catastrophe, Zane Gard, MD, and his family had moved to the small, friendly town of Sturgeon in May, 1980, to open a medical practice.

According to Dr. Gard's observations as he began to treat patients who were suffering from illnesses resulting from exposure to dioxin, "All small ground life died within 2-3 miles of the spill. Cattle on a farm 7-8 miles downstream died. The farmer who owned the cattle died within the first 6 months, another within a year and a half. A young Amish boy died of tri-lateral retinoblastoma (of which there have only been 9 cases reported anywhere in the world) and a young Amish man died of malignant lymphoma that same year. There was 10-15 times increase in flu-like symptoms, allergies and kidney infections (many were in young boys). The urinary infections always followed a rain. There was an increased number of cases of infectious mono diagnosed."

Dr. Gard and many other townspeople contacted the local public health department with questions about the dangers associated with the dioxin spill. According to Dr. Gard, "...the health department and the Monsanto Chemical Co. assured the townspeople that there was no danger to their health."

The Gards, all of them sick with a variety of illnesses consistent with other Sturgeon residents, left the town 18 months after the spill and returned to California where they could combine their efforts with other researchers to investigate the effects of toxic exposure to people. Dr. Gard and his wife, a PHN, hoped that their studies would allow them to develop treatments for toxic exposure.

To this day, the residents of Sturgeon suffer unprecedented numbers of cancers, tumors, and other serious illnesses and psychological disorders that are well above the national average. Many people have died. (see http://www.proliberty.com/observer/19990708.htm)

The dioxin molecule contaminate turned out to be one of the most insidious and deadly moleculres to enter into the human body.

Through the use of Hubbard's Purification Rundown, Gard and his family were able to become free of most of the effects of dioxin. Mightily impressed with this medical procedure, Dr. Gard begin offering his patients a sauna program similar to Hubbard's but added to the program the laboratory measurement of various toxins throughout the sauna time period. It soon became quite evident that as the otherwise incurable diseases reduced so did the laboratory profiles of the measured toxins.

Gard excitedly wrote up his case histories, including charts and graphs showing remarkable changes accompanying cures. He traveled about the US passing along the medical information that was so important to many patients. The Medical Association pounced upon Gard in full fury and cancelled his license to practice medicine. It isn't nice to cure people without using the cookbook rules established by the medical profession and the FDA — and this is particularly true when it is a large corporation, like Monsanto that is creating the disease and death! (Also see http://www.arthritistrust.org. Go to Research and then Research and Letters tab and find Zane Gard on the left hand side alphabetically.)

The last we'd heard of Dr. Gard was his move to Mexico where there seems to be more freedom to heal people.

February 11, 1986

Perry Chapdelaine
Executive Director

Dear Mr. Chapdelaine:

Thank you for your invitation to present the "Bio-Toxic Reduction Program" to your Foundation on July 16-19, 1986 in Santa Monica, California. As I mentioned, Giovanna DeSanti-Medina will also attend to help answer questions from the perspective of an individual who has successfully completed the program. She is case history # 2 on the information enclosed on the program and progress of those who have completed the program.

I am currently working on approximately 50 more case studies. It is expected that these will be completed shortly. We have had over 100 patients complete this program to date and have found an average improvement of 70-75% in these patients, which is remarkable when you consider the fact that most were severely disabled and failed other therapies. Many were considered untreatable. We have had program participants who range between the ages of 5 and 80. Thirty four patients have had peripheral neuropathy and all have improved. Those with arthritis have shown significant improvement after completing this program of detoxification (See case # 1 and # 22).

I hope you will find the enclosed material both interesting and informative. I look forward to presenting this information in July. If you have further questions, please feel free to contact me at (619) 583-5865.

Sincerely,
ZANE R. GARD, M.D.
Consultant/ Human Environmental Medicine, Inc. ZRG:gm
Encl.

Your diet, your job, your neighborhood or your hobby may be killing you. Chances are your mind will be the first to go. Ninety percent of the 150 million metric tons of toxic waste generated every year by American industry will be improperly disposed. It will end up in our beaches, in our drinking water, our playgrounds or abandoned in open fields, and eventually in our bodies. We're sitting on a time bomb that could explode in the next generation... or at the end of our own lives with birth defects, cancers, mental illness, and early senility.

A MEDICAL PROFILE :
Brain and Body Pollution
by
Zane R. Gard, M.D., E. Jean Brown, PHN, BSN,
Giovanna DeSanti-Medina
Copyright 1983 Zane R. Gard MD

"Toxic Bio-Accumulation and Effective Detoxification"

Today man no longer suffers the devastation of polio, cholera, smallpox, T.B., and typhoid epidemics. However, more insidiously he does suffer from high blood pressure, stroke, heart problems, cancers, allergy, obesity, and a barrage of mental illnesses that now reach epidemic proportions...trends which reflect the diseases of "industrialism." The past 150 years have been a time of incredible progress for medicine, science and industry. Because of these advancements we now enjoy longer, more productive lives. However, there are many who will inevitably pay a high price for our modern lifestyle. The "unnatural" by-products of our chemical technology have resulted in contamination of our "natural" resources. Though toxic substances have been in existence for centuries, today we are exposed to chemical concentrations far greater than were our ancestors. There is no single contributing factor which has impaired man's adaptability to the environment than that of our current widespread use and misuse of harmful chemical substances. EPA director, William Ruckelshaus, recently stated chemical pollution as the number one environmental problem.

Since 1965, over 4 million distinct chemical compounds have been reported in scientific literature. Each week over 6,000 new chemicals were added to the list between 1965 and 1978. As of 1981, of over 70,000 chemicals in commercial production, 3,000 have been identified as intentionally added to food supplies and over 700 in drinking water. During food processing and storage 10,000 other compounds can become an integral part of many commonly used foods. Directly or indirectly this toxic residue invariably works its way into our air, food, and water supplies...and ultimately into the human body. Add to the list of potential body toxins, radiation (x-rays, nuclear fall-out, computer terminals, powerlines, etc.), petrochemicals, industrial waste, medical and street drugs, tons of pesticides, herbicides, and insecticides, and the result is an incredible chemical avalanche to have befallen the human race in a relatively short time of evolutionary history.

It should not then be surprising that individuals who become environmentally susceptible or "maladapted" to one or more common chemical excitants are usually not the same thereafter. Current clinical, scientific, and governmental studies indicate a staggering increase in the incidence of environmentally-induced illnesses. Two major factors responsible for this outbreak are: discrepancies in established "safety" standards for "allowable" contamination due to inadequate toxicity data; and, the approved use of many toxic substances in this country which have been banned in other countries as known threats to public health. While many of these chemicals have unequivocally saved lives, property, and entire industries, most are not aware that millions of people have been and continue to be poisoned and countless others killed as a result of insidious chemical exposure. The toll on human suffering is incalculable at present as current statistical data does not accurately reflect non-occupational exposures, nor cumulative, interactive, or long-term chemical effects. However, it is estimated that at least 20 million Americans in the workplace alone are exposed to toxins capable of producing damage to the central nervous system even from minute concentrations. In the long run, everyone pays a price for unhealthy workers.

Noted researchist and clinical immunologist, Alan S. Levin, M.D., recently stated that, "The vast increase of chemicals in our environment, foods, end medicines, has greatly altered the body's ability to rid itself of toxins...these factors have changed the character of illness and disease so that the average physician can no longer rely on past case histories or text books but must depend on the immediate observation of the patient . The average citizen of the 1980's is biochemically and genetically different from the average citizen of the 1950's...so different, in fact, that ordinary texts and training are geared to treat people who no longer exist." Accordingly medicine has had to accommodate the "changing" patient. A convergence of toxicology, allergy/immunology, nutrition, and behavioral science, the field of Environmental Medicine has emerged. In an attempt to better understand man's complex interaction with his volatile environment, this interdisciplinary field focuses on the study of both endogenous and exogenous environmental factors as they relate to the physiological and psychological disease process.

When the body's homeostasis or "internal balance" is disrupted by toxic levels which exceed individual tolerance thresholds, an illness results in one form or another. Whether due to an acquired or genetic susceptibility (immune deficiencies, nutritional imbalances), direct environmental hazards (residential, occupational, recreational), other "passive" daily exposures (dietary, home, office, classroom), or a combination of these factors, the outcome of repeated chemical exposures is often a pathological state of "chemical hypersensitivity." Free radical damage which results in this "spreading phenomena" causes the patient to become hypersensitive not only to the chemical exposed to, but other chemicals, and in many cases leads to food sensitivities and other allergies. For those experiencing the degenerative process of chemical sensitization, daily life becomes a continual challenge as potentially offensive substances are omnipresent in both indoor and outdoor environments.

Some of the synthetic and natural toxicants capable of producing symptomatology in hypersensitive patients include industrial/ agricultural/ household chemicals, natural food toxins, drugs, and various inhalants (mold, dust, bacteria). Many incitants, present in liquid, vaporous, or solid form, appear as volatile or "harmless" while continuing to "out-gas" for an indefinite period of time. Chlorinated pesticides, many of which were developed in the 1940's, have been stated as the primary cause of environmental disease today. These include DDT, DDE, Dieldrin, Lindens, Heptachlor and Chlordane. Numerous common agents used in fumigants, solvents, lubricants, deodorants, and disinfectants can also have a significant impact over time. Chronic exposure to petrochemical derivatives such as formaldehyde end phenol found in anything from building materials, plastics, cosmetics, perfume, paint, hairspray, toothpaste, and adhesives to natural gas, can have ill effects on both hypersensitive persons and otherwise healthy populations.

Symptoms of chemical exposure and subsequent state of hypersensitivity may be obscure, particularly when polysystemic or delayed responses are involved, and therefore may be difficult to diagnose. The elusive maladaptive responses or "reactions" to this "chemical overload" range anywhere from fatigue, headaches, mental confusion, depression, and personality changes to hyperactivity, joint pain, breathing difficulty, and multiple allergies. Symptoms will depend largely upon which target organ, tissue, system is primarily affected in any given person. Routes of contact (i.e., the skin pores, respiratory system, or intestinal tract) will also have a significant bearing on the effects of an exposure. Initial symptoms may appear in the form of occasional nervousness, appetite changes, altered sleeping patterns, chronic yeast infections, or a number of apparent insignificant, unrelated symptoms at the onset of the condition. However, often these "subliminal" symptoms are merely early signs of impaired immune function or other biochemical changes, which ultimately may lead to chronic or degenerative disease states later on in life. Research has clearly demonstrated a high propensity for developing a physiological "addiction" to environmental chemicals, in which case symptoms may be either an exposure itself or a "withdrawal" response once the source is removed from regular contact. An illustration of "toxic bio-accumulation" may provide a means of understanding this disease process. Such compounds as DDT, PCP, PCB, THC, TCE, as well as other common pollutants and drug residues, have been shown to accumulate and remain in the body over long periods of time. Eventually the metabolizing of such compounds which are foreign to the biological system, leads to the accumulation of these oil soluble chemicals and their products into lipid (fatty) deposits throughout the body. Since almost every cell and virtually-every organ contain a "fat" component (even the brain), chemicals which are stored in the body pose a serious threat to both physiological and psychological health. Because these stored toxins can be released into the bloodstream during times of physical or emotional stress, any organ which is accessible to this residue is continually being exposed at low levels. The effect is much like a chronic exposure. This is why exposure to even minute amounts of toxic chemicals can be dangerous.

When the immune system over-reacts, conditions such as lupus may result; when it is suppressed, eventual cancers can develop. Studies in oncology show a marked association between PCB and DDE levels found in the body fat and an increase in the development of cancer. EPA studies suggest that virtually all U.S. citizens are carrying one or more toxic chemicals. It is becoming more apparent that almost all cancers are caused by adverse environmental factors. Environmentally persistent chemicals (such as pesticides) are designed to last over long periods of time, some having half-lives of twenty or more years. Many compounds which do not easily metabolize or breakdown within a short period of time are stored rather than readily eliminated from the body. This is one of the reasons cancers usually develop 20-30 years following a toxic exposure. This also accounts for the difficulty of determining long-term health risks involving newly marketed chemicals approved for public use.

Because liver "detoxification" enzymes can bioactivate certain substances to a more active state, a non-carcinogenic agent can become an active carcinogen through this metabolic conversion process. There is also growing concern over the effects of toxic substances which have not necessarily been determined highly carcinogenic, but have been classified as "week carcinogens" or certified "safe" for human use at low levels. Consideration must also be given to the toxic interactive effects of even minute chemical concentrations which are concurrently stored within body tissues. It may take decades to evaluate the full impact of many chemical substances widely used in this country today.

It has been shown that many chemical metabolites are more toxic than the parent chemical itself. Toxins or their metabolites (xenobiotics) stored within the nervous system may result in cognitive, intellectual, and mental impairments. Many clinicians without specialized training in Environmental Medicine may be unaware of the correlation between immune dysregulation and brain function. The immune system is a complex response system which protects the body against . . . pathogenic organisms and other toxins. The direct relationship of the brain and the immunity process had been established as early as 1961 at the University of Rochester, in New York, and has been confirmed by numerous studies since then. Recent scientific studies have shown immune dysfunction to occur upon exposure to chemicals even at low concentrations or at "sub-toxic" dose. Since the brain is the organ through which mental phenomena are manifested, any changes in brain chemistry caused by toxins which cross the blood-brain barrier, can produce wide range of neurologic or psychiatric symptoms, particularly if there is inflammation of actual brain tissue.

It has long been established that many routinely used chemicals are either CNS stimulants or depressants. It would appear an undisputed fact that toxic illnesses can frequently mimic mental disorders, however today chemical exposure is frequently still overlooked as an etiologic source of an altered mental state or "mental illness" in the clinical setting. Further complicating the diagnosis, these patients frequently demonstrate completely normal routine laboratory tests. This often leads to an erroneous assumption that a psychological illness is present. A thorough search of current scientific and medical literature provides vital information dealing with the underlying causes of many psychiatric, emotional, behavioral and functional brain disorders, to include learning disabilities.

Extensive laboratory studies of environmentally ill patients often show abnormal immune parameters, enzyme dysfunction, a malabsorption syndrome, hormonal disturbances, various viral and fungal infections, as well as elevated toxic levels, each of which plays a significant role in the body's ability to cope with toxic exposures. Recent diagnostic laboratory studies developed at the University Of New Orleans, utilize a sophisticated method of gas chromatography which can detect as little as one pert per billion of many common pesticides and numerous other volatile compounds in human serum. The Chlorinated Pesticide

Screening Test used on over 3,000 patients to date has routinely showed a correlation between chronic low-dose exposure to pesticides and adverse health effects. Perhaps for the first time in medical history, it is now possible to accurately quantify the presence of environmental incitants within the body and to measure their biological effects.

Many victims of an environmental disease are slowly dying or deteriorating in health following a chemical poisoning with the absence of any immediate notable symptoms. There are others who may have "adapted" to feeling irritable, depressed, fatigued, or may have never quite lived to optimal potential and attribute vague symptoms to "stress," the "flu" or some other superficial rationale. Unfortunately in these instances, unless appropriate medical management is instituted recovery from the chronic or long-term physical and mental effects of chemical exposure is remote.

Unquestionably major strides in improving environmental health will occur only when politics, science, industry, and medicine collectively make a concerted effort to address current public health issues dealing with chemical pollution. For those whose impending health problems simply can not wait far bureaucratic complexities, there will indeed be enormous consequences. An urgent issue facing not only the medical community but the nation as a whole, is how to increase man's tolerance for unavoidable ecologic stressors, rather than to rest in the hope of immediate environmental modifications or regulations. This is particularly true concerning the patient who is presently sufferlng from adverse health effects precipitated by both past and current environmental factors involving the use, manufacturing, distribution, transportation, and storage of toxic substances.

Though undoubtedly safer, less-toxic alternatives are available as an option in many industries, given the political and economic sanctions and special interests that dictate these choices. In the years to come it is likely that our society will continue to remain dependent on numerous toxic chemical sources. With increasing incidences of improper storage, illegal dumping, and accidents involving toxic substances, more and more unknowing victims of chemical exposure will fall prey to these unresolved ecologic threats. U.S. industry generates 88 billion pounds of toxic waste every year; 90% of which EPA estimates is improperly disposed of. Significant levels of this toxic residue ends up in America's drinking water. Experts now believe that the water we drink is becoming a threat to life itself.

In addition, a five year study by the EPA on "indoor pollution" concluded that the level of toxic chemicals ingested indoors are as much as 70 times higher than outdoors, making "the home more of a toxic waste dump than any chemical plants nearby." Most people spend 85% of their day indoors routinely breathing mild to severely contaminated air, in what may appear to be the "cleanest" of environments. Today there are no known demographic or geographical boundaries immune to these potential toxic effects.

The effects of environmentally-induced health risks are no longer isolated to any one sector of the population. High risk groups are not limited to those with known immune deficiencies, the chronically ill, young children, and the elderly, as previously thought to be the case. Chemical hazards can have adverse affects on human lives at any time from conception to old age. There is a wealth of scientific data which demonstrates that everyone becomes "hypersensitive" at some point in his/her ontogeny (during a traumatic or stressful period, as a result of hormonal changes such as puberty or pregnancy, following prolonged drug use, chronic infection or illness, surgery, etc.). There is little doubt that larger populations will predictably become increasingly intolerant of today's adverse environmental conditions unless the existing body burden of stored toxins is reduced.

Until recently the prevailing opinion was that once toxic substances became stored within the body there was little, if anything, that could be done for the individual exposed. In the past, various forms of detoxification have been considered for patients suffering from a toxic illness. These include fasting, colonic irrigation, the Ultrabalance Program, chelation therapy as well as numerous other nutritional approaches. In addition, the administration of various medications such as phenobarbital and cholestyramine, have been frequently used to reduce toxic effects. However, none of these methods consistently and safely reduce significant levels of stored toxicity. Medical management of these cases must also focus attention on the hypersensitive state of the patient. This often limits the choices of well-tolerated treatment approaches which will not add chemical sources to the body.

After 30 years of research, a medically managed detoxification program was developed to lower body levels of psychoactive drugs and to reduce the restimulative effects of drugs and other toxins. Today, the medically managed "Bio-Toxic Reduction Program®" is the only detoxification technique evidenced in current nutritional, medical, and biochemical literature which releases stored impurities from body reserves with complete proven safety. With therapeutic doses of vitamins, minerals, and oils, in conjunction with exercise and dry sauna heat, stored toxic residue are mobilized from the fatty tissue. Released toxins are then eliminated from the body by perspiration in the sauna and through the intestinal tract following daily doses of oil (which the body exchanges for contaminated fat). Because the oil is not absorbed into the intestine, the contaminants exit the body via fecal elimination and bile excretion. The precisely calculated protocol ensures that the recirculating toxins are flushed out of the system and to avoid re-entry into the bloodstream. For this reason, participants must complete the entire program. Close specialized medical supervision is required at all times.

Patients often re-experience initial symptoms of chemical exposure and frequently exude strong chemical odors as they undergo detoxification. These "manifestations" minimize as the program approaches the end. The efficacy of "Bio-Toxic Reduction" can be assessed in the terms of lowered toxic levels determined by pre- and post- program chemical analyses, as well as by the participants' general improved sense of well-being following the program. The duration of this out-patient program is about 21 days for less severe cases. This is a highly individualized program and results will vary with each participant.

Though the detox process does not "cure" specific symptomatology nor any particular disease entity, numerous scientific research projects and clinical cases clearly demonstrate the possibility of many general health improvements which may be otherwise unattainable without the reduction of bodily stored chemical residue.

This process is considered a vital component of a multifaceted approach to managing chemically-induced environmental diseases. Because nearly everyone is subjected to some form of chemical exposure in today's society, naturally participants can be "re-contaminated" following detox, however by lowering the toxic load the program enhances the body's own detoxifying mechanism (which may have become impaired due to a lifetime of chemical exposures). It therefore improves the body's ability to neutralize the effects of continued toxic exposure, particularly if "maintenance" therapy is adhered to. Research studies conducted by Dr. David Schnare, Ph.D., policy analyst for the U.S. Environmental Protection Agency, concluded that the individuals evaluated had experienced up to a 97% reduction of toxic levels through this procedure, and often continued to detoxify as long as four months following the program.

The principal author of this article, Zane R. Gerd, M.D., fellow of the American Academy of Environmental Medicine and medical consultant to Human Environmental Medicine, Inc., is one of the first physicians to implement this medical procedure as the main focus of a clinical practice. The need to research effective therapies for toxic exposure resulted from a personal desire not only to restore his own family's deteriorating health status following a dioxin spill in Missouri, but to provide a viable method of managing an increasing number of environmentally ill patients within his own private practice. The program literally saved his daughter's life. As a result of the success of the "Bio-Toxic Reduction Program,®" many victims suffering from the effects of chemical exposure, can now avail themselves of this unique program of detoxification long before an environmental illness becomes incapacitating. Interestedly, the program has also optimized the health status of those who had no "apparent" health problems. It has also been shown to increase tolerance thresholds for those with extreme sensitivities and has been well-tolerated by the environmentally ill.

Numerous case histories illustrate a high success rate for individuals completing the program who were previously disabled following acute or chronic chemical exposures. These patient profiles involving either significant reduction or total elimination of "fat stored" toxins have demonstrated various health improvements. A brief description of cases having completed the detox program include Vietnam veterans and other victims recovering from the effects of exposure to Agent Orange; police officers disabled after being sprayed with PCP who resumed full employment status; a lupus patient who regained immune response and joint motion; a paraplegic gaining improved muscle strength; asthmatics with elevated stored toxic levels, now void of measurable toxins and taken off medlcations; employees affected by the "sick building syndrome" as a result of poorly ventilated buildings (particularly new offices or those routinely sprayed with pesticides); residents recovering from chronic illness due to a toxic spill or living near landfills; individuals whose responses to medication ranged from paralysis and dyspnea to violent behavior now able to live "normal" lives after reducing stored levels of pharmaceutical drugs; health was restored in a young child poisoned by sugar purchased in a supermarket which was laced with numerous deadly pesticides; and many successful cases involving recovery from illness resulting from employer's failure to supply adequate safety precautions for workers exposed to hazardous materials. The continued success of this program will help to establish the relationship between the accumulation of toxins, senility, mental illness, and criminal behavior. Further studies are being done on the incidence of birth defects ln offspring of parents heavily exposed. There is currently considerable documentation available an the benefits of the "Bio-Toxic Reduction Program" in drug/alcohol rehabilitation.

Few today question the link between carcinogens and other toxic chemical exposures to the development of cancer, birth defects, respiratory disease, and mortality. There is a need, however, to fully understand how elusive daily harmful exposures - within the home, workplace, and from dietary intake — can destroy the quality of life long before a serious illness develops. Tragic accounts of chemical poisonings that reach our nation's headlines are well publicized. But what about the silent suffering of our time . . . the anguished suicide victims who were unknowingly unable to "cope" with the environment; for the innocent children plagued by deformities or mental retardation; the tragedy of unsuspected chemical victims confined to locked mental wards or prisons; for many chronically ill who are held captive by ignorance or lack of awareness on chemical pollution...it may be too late. For those of us knowlegable of the potentially treacherous effects of chemical exposure and the available alternatives . . .we are far from "helpless." For many, the choices available today will make it possible for man to live in harmony with his ever-changing environment

While millions of federal dollars are allocated to "Superfund" clean up efforts, very little, if anything, has been done to "clean up" the toxic residue lodged within the human host itself. The reality is that needless suffering and health losses will continue to occur simply by consuming toxins in the food we eat, in the water we drink, and in the air we breath — the essential components of life itself. Without question, the legal, social, and medical implications are astounding. Critics who feel that concern over chemical use is disproportionate to any imminent danger can not fully comprehend the situation without witnessing the actual nightmare of toxicity. The threat of destruction of our nation due to chemical insults has been stated by authorities as second only to nuclear war. The broad spectrum of environmentally-induced human maladies only confirm this threat. Individual attempts to overcome these challenges may prove to be the only immediate relief in sight. Though the environment may not be improving, fortunately medical approaches dealing with the residual problems have. Reducing bio-toxic accumulation can be looked upon as powerful ammunition for a raging battle over which we may have at least some control.

National campaigns to "save-the-whales" and other endangered wildlife indeed have merit as today entire ecosystems are threatened. But considering the magnitude of the pollution problem in view of human survival, any effort to preserve the human species should not be underestimated.

REFERENCES

Ader, Robert., PSYCHONEUROIMMUNOLOGY (New York: Academic Press, 1981)

Calabrese, M.D., Edward J., POLLUTANTS AND HIGH-RISK GROUPS: The Biological Basis of Increased Human Susceptibility to Environmental and Occupational Pollutants (New York: John Wiley and Sons, 1982)

Green, M.D., Mayer., "Allergic to Everything 20th Century Syndrome". JOURNAL OF THE AMERICAN MEDICAL ASSOCIATION, Vol. 253, No. 6, Feb. 8, 1985

Hayes, W.J., PESTICIDES STUDIED IN MAN (Baltimore: Williams and Wilkins, 1978)

Imperato, M.D., Pascal J., ACCEPTABLE RISKS (New York: Viking Penguin, Inc., 1985)

Hunter, Beatric Trum., CONSUMER BEWARE (New York: Simon and Schuster, 1971)

Levine, M.D., Alan S., THE TYPE 1 /TYPE 2 ALLERGY RELIEF PROGRAM (Los Angeles: Jeremy P. Tarcher, Inc., 1983)

Levine, Ph.D., Stephen A., "Biochemical Pathology Initiated by Free Radicals, Oxidant Chemicals, and Therapeutic Drugs in the Etiology of Chemical Hypersensitivity Disease". JOURNAL OF ORTHOMOLECULAR PSYCHIATRY, Vol. 12, Third Quarter, 1983

Luster, Michael, et. al., "Immunological Hypersensitivity Resulting from Environmental or Occupational Exposure to Chemicals: A State-of-the-Art Workshop Summary". FUNDAMENTAL AND APPLIED TOXICOLOGY, 2:327-330, 1982

Matsukura, M.D., Shigeru., et. al., "Effects of Environment Tobacco Smoke on Urinary Cotinine Excretion in Nonsmokers," NEW ENGLAND JOURNAL OF MEDICINE, Vol. 311, No. 13, Sept. 1984

Regenstein, Lewis., AMERICA THE POISONED (Washington, D.C.: Acropolis Books Ltd.,1982)

Saifer, M.D., Phyllis., DETOX (Los Angeles: Jeremy P. Tarcher, Inc.,1984)

Schnare, Ph.D., David W., et. al., "Evaluation of a Detoxification Regimen for Stored Xenobiotics". MEDICAL HYPOTHESIS, Vol. 9, 1982

Schnare, Ph.D., David W., et., at., "Reduction. of Human Organohalide Body Burdens - Final Research Report". Prepared for Advancements in Science and Education, Los Angeles, Ca. July 1983

U.S. Department of Health, Education, and Welfare., National Institutes of Environmental Health Sciences, HUMAN HEALTH AND THE ENVIRONMENT (U.S. Government Printing; DHEW Pub. No. NIH 77-

1277,1976)

Vas, J. 0., "Immune Suppression as Related to Toxicology". CRITICAL REVIEW TOXICOLOGY, Vol.5, 1977

Zamm, M.D., Alfred V., WHY YOUR HOUSE MAY ENDANGER YOUR HEALTH (New York: Simon and Schuster ,1980

• Copyright 1985 Zane R. Gard M.D.

CASE HISTORIES: Bio-Toxic Reduction Program

Formerly from Human Environmental Medicine, INC.,
San Diego, California

CASE #1: A 32 year old female was diagnosed as having lupus erythematosus at age 15, in May 1971. It has been noted that the onset of her condition was while living in Denver, Colorado, which is extremely polluted. Her chief complaints consisted of pain and swelling of her joints with 30% motion of hands and fingers, constant sinusitis, frequent ear infections, headaches, fatigue, extreme chemical sensitivities, pre-menstrual syndrome, and frequent vaginal yeast infections. Her medical history revealed eleven surgeries, including a sinovectomy of the right hand, hymenectomy for control of vaginitis, appendectomy, and a spleenectomy related to lupus complications.

She was on Predisone for several years, but this was terminated following the spleenectomy. Serious ear, nose, throat problems followed the surgery. Routine administration of anti-biotics subsequent to her surgeries intensified the vaginal moniliasis.

In 1979 she suffered a lupus flare-up and was placed on Prednisone once again. After moving into a mobile home in 1980, she suffered from insomnia, back pain, myofacial syndrome, dizziness, tendonitis, itchy ears, muscle weakness and spasms, and an increase in fatigue, headaches, ear and sinus infections with some blurred vision, depression, and mood swings. She also became aware of more food and chemical intolerances.

By 1984, her over-all condition deteriorated drastically and she tried almost every anti-inflammatory drug available as well as gold shots, with no relief. She was encouraged to try an anti-cancer drug which had numerous side effects. At this point, she sought alternative modes of therapy.

In 1984, she was diagnosed as having Sjögren's syndrome, mucocutaneous Candidiasis, multiple allergies, hearing deficit, hypertension, and latent tetany. Following placement on a yeast free diet and Nystatin therapy, the patient began to experience more energy and was able to isolate offensive foods. She was also able to discontinue the Prednisone. A fat biopsy indicated elevated levels of chlorinated pesticides. She was then place on the Bio-Toxic Reduction Program. She experienced joint swelling and pain while detoxifying which ultimately subsided. Her headaches disappeared completely within a few days of therapy. She began hallucinating as a response from the release of body stored analgesics and anesthetics.

Upon completion of the program, which lasted 68 days, she had 100% motion of all joints, with no inflammation or soreness. The myofacial syndrome had cleared, she was experiencing no muscle spasms or tenderness. Follow-up allergy treatment, Gamma-globulin end thymosin injection therapy and "maintenance" detox therapy have been instituted as needed. Though she still has numerous environmental sensitivities, the detoxification therapy has allowed her to become active in church and community affairs and has considerably improved her ability to function on a daily basis. She is at least 90% better than her previous condition. She is currently on no medications.

CASE #2: This 30 year old married female, native of San Diego with two children was evaluated in 1983 for recurrent asthma, chest pain, headaches, dyspnea, congestion, and headaches. Childhood medical history is relatively unremarkable with the exception of asthma, allergies, and enuresis. Past history indicates that she had suffered from a vaginal yeast infection at the age of 18, which was associated with a vague "altered mental state," heart palpitations, and anxiety states. However, this was diagnosed seven years later as Candidiasis. Frequent visits to the emergency room resulted in prescriptions of Valium and referrals for psychologic counselling. As a senior in college, she was unable to continue her studies due to short attention span, poor concentration and retention. During the middle of her second pregnancy, she began to experience severe confusion, restlessness, and hyperactivity. Her yeast infections were aggravated by each pregnancy and appeared to have exacerbated her symptoms.

Shortly after the birth of her second child, she experienced prolonged bouts of depression, severe anxiety, feelings of unreality, light headedness, appetite changes, insomnia, memory problems, suicidal obsession, high fevers, nightmares and a constant sharp pain to the right side of the head She began to experience tingling sensations of the scalp, seizure-like activity and temporary paralysis of the arms upon arising.

By age 25, she was incapable of caring for herself and her children without assistance. This patient had seen approximately 45 health practitioners within a ten year period. Earlier diagnostic impressions were that of a major depressive disorder/mixed personality disorder characterized by histronic and borderline components.

In 1980, she was referred for admission to the county mental health facility due to prolonged suicidal states. Her condition was diagnosed between 1979 and 1981 as consistent with a schizophreniform or manic depressive disorder. She was treated accordingly with a combination of psychotherapy and several different psychotropic medications The treatment failed to produce positive results.

In 1981, a nine month series of allergy shots regulated her menstrual cycle for the first time in eight years.

In 1982, she was evaluated by a specialist in Environmental Medicine, who found her extremely chemically sensitive. Laboratory studies confirmed abnormal immune parameters as well as an irregular EEG. Following his recommendations, removal of known chemical sources from the home, removing sources of natural gas, avoiding tap water, and using a filtering mask, produced dramatic and immediate relief of symptoms.

In 1984, a fat biopsy detected elevated levels of chlorinated pesticides as well as other minor levels of toxic agents. She underwent the Bio-Toxic Reduction Program for 43 days. A gradual improvement of her condition was associated with decreases in levels of stored toxicity as verified by a follow-up fat biopsy. While detoxifying she experienced several days of asthma, "attacks of panic" similar to that of ten years prior, as well as severe irritability, depression, intense head pain, and restlessness. She also experienced the side effects of the numerous psychiatric medications which were terminated three years prior to the program.

Following the detox therapy, she no longer suffers from reoccurring asthma. The program improved her over-all sense of awareness, the chronic eye and "stabbing" head pain is gone; she has far fewer colds, fevers, ear infections, and flu-symptoms; and it has greatly improved her chemical tolerance threshold. Her ability to function consistently on a daily basis has dramatically improved A follow-up EEG after completion of the program was completely normal. After being totally disabled for three years, she is now involved in a vocational rehabilitation program. It is now known that she lived within a mile from a county landfill for 18 years, which stored toxic chemicals for local industry for nearly twenty years. The San Diego County Public Health Dept. recently launched a study on the high incidence of cancer in that neighborhood. Though possible damage to the central nervous and immune systems still confine her to many dietary and lifestyle restrictions, this was one of the most significant breakthroughs in her health restoration. She is 80% improved since completing the program and has required no medication nor psychotherapy since appropriate diagnosis and medical management of her condition.

CASE #3: This 50 year old white female was first seen on May 16, 1984 complaining of constant pain and pressure in her sinuses radiating to the top of her head, as well as fatigue and post nasal drip. She became aware that her headaches were always worse at work. A history of her present illness indicates that she was relatively symptom free at the time she was employed as an accountant in a new three-story office building in May 1983. Her suite was the only completed office at the time. By October she noticed that she easily tired and developed dark circles under her eyes. She then developed upper respiratory infections and finally sinus pain. In December, her menstrual cycle ceased and by May 1984 her hormone imbalance caused a problem with her uterine fibroids. She began having symptoms daily. Physical examination revealed white coating on the tongue, suggesting Candidiasis as well as a notable myofacial syndrome. Prior to her coming to the detox center, she was placed on Estrogen, Erythromycin, Sudafed, muscle relaxants, and Sodium-selinate, however there was no improvement in her condition.

The patient was placed on candida therapy. Following the Bio-Toxic Reduction Program, this patient experienced an increase in energy levels, a tremendous improvement in her social life, is gradually becoming less sensitive to the chemicals in her environment. During the detoxification program, she re-experienced the symptoms which occurred at the onset of her illness.

In August 1984, the State Dept. of Occupational Safety and Health determined that the air conditioning system was 100% closed, causing the same air to recirculate, which was responsible for numerous respiratory diseases prevailing in that particular office.

CASE #4: This 54 year old white male was first seen at the Clinic on May 25, 1983. His chief complaints were headaches, difficult concentrating, cloudy thinking, depression, a 'tight band' around his head, neck and thoracic spasms, swelling in the fingers, and scrotal rash. His medical history revealed hypoglycemia, myofacial syndrome, mucutaneous Candidiasis, and extensive allergies. He did improve somewhat on the standard protocol for Candidiasis and allergy treatment He also underwent chelation therapy prior to his visit to the clinic, however it was unsuccessful in relieving his symptoms.

This patient underwent the detoxification program and feels 95% better then before. Though he still reacts to certain foods and chemicals, his reactions appear less severe. The patient stated that professionally and socially, this program was the most important phase of his recovery. He noted that he has tripled his business since completion.

CASE #5: This 29 year old female was first seen on February 3,1983 for allergy evaluation. She was on Nystatin therapy far Candidiasis and was improving. She was still feeling depressed (particularly premenstrual), lethargic, extremely chemically-sensitive, moderate food allergies, vaginal yeast infections, loss of libido, cystitis, abdominal bloating. Adherence to Candidia protocol resulted in an over-all improvement of her condition.

In August 1984, she began to experience lower thoracic and upper lumber pain, tightness in chest and minor dyspnea.

At the conclusion of a 33-day, detoxification program, she was more alert, free of depression, and was feeling good "all of the time." She noted dramatic improvement in energy levels, and her back pain and muscle spasms had totally disappeared. This patient has improved 90& over her previous condition.

CASE #6: This 39 year old female was first seen on July 27, 1983, complaining of extreme fatigue, depression, hypoglycemia, hypertension, headaches, prolonged flus and colds, abdominal discomfort, marked confusion, and joint pain. She had polio at age 8. Family history indicates that her mother had lupus and numerous allergies. One sister has lupus. She had a high carbon tetrachloride exposure at age 25 and lost 50 lbs in one month's time following this incident. She has had difficulty since this time. There is evidence of liver damage related to this exposure.

The patient underwent 51 days of detoxification. Following the program, she no longer suffered from nausea, chest or neck spasms, and she feels her mind is sharper and clearer. After a period of disability prior to detoxx, she is now working full time.

CASE #7: This 52 year old male was first seen on March 8,1984, complaining of chest tightness, wheezing, coughing, post nasal drip, nasal congestion, irritability, depression, digestive problems, craving of sweets, insomnia, and mood swings. Patient indicates that these symptoms began while working with a Kodak activator from 1973 to 1975. He worked with a considerable amount of electronic equipment such as TV cameras, lights, etc. which were in a poorly ventilated 'room. Allergy history indicates intolerance to petrochemicals and hydrocarbons such as perfumes, hairsprays, insecticides, and any scented products.

This patient was on detoxification therapy for 63 days. There was a 95% improvement in his condition and now feels that he is better able to cope with his highly stressful jab.

CASE # 8: This 25 year old white male was first seen on Jan 2, 1985 feeling pressure and soreness in his sternum, eye pain, nasal congestion, constant headaches, memory problems, difficult concentrating, and numerous chemical sensitivities. This patient was relatively symptom free prior to his employment for a pesticide service, three months prior. Safety precautions were not followed as he was to carry pesticides inside the cab of his truck and was not given protective clothing. The company physician advised him to remain working at his position despite his condition. A chlorinated pesticide screening test indicated elevated levels of Penta, in addition to minor levels of other pesticides.

Within three days of the Bio-Toxic Reduction Program this patient's headaches were gone. During detoxification, the patient stated that he could taste and smell the chemicals that he was previously working with. His mental confusion had cleared, his energy levels returned, and his chest pain had diminished and he was no longer having memory problems. Prompt treatment avoided the possibility of becoming totally disabled from this exposure. The patient was able to find work immediately following the program, provided he avoided close chemical contact.

CASE #9: This 30 year old white male was first seen in this office on March 7, 1983. Patient complained of inability to concentrate, excessive fatigue, headaches, irritability, depression, lack of mental and physical energy, insomnia and nightmares. He has had difficulty with headaches for 22 years. These symptoms became considerably more severe in 1981 when he was stationed on an aircraft carrier. He states that the water tasted like it had gasoline in it. The water supply for the ship was pumped in using hoses that were used to pump fuel. From this time on he began to develop sensitivities to other chemicals. Following this time, he suffered from vertigo, post nasal drip, and daily headaches after drinking the contaminated water. A fat biopsy revealed elevated levels of PCB and DDE

After completing the Bio-Toxic Reduction Program he was able to tolerate far more chemicals than before. Someone entering the room with perfume did not cause him to lose his concentration as it would previously; he could also take his young child on an outing without the usual irritability and depression. He was even able to do some painting around the house, which he was certain he'd never be able to do again. Though still affected by food sensitivities, his reactions are less severe. This patient is approximately 85% improved

CASE #10: This 28 year old female was first seen on June 6, 1984, complaining of chronic sinus congestion, pressure in sinuses and temples, and marked depression. Onset of depression was at age 13. She had undergone psychotherapy since 1978 and was treated with various anti-depressants with no improvement, however with gradual increase in her depression. Various medications were causing difficulty with her motor functions as well as minor confusion and poor memory recall. She would frequently lose her balance and fall. Medical history reveals frequent yeast infections, pre-menstrual tension, food and chemical allergies, hypoglycemia. Her diagnosis was as follows: multiple allergies, myositis, latent tetany, exogenous obesity and severe mental depression. She lost 9 lbs on the candida diet and her depression improved as well. However, constant food cravings were still a constant threat. She still suffered from confusion and feelings of frustration and anger.

After completing the detoxification program she felt much more energetic and required far less sleep. She was able to run for nearly a half hour each morning. The continual feelings of sadness and hopelessness no longer persisted. Improvements in concentration were phenomenal; she was able to work between 6-9 hours without any problems. The patient no longer required the anti-depressants and all motor skills returned since discontinuing the medications. Though she is still working on her weight problem, the obsession with food is far less severe following the program.

This participant wrote in a summary letter, "I am a different person since completing the program. I feel I am finally getting well. The difference is like night and day. It literally saved my life."

CASE #11: This 40 year old white male was first seen on October 25, 1984 with chief complaints of abdominal pain, pyrosis, chest congestion, headaches, mood changes, memory impairment, nausea, insomnia, and generalized malaise. These symptoms were directly related to chemical exposures where he had been employed in service and sales of marine equipment until August of 1982. Seventy percent of his work involved repairing inflatable boats. It is noted that this patient was free of any neuropsychological problems before his exposure. He was routinely exposed to Toluene and Benzene, two of the twenty-nine volatile compounds, including various hydrocarbons, paint thinners, epoxy thinners, gasoline, epoxy resins, ammonia, varnish, latex, and chrynal acrylic adhesive. The containers were not labeled as to contents or dangers of contact The company owner failed to follow through with an initial agreement to provide the necessary safety equipment and required air filtration system. Initially the symptoms occurred only intermittently approximately once or twice per week beginning in April 1983.

By May 1983, he was working in excess of fifty hours per week, however only minor respirator equipment was provided. It was not until Sept. 1983 that he associated the severity of his symptoms to the days he was heavily exposed and that he felt some relief on weekends. Finally, he was able to make specific correlations to his occupational exposures. By October, the symptoms progressed in intensity and frequency and he felt ill most of the time.

In January 1984, he was no longer able to work due to nausea, vomiting, disorientation, memory impairment, and severe anxiety, depression, chest pain, congestion, and shortness of breath. A gastroenterologist determined that he had a severe reflux esophagitis thought to be caused by the toluene exposure. He also felt that the toluene was responsible for psychiatric and neurologic deficits. Examination revealed cerebellar dysfunction. Referrals to other specialists led to admission to the Alcoholism/Chemical Dependency Center in January 1984, where he was treated like a drug addict.

A pulmonary specialist diagnosed his condition as 'occupational asthma' related to an organic solvent. Subsequently a neurologist determined that his mental depression was not occupationally caused, but that the asthma was likely to be environmentally-induced. The patient was placed on numerous psychiatric medications, which did not relieve his symptoms. His chemically-induced depression had left him dangerously suicidal.

Because Toluene is fat soluble it accumulates in body fat with repeated exposures. The primary toxic action of this compound is on the central nervous system. Results of a General Volatile Screening Test revealed extremely high levels of Toluene measuring 39 ppb (of which "0" is the norm). There was also evidence of other body stored toxic levels.

This patient began the Bio Toxic Reduction Program in April of 1985 and completed the program in 52 days. He exuded very strong chemical odors while detoxing in the sauna. His headaches, respiratory difficulties, memory and thinking problems, personality disorder, and over-all health has improved by 85%. The suicidal feelings dispersed upon completion of the program. He attributes detox with saving his life. By the 29th day into the program, the serum chemical analysis returned showing no toluene detected whatsoever. He now feels physically able to return to work and is currently seeking employment in a 'safe environment'.

CASE #12: This 46 year old female came in with a demyelinating process of the central nervous system, possibly secondary to Sodium Pentothal anesthesia, as indicated by history. She had become paralyzed 23 years ago when she was given Sodium Pentothal at the delivery of her second child. A form of paresthesia remained for over 8 years following. She was told she was allergic to Sodium Pentothal, therefore wore an alert bracelet.

In January of 1982 she was again given Sodium Pentothal, even though the physician was informed of her former reaction. The paresthesia which resulted from this exposure has been far more damaging. She describes the bilateral dysasthesias of her hands as "feeling like they are coated with sandpaper" — which impairs her fine movements. During her initial 21 days on the Bio-Toxic Reduction Program she was able to once again "hold a pencil" and even "write, with a better than first grade appearance." She can now button her own clothes, do her own hair, and is beginning to play the piano again.

The Neuropsychiatric Institute in La Jolla agreed that her problem was most probably "Peripheral neuropathy, with no indication of Multiple Sclerosis." They were also impressed with the marked progress she has made since starting the program. (It is important to note that the abnormal EEG tracings that have been reported on several patients prior to the Bio-Toxic Reduction Program, all become normal following the program.)

CASE #13: This 26 year old female complained of aching feet of three years duration. Pain on the bottoms of both feet of two years duration. Pain below ankles of 16 months duration and soreness of the achilles tendons of one month's duration. Patient was seen and treated by numerous physicians, all of which felt she might be developing bilateral plantar fascial tears. Neurology evaluation was reported as negative. Her environmental history indicated the inside of her home was sprayed frequently for flea control. History also indicated developing paresthiasis of her feet. Physical examination revealed a well nourished white female in fair health. Abnormalities noted were evidence of possible candidiasis in her mouth, cervical and inguinal adenopathy, myofacial syndrome and decreased dorsalis pedis pulses.

Laboratory evaluation revealed normal SMA 24, CBC, and urinalysis. Urine for formic acid was negative. Anti-candida was reported and negative. Cellular report was abnormal with an increase of lymphocytes, OKT11, OKT4, and OKT8 cells and a decrease of Surface IG, natural killer cells and total B cells with a H/S ratio of 1.5. The "Serum" General Volatile Screening Test revealed p.p.b. of Toluene 16.4; Ethyl benzene 10.9; Xylenes 42.1; Trimethylmebenzene 1.2; Chloroform 1.0; 1,1,1 TriCiethane 4.3; Trichloroethylene 0.3; and Dichlorobenzenes 1.8. p.p.b. of Chlorinated Pesticide Screening Test revealed DDE 11.7; Heptachlor Epoxide 0.5; trans-Nonachlor 0.2; and HCB 0.6.

Final diagnosis: 1. Immune Deficiency Syndrome secondary to Toxic levels of DDE, Aromatic and Halogenated Hydrocarbins. 2. Myofacial Syndrome. 3. Paresthesia of feet 4. Cervical and Inquinal Adenopathy.

To this date the patient hasn't undergone therapy, she is waiting approval from Insurance Co. The chemicals she is carrying can safely be removed by the Bio-Toxic Reduction Program.

CASE #14: This 66 year old patient complained of numbness of hands, arms, legs and feet that started about one year before his first visit. He had paresthesia of fingers, left forearm and increased sensitivity to hot and cold with tremors. He had undergone neurolgical evaluation including nerve biopsy which revealed "degeneration from an unknown cause." Various therapies were used with no improvement, including 40 chelation treatments, therefore he was referred to us for the Bio-Toxic Reduction Program.

Occupational history revealed chronic low exposure to volatile hydrocarbons. History also revealed exposure to Clordane.

346

Laboratory evaluation revealed a normal CBC and SMA 24 other than an elevated BUN (28). The Anti-Candida report was within normal limits. The Immune Profile was abnormal with the following increased: WBC 10600, and natural killer cells 24%, and the following decreased: Lymphocytes 11%, Total T Cells (0KT11 921 per cc.), and Total B cells 105. H/S ratio was 1.2 This indicates a relative and mild absolute lymphopenia resulting in a mild decrease in the absolute number of T and B cells. The abnormal H/S ratio is associated with diminished in vitro T cell Function. The General Volatile Screening test revealed Toluene 0.3 p.p.b. (Serum), Ethyl benzene 0.3, Xylenes 0.3 and Tetraclorethylene 0.3. The Chlorinated Pesticide Screening Test revealed: Dieldrin 0.3 p.p.b. (serum), Beta BHC 0.7, DDT 0.2, DDE 10, Heptachlor 0.8, trans-Nonchlor 0.4, and HCB 0.7.

Evaluation led to the diagnosis of 1) Generalized Arteriosclerosis, 2) Myofacial Syndrome, 3) Polyneuropathy of Extremities, 4) Stasis Dermatitis of left ankle, 5) Chemically Induced Immune Deficiency Syndrome.

Patient was placed on the Bio-Toxic Reduction Program and Electro-Acuscope therapy which resulted not only in a general improvement of his general symptoms, but marked improvement in his peripheral neuropathy including return of his strength and grip to normal. His tremor has markedly improved as well as his dexterity. The circulation to his feet has improved to where the skin color is essentially normal and the stasis dermatitis has cleared. His neurologist has released him from further care. Patient is still chemically sensitive, however this is gradually improving, and he is back working part time and enjoying every minute.

CASE #15: This 47 year old Caucasian female was first seen in July of 1985 following acute and chronic insecticide exposure which began in 1977 when a helicopter passed over her house so low that she thought it was crashing and she ran outside only to be drenched with pesticides which she did not wash off her body for approximately one hour. From this time on the spraying occurred approximately every two weeks until a Court injunction was granted which stopped the spraying.

Her symptoms gradually became more severe after each exposure. Her symptoms at the time of her first visit consisted of extreme sensitivity to any type of chemical exposure such as cigarette smoke, petrochemical derivatives, insecticides and auto exhaust fumes. On exposure, she develops vertigo, a dry throat, muscle spasms, paresthesia, and weakness of the lower extremities. At night she develops not only weakness , but myoclonic twitching. In the past she has passed out when exposed to cigarette smoke. Dyspnea develops following exposures. She develops headaches in the mornings which are dull in nature. The myoclonic twitching is made worse with each exposure.

Laboratory evaluation revealed the CBC and SMA 24 to be basically normal. Urinalysis was basically normal. Immune Profile abnormal with a decreased hemolytic complement to 0 (normal 70-150), an increased lymphocyte count to 47% and a decreased natural killer cells to 10%. The H/S ratio is decreased to 1.5. On the Volatile Screening Test the Serum showed p.p.b. of Toluene 0.3 — The Chlorinated Phenols measured 8 p.p.b. Penta — 2,4, D was 3.6 and 2,4 DB 5 p.p.b.; The Chlorinated Pesticide Test showed DDT 0.3 p.p.b., D.D.E. 11.7 p.p.b., Heptachlor Epoxide 0.3 p.p.b., trans-Nonchlor 0.4 p.p.b., and HCB 0.5 p.p.b. Chlorinated Pesticides Test on the foliage on his property revealed DDE, DDT, DDD, PCP, Dieldrin, DHC, Lindane, HCB, Endrin, and HE.

This evaluation led to the final impression of: 1) Chemically induced immune deficiency, 2) Peripheral neuropathy, 3) Pesticide poisoning, chronic, 4) Latent tetany, 5) Candidiasis, 6) Depressive reaction to physical illness.

This patient has not started therapy yet, but is scheduled. This case is an excellent example of pesticide poisoning and the disability that follows.

CASE #16: This 30 year old white female had a nine month history of what patient thought was flea bites on legs. History revealed patient hadn't felt well for approximately 10 years, with gradual onset of flu like symptoms, headaches, muscle twitching and spasms (severe at times), fatigue, depression, irritability, highly emotional, occasional difficulty thinking and remembering, and chemical sensitivity with recent onset of a generalized allergic pruritis especially on face and neck.

Patient was first treated with standard allergy evaluation and therapy with no improvement other than temporary with steroids. Further history revealed that her symptoms became worse after moving into her present home, therefore laboratory evaluation for fat stored chemicals was performed on her which revealed a high level of "Penta."

Her home was checked and though there was residual penta in the home it was felt, by the laboratory, this amount should not be a contributing factor. With further investigation it was discovered the town in which she had lived as a child has a potential problem. The town has been noted as having levels of "toxins," and at this time most of the classmate she had, either have a serious illness, or had already died from "cancer." Several of her close friends died in their 20's of cancer. There has also been a number of miscarriages as well as stillbirths. Further investigation is being done on the town.

Laboratory evaluation: EKG, CBC, SMA 24, Thyroid profile and Urinalysis were within normal limits. Mineral Analysis was abnormal with some deficiencies but no toxic mineral levels noted. Anti Candida report revealed IgG 288, IgA 444 and IgM 286 (normal under 100). Serum tests for Chlorinated Phenols: Penta 49 p.p.b.; General Volatile: Toluene 0.6 p.p.b., Ethylbenzene 0.4 p.p.b., Xylenes 1.0 p.p.b., Trimethylbenzenes 3.5 p.p.b.,1,1,1, Trichlorethane 0.3 p.p.b., Chlorinated Pesticides: DDE 2.1 p.p.b., Heptachlor Epoxide 0.3, p.p.b., and HCB 0.2 p.p.b..

The patient was placed on the Bio-Toxic Reduction Program and showed almost immediate, improvement of her severe pruritis and generalized dermatitis. Her headaches became worse before they finally cleared. At approximately 21 days of therapy the patient noted an increase in her muscle twitching and after a short time in the sauna the Jacksonian seizure activity would start. At times this was severe requiring medical attention before the seizures would subside. All laboratory values were normal during these seizures. Myoclonic muscle twitching, Petit Mal, Jacksonian and occasionally Grand Mal Seizure activity are the "Hallmark" of "Chlorinated Pesticide Poisoning." (Chlordane has been the most common cause in our patient load.)

It was necessary to discontinue her program from time to time until the seizure activity would subside. It was noted that during her seizure activity her darkfield cell analysis revealed crystals which were believed to be evidence of a chemical in her blood. This has not been observed at other times in her blood. Her Penta level, when starting the program was 49 p.p.b., at three weeks 20 p.p.b., and none by the end of the fourth week. She is far from being free from any problems, however, she is markedly improved and there are fewer "bad days" now. The headaches are only occasional (usually stress or exposure related). The dermatitis and balance of symptoms have totally cleared. She will remain under maintenance therapy due to her weakened immune system. She is still very sensitive to chemical odors and mold exposure. With time these symptoms will become less noticeable until they disappear.

CASE #17 This 40 year old Caucasian female was first seen on Oct. of 1983 with a 20 year history of progressive symptoms as follows: Menstrual irregularity, premenstrual tension and cramping, constant vaginal candidiasis, frequent urinary tract infections, urethritis, muscle aching and cramping with spasms, numbness of hands and feet at night, chemical sensitivity and inability to perform even light house work. Symptoms were gradual in onset becoming more severe yearly. Patient became unable to perform even light housework shortly following the tenting and treating of her home with Chlordane in 1980.

Patient had numerous evaluations and therapy none of which diagnosed her condition, or helped her until in 1983 she was treated at Meadowlark where she was placed on a fast, followed by a vegetarian diet which offered some improvement. Their evaluation noted elevated copper and mercury levels. Laboratory evaluation was normal for CBC, SMA 24, thyroid profile and urinalysis. her fungal hypersensitivity panel revealed IgE normal, but IgG 223, Fusarium 498 and Phoma 231. (above 100 elevated) Candida anti-bodies were IgG 359; IgA 146 and IgM 65. It was recommended she have pesticide levels performed, but due to finances this was deferred. Patient was placed on a yeast free diet and anti-candida program which helped her recurring urinary tract infections and candidiases, however her general condition was not improving, therefore started allergy therapy which also failed to make any improvement. Patient continued to require frequent antibiotics for urinary tract infections and noted that frequently the eating of beef, chicken or fish was followed by return infection within 2- 4 days.

On Oct. 18, 1984 she was started on the Bio Toxic Reduction program. Her CBC, SMA 24, EKG and urinalysis were within normal limits with exception of uric acid of 8.3 and CEA 6.8. Laboratory was following a three week Ultrabalance diet. Pt. declined the Chlorinated Pesticide Testing therefore it was not done at this time.

She almost immediately began to feel better in spite of many manifestations. The myoclonic muscle twitching and Jacksonian spasms were becoming more frequent, therefore she requested the Chlorinated Pesticide test be performed. This was drawn on Nov.12,1984 and revealed: Dieldrin 0.1 p.p.b., Beta- BHC 0.2, DDT 0.3, DDE 20.4, Heptachlor Epoxide 0.4, trans-Nonachlor 0.2, and HCB 0.2. Patient developed a strong odor of chlorine in spite of all laboratory being normal and had a marked increase in myoclonic muscle twitching and Jacksonian spasms therefore program was temporarily discontinued.

Condition slowly improved, however on Dec. 8 she called after developing muscle spasms again after exposure to chlorox when cleaning sinks again even though advised not to do this.

On 3-14-85 the Chlorinated Pesticide screening test was repeated which revealed: Dieldrin 0.2 p.p.b., Beta-BHC 0.2, DDT 0.3, DDE 10, Heptachlor Epoxide 0.3, trans-Nonachlor 0.1, and HCB 0.4. This indicated the BTR program was not completed, however the elevated DDT also indicated a possible continuing exposure. A General Volatile Screening Test revealed Xylene 0.5 p.p.b. and Tetrachlorethylene of 3.2. This is very high considering the time on the BTR program as these usually are quickly reduced and eliminated.

On 6-26-85 the Toluene was 0.3, no Xylene measured and the Tetrachlorethylene was reduced to 0.5.

On 8-2-85 a repeat Chlorinated Pesticide Screening Test revealed further exposure: Beta-BHC 0.4 p.p.b., DDT 0.5, DDE 20.5, Heptachlor Epoxide 0.6, trans-Nonchlor 0.3, and HCB 0.9. These levels may have increased due to exposure to pesticides being used in the State Parks. On at least two occasions the area was sprayed just prior to their arrival at the campsite. Their vacation took them across the States, and they slept out in State Parks most of the trip.

Patients' condition gradually improved, however, the urinary tract infections and vaginal yeast infections increased as toxic pesticides levels became elevated again. Patient was placed on a fast again in June of 85 at Meadowlark following which she developed signs of adrenal exhaustion and had to be treated accordingly.

In Oct. 85 the patient completed 2 more weeks of BTR therapy, however toward the end her myoclonic muscle twitching and Jacksonian spasms returned. The laboratory work was essentially normal, however this time it was noted that her serum phosphorus was decreased to 1.9. Seizure activity was relieved in the sauna. Her history clearly indicates that this activity slowly started after her home was treated with Chlordane in 1980.

On Nov.11, 1985 a repeat Chlorinated Pesticide Screening Test revealed a decrease in levels to: Aldrin 0.1, Beta-BHC 0.1, DDT 0.2, DDE 7.6, Heptachlor Epoxide 0.4, trans- Nonchlor 0.1, Endosulfan I- 0.1, HCB 0.4. Fat stored chemicals come out in the same order in which they are originally stored which explains a variation in testing as BTR progresses.

Patient is doing extremely well now. Though not totally recovered, she is now able to do her house work, shop, and is not having the recurring urinary tract infections or yeast infections. They have had their home tested and discovered this is not the exposure source. They are using bottled water and organically grown foods. She will be rechecked to insure she is not being re-exposed in the near future.

CASE # 18: This 33 year old Caucasian female from Imperial County came in with multiple complaints. She is very concerned over the "New River" that flows through Imperial County. There are several towns in its path, they happen to live in one of them. From El Centro (population approximately 24,000), Brawley and Holtville (population approx.7000 each), Calipatria (population 2000) Niland (population 1000) "New River" goes directly into the Salton Sea. The South end of the Salton Sea is dark and murky where the water enters. The other end is relatively clear. There are fish in this water, which are caught and eaten by the local people. The river originates in Mexico which gives them no control over the use of this "River." It is known to contain Raw Sewage, Raw Chemicals etc. There have been several attempts to put up some type of "Filter system - so far none effective.

An officer from the Police Department in Calipatria fell into the water 2 years ago, and has not been well since. He told them "The River holds all the diseases of the world." Also they report that any animal drinking from that water has died. The children in the area think the water has "Snow" on it, for there is "Foam-floating down the river all the time." The School children have constant colds and infections. It is reported that many children in the school are using inhalers in order to breath. There are "reportedly" several cases of "Crib Deaths" or SID each year. Patient's main complaint was that of constant "Flu like symptoms," headache, and a fear of having a complete "Breakdown"... She is in the process of moving, and starting the Bio-Toxic Reduction Program.

Laboratory findings from 12-3-85 showed mild chemical hepatitis; "Humoral report shows the percent of T suppressor/cytotoxic is at the upper limit of the expected range. Expansion in this T cell subset may be seen with antigen challenge." The General Volatile Screening Tests with serum levels in p.p.b. as follows: Toluene .6; Ethylbenzene 5.1; Xylenes

23.1; Chloroform .9; Dichloromethane .6; Tetrachloroethylene 1; Dichlorobenzenes 2.7 — The Chlorinated Pesticide Screening Test: Beta-MC .1; DDT .1; DDE 3.4; Heptachlor Epoxide .4; Trans-Nonachlor .1; HCB .2.

CASE #19: This 67 year old patient from Santa Marie, California was referred to me by a Physician at the Sansum Medical Clinic with what he felt was "Chemically induced Cirrhosis of the Liver." Unfortunately this patient is too far along for us to give her any help. We hate to report we are too late to reverse any of the damage that has been done. The outlook is very grim. When her laboratory work was done, we received immediate calls from the laboratories regarding the ranges. Copies of all findings are enclosed, as well as the ones shown here: General Volatile Screening Test Serum levels in p.p.b: Benzene .3; Toluene 55.6; Ethylbenzene 27.1; Xylenes 178.2; Trimethylbenzenes 1.4; Chloroform 1.1; Dichloromethane 2.9; 1,1,1-Trichlorethane 15.4; Tetrachloroethylene 3.7; Dichlorobenzenes 14.9. This report was given to Senator Wilson, and prompted a visit to the area. A complete investigation is under way at this time in regards to the potential danger.

CASE #20: This five year old (hyperactive) male child was seen for evaluation following the home being treated for fleas with DURSBAN/DIAZINON on two occasions. The mother reported she had taken her son to several Physicians for his constant "twitching" and was told this was "normal." She was not convinced, since he had never had any of these symptoms until after the home was treated for fleas. She also reported the animals became ill, and one died. The dog developed tremors and had to be put on "allergy medication." The dog improved when they moved to another location, but became ill after a visit to the Pet Hospital and exposure to flea dip area.

Mother reports almost constant muscle jerking when he sleeps. He also has what appears to be Petit Mal. All initial laboratory findings were normal, including a cholinesterase. However, on 10-22-85 the General Volatile Screening Test showed the following serum levels in p.p.b.: Toluene 23.8; Ethylbenzene 6.6; Xylenes 111.4; 1,1,1-Trichlorethane 7.2; TetraClorethylene 1.9.

The whole family started on the Bio-Toxic Reduction Program. In less than 30 days a repeat General Volatile Screening Test showed only two low levels remaining: Xylenes 1.2; TetraclorEthylene 0.4. Patient is now sleeping quietly through the night. Is less hyper and easier to handle.

CASE # 21: This 30 year old mother of the above child was having difficulty dealing with not only her son's problems, but her own constant headaches and flu like symptoms. She also was troubled by Petit Mal and Jacksonian Seizures on occasion. The General Volatile Screening Test showed the following: Toluene 18.6; Ethylbenzene 5.1; Xylenes 90.6; 1,1,1-TriClEthane 6.0; TetraclEthylene 1.5. There were also 1.7 p.p.b. of PCB's.

Within less than 30 days the repeat GYST showed the following: Toluene

0.5; Xylenes 0.3; Styrenes 0.7; Chloroform 1.6; Dichloromethane 0.3; 1,1,1-TriclorEthane 0.4; TetraclorEthylene 0.6. Nothing else was detectable.

These cases demonstrate the ability to remove extremely high levels of Toxins, safely. We will have a re-evaluation on these cases in the future. At the last visit they were both doing well.

CASE #22: This 28 gear old white female was first seen on May 7, 1985. Her chief complaint was intermittent swelling of joints of fingers. Onset six years ago. Occasional problems with toes and right knee.

The onset would usually start with a tiny red dot at the joint of one or more of her fingers. Within 24 hours the joint, or joints would be swollen and painful. She has been to specialists in Internal Medicine, Orthopedics, Endocrinology and Rheumatology. All laboratory work has been within normal limits. No evidence of arthritis. Routine laboratory work at our office produced the same results. The Immune Profile indicated the T cells diminished, the Anti-Candida was elevated in the IgG (191) and IgM (253), and the Antinuclear titer was positive. She was started on the Anti-Candida Program and seemed to respond favorably. The joints were less "stiff" and there was no noticeable swelling. The sensitivity to certain chemicals and foods was increasing.

On the third of December she came in with a severe flare of both hands and feet. The proximal joints on three fingers of the right hand were triple in size, blueish in the center extending half an inch on either side of the joint ending in bright red. The left hand was similar, but lesser in involvement. A serum biopsy was scheduled followed by an injection of Precortin and Decadron. The injection had no effect on the inflammation. The General Volatile Screening Test brought some alarming results. Toluene 59.1 p.p.b.; Ethelbenzene 47.1 p.p.b; Xylenes 256.9 p.p.b.; Chloroform 3.7 p.p.b.; 1,1,1-Trichloroethane 16.2 p.p.b.; Tetrachloroethylene 5.8 p.p.b.; Dichlorobenzenes 8.7 p.p.b.. The Chlorinated Pesticide Screening Test showed .1 p.p.b. of DDT indicating slight recent exposure. DDE 1.1; Heptachlor Epoxide .4; trans- Nonachlor .1 and HCB .3 p.p.b.

She has just started the Bio-Toxic Reduction Program and we shall watch with interest as she proceeds through the program. Pictures will be taken periodically to further evaluate the progress.

Lawyers Treat Symptoms, Too!
by
Anthony di Fabio

You are a young boy or girl who wishes to grow up to be a health professional, a medical doctor. You want to help folks. You successfully pass seven years of higher education and receive your degree. Now you're ready to help folks, right? What you've never been told through nearly a generation of formal education is that your chief method for helping folks must use cook book recipes designed primarly by pharmaceutical companies with a huge vested interest in patented medicines.

Helping folks to achieve wellness is not the game -- and you've never been told this fact!

You're a bright, sincere want-to-help person. A patient comes to you with serious medical problems, one that no cookbook recipe will cure. What do you do?

If you truly want to help folks you'll research the literature, both professional and unprofessional literature. You'll look for something, anything, to solve this poor patient's instransigent problem.

Eureeka!

You've found it!

You explain to your patient what you've found, that its not "the customary cookbook treatment" but you think it's worth a try. You have the patient sign forms giving permission to use this treatment and that s/he knows that it is not a "customary" treatment.

Eureeka! Again.

Your patient gets well in the face of all the cookbook literature that carefully explains there is no cure and you should be giving symptom relief treatments only -- as described by the accepted cookbook.

Wow! You got an "incurable" well, so now you're ready to accept others that come to you with the same condition via referral.

One of this foundation's founders, Jack M. Blount, M.D. cured 11,000 people of so-called uncurable rheumatoid disease before he died.

Dr. Blount also cured this writer of Rheumatoid Arthritis more than a quarter of a century ago!

But everyone knows that rheumatoid arthritis is uncurable, so Dr. Blount must have been a kook, a person who practiced medicine without following the "accepted procedures."

Thousands of right thinking, right acting doctors have had their licenses revoked, or been fined and placed into a legal straight jacket, or been otherwise hounded by those who would support the pharmaceutical company's cookbook rules that sell damaging patented chemicals.

354

Just in this book alone I can name Jonathan Wright, M.D., for example, who has several times been hauled into court because he refuses to use pharmaceutically inspired cookbook rules. Then there's Stephen B. Edelson, M.D who was helping ladies who'd made the mistake of getting silicon implants for their breasts and now suffered from "incurable" diseases. And, of course, Zane Gard, M.D. who solved the problem of extremely damaging agent orange affecting himself and family, and now passed on his knowledge to others seriously affected by similar environmental toxins. Edelson gave up his license and retired. Gard moved to Mexico where he could practice medicine without being controlled by agents of the pharmaceutical companies. Wright spent tens of thousands of dollars defending himself from improper, false and certainly bordering-on-evil charges.

One year, this author identified more than 100 excellent doctors who suffered from the same persecution, their only crime being that of not practicing cookbook medicine.

Over time, thousands of truly caring doctors have lost their licenses or have been strait jacketed.

I got to thinking about some of the legal implications of our present social disgrace and, while I'm not a lawyer, I wanted to share some thoughts. Perhaps I'm wrong, but at least these ideas are worth thinking over.

As a doctor your game is to treat sick people. But what do you do when the cookbook crazies come after you? Your very first step is a quick visit to your nearest sympathetic legal eagle, your attorney.

Just as all doctors are not equal (no matter how their state license reads), neither are all lawyers equal (no matter how their state license reads).

And, just as your friendly neighborhood medical doctor must also earn a living, so must your emphathetic attorney. Conflicts between self-survival and solving the client's problem can easily ensue in both instances.

Although qualified to do otherwise, and as your family doctor usually draws upon a specific population or practices jointly with particular hospitals, so does the lawyer draw from those of specific need and also normally practices as an officer of the court under particular jurisdictions.

There are many distinctly Machiavellian tactics used by governmental authorities to "get" alternative/complementary practitioners.[2] For now, keep in mind that, no matter how clever your friendly neighborhood lawyer, s/he is not really prepared for the depth and extent of the tactics that will most likely be employed.

Let's set up one of the most common ploys by State and Federal officials:

John Doe, M.D. is well known for his expertise in treating cancer. By word-of-mouth patients flock to his medical center where not only are their tumors put into regression and cancer spread is halted, but each patient is taught metabolic nutrition and change of life-style so that when they return home they sustain their gains.

A member of the Quack, Quack Busters organization — or an equivalent sub-species — gets wind of the fact that Dr. Doe is not using FDA and State Medical Board "approved" radiation, surgery, or chemotherapy, and so he has secretly reported John Doe to the State Medical Board.

Digressing briefly from John Doe's tribulations, let's address this so commonly used tactic, "you're not using FDA 'approved' procedures."

Remember, Federal law normally trumps state law!

Ray Evers, M.D., (deceased) often cited as the father of chelation therapy, lost several fortunes defending from the multiple evil empire, but finally succeeded in bringing his case before the United States Supreme Court. Derived from rulings in his favor is a paragraph from the "Foreward to the 50th Edition," *Physician Desk Reference* (1996: the only copy available to me):

> "The FDA has also recognized that the FD&C [Food Drug and Cosmetic Act] does not, however, limit the manner in which a physician may use an approved drug. Once a product has been approved for marketing, a physician may choose to prescribe it for uses or in treatment regimens or patient populations that are not included in approved labeling. The FDA also observes that accepted medical practice includes drug use that is not reflected in approved drug labeling." [See United States v. Evers, supra, 643 F.2d at 1048, quoting 37 Fed. Reg. 16503 (1972).]

Two observations can be made from the above quotation:

1. State (and FDA) insistence on drug use only according to "FDA approval," is not the law of the land.

2. Since most state constitutions do not address this specific legal point, then accusations against you for so doing should immediately be removed to Federal jurisdiction — not to be heard in any State court, although, within limits, State Courts are jurisdictionally capable of hearing both Federal and State constitutional deprivations.

Federal preemption over state law consists of two types:

"Express preemption" occurs where Congress says within the statute 'we hereby preempt.' Here, federal laws are explicitly precluding state and local regulations.

"Implied preemption" has, within itself, three sub-categories: conflicts preemption, preemption because state law impedes the achievement of a federal objective, and preemption because federal law occupies the field.

An apparent conflict preemption in the State of California, for example, when treating cancer, mandated by law that licensed physicians use only "approved" methods, which interprets to mean radiation, chemotherapy or surgery. I understand this California law has been changed since this article was written, but before its change, one of the finest doctors I knew was sent to prison for six years for violation of the law. Even though his patient had come to him and asked that the "cut, slash and burn" treatment for her breast cancer not be used and even though she signed a disclaimer, that she was only to be treated to strengthen her immune system, even though all of this, the State of California sent this world renown doctor to prison for six years!

So, how does one reconcile the Supreme Court's prior, strong statement that the physician has carte blanche to use treatments he deems necessary with this blanket State usurpation of physicians' legal and professional right to choose and patients' freedom-of-choice rights?

Probably Federal case law — those court cases testing the conflict between these diametrically opposed directions — is or will be complex and circuitous, depending upon specific litigagous details before reaching a direct confrontation.

Presumably the Federal Government's power to determine what constitutes "safe and effective" drug use does, however, trump California's law on the liberal use of marijuana, or even that of Colorado's liberal marijnuana stance!

Conflicts between State and Federal law are complex and often settled in favor of the State provided the Federal Court can find a way to do so. Numerous preemption cases follow no predictable jurisprudential or analytical pattern.[9]

But, back to Dr. John Doe:

The quack, quack buster has complained to the state medical board in secret. After due hurrumphing, members of the state's distinguished set of political appointees, the medical board, turns the quack, quack busters' pseudo complaint over to the attorney general office.

No copy will go to Dr. Doe so that, at this point, John Doe doesn't know who is complaining about him, or what the complaint is about, or even that a complaint exists. We can all be assured, however, that it will not be one of Dr. Doe's patients!

The State attorney general office is an extremely busy place. Who gets the assignment to go after John Doe is pretty much a matter of office economics and personnel availability. Let's say that Jim Dumdum gets the assignment.

The probability is very high that Jim Dumdum is young, relatively unfamiliar with the real world of legal eagleing, and that he's immersed himself in nothing but overly bloated legal language and definitions for 6 or 7 years, just like a medical doctor has done in medical territory. Assistant Attorney Dumdum most likely has never heard of alternative/complementary medicine, but does know all the State laws and regulations so far as he can find them in the encyclopaedia of laws named after his state; i.e. [State] Code Annotated, called [S]TAs.

A small group of men, the medical board, a quasi-state political-appointee agency, has declared that John Doe has probably done wrong, and therefore, as a defined function of the attorney general office, Jim Dumdum has been called upon to defend his state's citizens from alleged gross evil.

So far as Jim Dumdum is concerned, he must represent "the people" (all the remainder of the people in your state, including those who think you're a really swell doctor) and he must attack you.

So, at this point Dr. Doe might receive a letter from an official directing him to come in and justify himself. Depending upon the state, he must report to any one of a variety of official offices: State Medical Board, State defined Administrative Review Board, Attorney General Office, or, perhaps, even before a Court of Law.

Dr. Doe's best strategy, of course, is to seek professional legal assistance. But, not really knowing what's to be charged, or even the nature of declarations against him, he's in poor condition to discriminate between attorneys — State or Federal — and whether or not Constitutional rights are involved.

Most family neighborhood lawyers make their living in the nearest State courts and will almost invariably lean toward State courts or toward administrative law jurisdiction. (Note: Unless the coming fight at a lower court [or administrative review] level — John Doe's counter-assertions — includes constitutional claims, such as violation of constitutional rights, higher state courts will not review violation of constitutional rights claims, and John Doe will be precluded at any further step from claims of violation of constitutional rights at higher State Courts. However a claim in Federal Courts might still be permitted.)

If rights assigned to Dr. Doe by the Federal Bill of Rights have been violated, or are believed to be violated by the State processes, then Federal Courts should be the first and only recourse, although similar claims are permitted in State courts, especially when State law includes similar rights.

[Although some States have reserved stronger rights to the people, some weaker, and some about the same, it's in Federal Courts where thousands of Federal case histories — legal guiding lights -- abide, and are most easily understood. And it's the Federal judges who are most familiar with those cases.]

So, let's say that the next State action is the coordinated frontal attack on Dr. John Doe: (1) Distorted newspaper reports about Dr. John Doe, in efforts to discredit and slander him ("poisoning" the judge or jury pool); (2) Ousting of Dr. Doe from hospitals, based on innuendo and rumor; (3) Appearance of armed government agents in the waiting room with announced intention of arresting Dr. Doe or his personnel; (4) Collection of all the patients' personal medical files; (5) Ripping out of the hard drive from the good doctor's computer; (6) Searches thru drawers, offices and, yes, even outside garbage containers for either evidence or objects that can be construed to be evidence. (Dr. Jonathan Wright was exposed to all of the above. His primary crime at the time was refusing to use American vitamin and mineral shots for his sensitve allergy patients. He'd been ordering them from Europe where the vials did not contain preservatives that affected his patients.)

Notice!

Probably no warrant, or other identification has been provided during this obvious violation of constitutional rights in the name of "protecting the public."

By this time it hasclearly occurred to Dr. Doe that he needs professional legal advice. Where does he turn? To the lawyer he knows best, perhaps one who has in the past handled his auto accident, civil contracts, or covered another type of domestic dispute.

Will the attorney refer him to a Constitutional expert? Usually not. The attorney will quickly pull out his encyclopaedic [S]ACAnnotated and read up on all of the State's administrative and other pertinent law, preparing himself for a charged battle of wits — in a somewhat biased arena.

What Relief Will Dr. Doe's
State-Oriented Attorney Seek?

Most likely Dr. Doe's attorney will seek both Declaratory and Injunctive Relief from State violation of Due Process Rights.

Declaratory relief is primarily relief from confusion created by statute, by interpretation, or by actions of the law. It's a statutory remedy for "the determination of a justiciable controversy where the plaintiff [Dr. Doe] is in doubt as to his legal rights."[8]

The theory is that an early resolution of Dr. Doe's legal rights will resolve some or all of the other issues in the case.

Injunctive relief would be a court order in favor of Dr. Doe "prohibiting the State from doing some specified act or commanding someone to undo some wrong or injury."[8]

At the core of injunctive relief is a recognition that monetary damages cannot solve all problems. An injunction may be permanent or it may be temporary. A preliminary injunction is a provisional remedy granted to restrain activity on a temporary basis until the court can make a final decision after trial. It is usually necessary to prove the high likelihood of success upon the merits of one's case and a likelihood of irreparable harm in the absence of a preliminary injunction before such an injunction may be granted;

otherwise the party may have to wait for trial to obtain a permanent injunction.

Temporary injunctive relief would be applicable, for example, in prohibiting the State from withdrawing Dr. Doe's license until the full facts of the case can be heard.

Such judicial determinations [remedies] to be won as outcomes of Plaintiff's State trial would be based upon an itemized listing of claims and counter-claims between the State and the Defendant, Dr. Doe.

As we are assuming for the sake of this article that Constitutionally guaranteed due process rights have, in fact, been violated by State or Federal employees under color of law, it is mentioned only in passing that the judicial body hearing the State's additional complaints will also hear Plaintiff's point-by-point rebut to them when and if the court decides it is appropriate to hear them.

Since all State Constitutions also include Federal guarantees of Constitutional rights, including rights to due process, the really bright attorney will also seek an award of attorneys fees and costs pursuant to U.S.C. Title 42 Section 1983 — violation of Plaintiff's rights under color of law.

This is the point where relief sought reflects "customary" practices based upon the experiences of the Plaintiff' regional attorney. He "knows" that if he can get the local judge to provide Declaratory and Injunctive relief, and to declare violation of due process rights, he's got the Plaintiff "saved."

If he can also get "attorney" fees, he's reached the Leprechaun's pot-o'-gold — and he's become Dr. Doe's real savior!

John Doe's attorney, being a very good one, will have inserted in his multiple answer to charges the assertion that Dr. Doe's rights have been violated pursuant to U.S.C. Title 42, Section 1983. It's highly doubtful — in the writer's opinion — that the really generous pot-o'-gold — monetary penalties and punishment to governmental violators of due process rights as provided by Title 42, Section 1983 — will be reached at this State trial level.

A rule just now invented is this: The amount of dollar award siphoned from wrong-doing State employee pocketbooks is indirectly proportional to the distance t he wrong doer official is from State Courts.

Unfortunately (or fortunately), State Court, Judges and State licensed lawyers are mostly creations of the State, not the Federal Government. They're more responsive to the sensitivities of State officialdom and State tax-payers. (Being accused of "raiding" State coffers or administrative officials pocketbooks reflects badly on "professionalism" and can affect the number of votes the judge receives on his next election to office.)

Also Constitutional issues are most often strongly and/or completely entertained at the appeal levels, not the State trial court levels — and this writer, probably along with Dr. Doe's attorney — is of the opinion that monetary penalties based on U.S.C. Title 42, Section 1983, even if reached at this State trial court level, will be of minimum restitution for Dr. Doe.

There will almost certainly be reluctance to haul specific State or Federal Administrative personnel before the trial court. Consider this second general rule (also just now invented): Subpoenas — a court order to appear as a witness — for individual State or Federal officials at trial court are issued in inverse proportion to the height of the administrative level!

State subpoenas have absolutely no power across State boundaries. Federal authorities — those administrators who, along with others, may be most likely to have initiated your local judicial problems — such as those located in Washington, D.C. at the FDA, cannot be reached via State Subpoena.

Federal Court, when necessary, can reach across all American boundaries!

In a 1970s Tennessee State University violation of due process rights a college professor, Chapdelaine, had received a project director's grant of half a million dollars from the National Science Foundation to help develop computer assisted instruction — quite a generous project grant in those days. From the very moment the grant arrived school officials tried every imaginable Machiavellian tactic to control the funding or the project's findings. Eventually they fired the professor without cause although he held tenure both by virtue of contract as well as State Statute.

"Holding tenure" simply means that prior to discharge the professor has a right to an unbiased hearing, and that his firing must be based upon a set of objective standards which were in violation by the professor.

This "due process" hearing was denied at all State levels — College up through the Commissioner of Education.

Clearly, explicitly defined due process rights were violated.

After long, diligent search Chapdelaine at last found legal representation.[11] As a generality, lawyers did not want to tackle a strong, local power structure, thus the "long, diligent" search for representation. Since this was the first time that State officials had been challenged to implement their own tenure laws — even though it was held that Tennessee's constitutional bill of rights was stronger than those of the Federal Government — stiff legal resistance was expected and did occur, the State Attorney General Office, of course, eagerly "protected" the citizens of the State of Tennessee.

The fight finally reached the Supreme Court level (highest) where Chapdelaine's claim was fully vindicated, he had, indeed, tenure rights both by contract and by State statute.

So, what was the State remedy?

Did the Department Head, the Dean of Arts and Sciences, the Dean of Faculty, the University President, and/or the Commissioner of Education suffer any penalties?

None whatsoever!

Plaintiff's award was simply a years' pay plus interest — no reinstatement, no objective, unbiased hearing judged by explicit standards as promised both by Statute and Contract law given "tenure" — and also a continuation of an underhanded employment blackballing for equivalent teaching positions and other possible State benefits such as illegal denial of desperately needed food stamps (ten children).

As there was legal judgment against but no penalty against those who had violated the law all personnel at all administrative levels were free at any future time to deny others a fair and objective hearing!

The attorneys who represented Chapdelaine were pleased, of course. They'd won a precedent case as well as one-third of the award. Further, their names could now be found associated with a precedent setting "key" case. A key case is one that is referred to and quoted as a major guiding light thereafter.

But, more a slap-in-the-face to Chapdelaine than a great victory was the automatic change in the style of the case. Whereas it had begun as Chapdelaine versus the State of Tennessee and Tennessee State University, President Torrence, et. al., the style was changed, now becoming State ex. rel. Chapdelaine v. Torrence [532 S.W. 2d 542-550 (Tenn 1976)]. (This means "State of Tennessee on the relation of Chapdelaine.")[10]

Since the State is sovereign, it can do no wrong! Therefore, on the State Supreme Court declaring Chapdelaine the winner — and after all of his lawyer's fight and his own pain and deprivations against the State's unlimited funds — the State joined the Plaintiff so that the end results published in the Tennessee case histories appear to say that the State of Tennessee had all along agreed with and had joined the plaintiff!

It was all along the University President's and "et. al." fault, not the State's!

President Torrence and his co-conspirators, of course, retained their jobs and salaries, and were totally free to deny another professor his/her constitutional rights!

So why would Dr. Doe's exceptionally bright local attorney bother to include U.S.C. Title 42, Section 1983 in his State trial court pleadings?

In this writer's opinion the reasons Dr. Doe's bright attorney included a Title 42, Section 1983 claim at the State trial level was primarily twofold (1) if it were not claimed at the trial court stage, it could never be reviewed at State appeals stages if it were decided to appeal; (2) as a commonly used pressure to the other side, to get the due process violaters to look at the possible personal penalties their misbehavior might lay on them — a kind of subtle warning, as it were. Many filings in State courts add on a Title 42, Section 1983 claim, but it is my personal opinion that both these attornies and their judges pass it off as a kind of often observed legalese boiler plate, but not a paragraph that's truly intended for judicial action. In my opinion, it's only in Federal Court the paragraph is taken seriously.

The Problem: Treating Symptoms

When Dr. Doe's lawyer wins this case (Declaratory and Injunctive relief and some costs) and Dr. Doe returns to his alternative/complementary practice, the basic problem of State and Federal supported and funded suppression has not been solved, nor will the proper and complete remedy have been provided by the State trial court.

But, Dr. Doe's lawyer saved Dr. Doe's bacon!

Right?

We're all happy for Dr. Doe, if he wins Declaratory and Injunctive relief as well as some costs — but those evil ones are still lurking behind the legal shadows of State or Federal protection (under color of law) — and they're ever so free to go after Dr. Jane Doe (or you) next in the same manner, using the same violation of due process rights.

By the same historical experiences, many other denials of due process rights are suffered by Americans in many other fields of human endeavor by various city, state or federal employees.

One cannot obtain a permanent injunction against an act that has never been performed! Prior restraint is often considered a particularly oppressive form of censorship in Anglo-American jurisprudence. Realistically, to ask for a prior restraint against individuals in a Governmental agency would be asking for a violation of rights guaranteed by the U.S. and State Constitutions at the same level as has already been applied to Dr. Doe.

In a manner of speaking, Dr. Doe's lawyer has done everything he set out to do. He's protected his client's rights, brought in some money, and slapped one of the State or Federal governmental bodies on their non-tender wrist.

Dr. Doe's attorney is not in business to crusade against bad governmental departments! Or bad governmental employees!

He's done his job! He's pulled his client out of a deep, dark hole!

But, where it has cost John Doe, M.D. perhaps $500,000 or more and loss of patients and reputation during and for his adequate defense, it has cost those who've made the decisions to violate his basic rights absolutely nothing! In fact, they continued to collect their monthly salary during the many months of altercation — and the court's slap on the wrist to the whole department is absolutely meaningless — of zero effect — against those individuals who violated Dr. Doe's Constitutional rights!

Further, unknowingly, all of the tax payers in the state have pooled their resources to pay State costs for this legal farce — whether they wanted to or not!

In Dr. John Doe's case, where obvious due process rights have been violated by State functionairies, no one has been held accountable, except the held-in-ignorance tax-payer.

Like mainstream cookbook medical doctors, John Doe's lawyer has just treated a symptom, not a cause!

The Solution:
U.S. Code Title 42, Section 1983,
Civil Action For Deprivation of Rights

This Civil Rights Act provision was formerly enacted as part of the Ku Klux Klan Act of 1871 and was originally designed to combat post-Civil War racial violence in the Southern states. Reenacted as part of the Civil Rights Act, USC Title 42, Section 1983 is today the primary means of enforcing all constitutional rights.This Federal Act is powerful and wide in scope. It reads:

"Every person who, under color of any statute, ordinance, regulation, custom, or usage, of any State or Territory or the District of Columbia, subjects, or causes to be subjected, any citizen of the United States or other person within the jurisdiction thereof to the deprivation of any rights, privileges, or immunities secured by the Constitution and laws, shall be liable to the party injured in an action at law, suit in equity, or other proper proceeding for redress, except that in any action brought against a judicial officer for an act or omission taken in such officer's judicial capacity, injunctive relief shall not be granted unless a declaratory decree was violated or declaratory relief was unavailable. For the purposes of this section, any Act of Congress applicable exclusively to the District of Columbia shall be considered to be a statute of the District of Columbia." [U.S. Code as of: 01/19/04]

This act clearly states that any government official — Federal, State, County, City — who deprives a citizen of any of their constitutional rights, such as due process, under color of law, can be held personally responsible!

"Under Color of Law" is the kicker!

To utilize a state office or state regulations to deliberately violate a citizen's constitutional rights is the "color of law' requirement.

It happens persistently and everywhere and will never be stopped until judges start reaching into the officialdom's pockebooks!

In other words, assuming Dr. John Doe's due process rights have indeed been violated, then every Federal or State or City employee who entered into the end-game of "getting John Doe" is liable for personal financial penalties.

Bluntly, John can reach into each responsible person's pocketbook and pull out a substantial amount of money for his own inurement! Such an action, it is believed by former lawmakers, as well as by this writer, should serves as a huge barrier to the willy-nilly "going after doctors" that now exists.

Advantages to this legal approach are clear: (1) Wasted taxes and court time is lessened; (2) Good doctors are saved; (3) Suppressive or outright ignorant civil functionairies are identified and suppressed in turn; (4) Governmental agencies begin operating as Congress intended.

In Monroe v. Pape 365 U.S. 167 (1961) six black children and their parents brought a Title 42, Section 1983 action in federal district court against the city of Chicago and thirteen of its police officers for damages for violation of their rights under the Fourteenth Amendment. They alleged that, without warrant, the police officers broke into their home in the early morning, routed them from bed, made them stand naked in the living room, and ransacked every room, emptying drawers and ripping mattress covers; that the father was taken to the police station and detained on "open" charges for ten hours while he was interrogated about a two-day-old murder; that he was not taken before a magistrate, though one was accessible; that he was subsequently released without criminal charges being filed against him.

Were the police officers and the city of Chicago liable under Title 42, Section 1983 for what was done to the plaintiffs?

According to the U.S. Supreme Court, police officers acting illegally and outside their scope of authority may be liable under Title 42, Section 1983 despite the requirement that the officers must have been acting under color of state law. The statutory words "under color of any statute, ordinance, regulation, custom, or usage, of any State or Territory" contained in 42 U.S.C. 1983 do not exclude acts of an official or police officer who can show no authority under state law, custom, or usage to do what he or she did or who even violated the state constitution and laws. The city of Chicago, however, was not held liable, because the Court ruled that Congress did not intend to bring municipal corporations within the ambit of Title 42, Section 1983. This ruling was later overturned by the Court in Monell v. New York City Department Of Social Services, 436 U.S. 658 (1978).

Monell virtually opened the floodgates of the courts to civil rights (or Title 42, Section 1983) litigation. Prior to this, it was difficult to hold public officials liable under Title 42, Section 1983 because of the requirement that they must have acted under color of state law. Most civil liabilities, however, stem from the abuse of power or authority by the police, and such actions were considered outside the color of state law. Monell changed all that. Now police officers can be sued under Title 42, Section 1983 if what they did arose out of a "misuse of power possessed by virtue of state law and made possible only because the wrongdoer is clothed with the authority of state law." An officer who abuses his or her authority can now be sued under Title

42, Section 1983 as having acted under color of state law. Under <u>Monell</u>, the term "under color of state law" is not synonymous with "acting within the scope of authority." An officer can act outside the scope of authority, or even illegally, and still be sued under Title 42, Section 1983 as having acted under color of state law.

Of course, what applies to officers also applies to all other State employees! Indeed, all governmental employees, Municipal, State and Federal, can be held personally responsible!

How Many Cases Have Been Decided Under U.S. Code Title 42, Section 1983?

This writer has spent hours thumbing through the thousands of cases recorded at the Federal District Court and U.S. Supreme Court levels. They cover almost every abuse of power that one can imagine. Clearly the Congress and President were wise back in the 1800s when this law was first adopted and also later when revised by its broadening.

Wiser, still, would be any alternative/complementary doctor who, on experiencing violation of constitutional rights, under color of law, aims directly for the Federal Courts, and, together with proof, who also invokes U.S.C. Title 42, Section 1983!

In a violation of constitutionally guaranteed rights, U.S.C. Title 42, Section 1983 is the only remedy in law that (1) optimizes the opportunity to confront the actual personage behind claims against you; (2) opens an opportunity to learn who are the actual hidden third parties (quack, quack busters, for example); (3) punishes (reaches into the pocket-book) of the guilty parties, especially governmental employees. The specific administrative individuals who've made the decisions against you can be ascertained, and confronted!

State administrative law and/or medical board reviews or State judicial hearings generally, deliberately or by habit or ignorance, deny or minimize the opportunity for all of the above.

Most important of all, the offenders are punished through their pocketbooks and the word would swiftly pass to other officials thus causing city, state and federal employees to carefully consider their future actions. In other words, what's needed is a system that brings about a state of personal responsibility among officialdom!

The FDA is Not All Bad

The FDA as a protective institution is not all bad!

It's easy to condemn the whole of this organization without identifying specifically who, in the organization, is responsible for specific decisions.

News media practices inadvertly condition us to accept glittering generalities, a method of condemning the whole without pinpointing decision responsibility.

To some extent we all swing blanket blame: "The FDA did so and so." "The AMA is no good." "The ADA is harmful," "The State Medical Board is corrupt!," etc.

Only specific people employed by these organizations have made specific decisions that affect health professionals placed in constitutionally impermissive jeopardy!

U.S.C. Title 42, Section 1983 permits one to determine who these specific people are, how they did it, why they did it, and provides penalties for what they did!

Well meaning Congressmen, responding to one pressure group or another, try their best to pass laws that — even when against our will — protect us from harm.

Sometimes their watchdog efforts pay off!

Consider the case of thallidomide. Thallidomide was synthesized by Chemie Grünenthal at Stolberg, Germany in 1953. Touted as an ideal morning sickness remedy, it was used throughout Europe and other parts of the world under numerous tradenames, primarily for morning sickness with pregnant women.

FDA's Frances Kelsey, new to her job, and for perhaps good reasons — although some say bumbling bureaucracy — denied persistent requests for approval in the United States.

An estimated 8,000 to 12,000 infants were born with deformities caused by thalidomide. Of these, only 5,000 survived beyond childhood.

The medication never received approval in the United States at that time, but 2.5 million tablets had been given to more than 1,200 American Doctors during Richardson-Merrill's "investigation," and nearly 20,000 patients received thalidomide tablets, including several hundred pregnant American women[7]. Seventeen American children were born with thalidomide-related deformities, by best estimate. (As thalidomide is not a mutagen, these defects were not passed on.)

Primarily because of this world-wide tragedy — and faulty method of ascertaining drug utility — Tennessee's U.S. Senator Estes Keauver, resurrected and had rewritten a new FDA function, signed into law by John F. Kennedy on October 10, 1962, The Kefauver Harris Amendment which demanded that pharmaceuticals pass both a "safety and effectiveness" standard. Until this law was passed a new drug had only to be safe for human use.

Because of thalidomide tragedies FDA's "safety" requirement was increased to "safe and effective!"

Whoa! Wait a minute!

If thalidomide was effective for its touted useage — and it certainly was as a sleep agent — then what form of circumulative illogic added to our protective requirements an "effective" standard?

Let's see: Thalidomide was one of the best sleep tablets ever constructed. It was surely effective for its labeled purpose. But it was not safe for babies in the womb and therefore should not be taken by pregnant women.

So, apparently Congress's reasoning was that our laws must extend to insure that drugs are effective -- although the problem with thalidomide was that it was not safe for a certain class of people.

Or is this the way Congress always works?

Note that thalidomide was perhaps one of the best-ever solutions to morning sickness. It was definitely "effective!" It just wasn't "safe" for its intended purpose!

There can be absolutely no doubt — whether bumbling or shrewd science — Kelsey (and the FDA) saved thousands of American tears!

But wasn't this new standard deceptively installed by whipped-up emotion? Wasn't this a matter of charging after one bull, and goring another?

Did the Kefauver-Harris bill based on whatever distorted type of logic really become a significant force for good?

The Symptomatic Nature of the
FDA's Safety and Effectiveness Standard

No one wants to intake food or drugs that are unsafe. But safety is relative! Too much water given to a drowning women — or even voluntarily drunk — can be very unsafe. Tolerating temporary but painful side-effects while actually healing an intransigent disease can become an accepted standard of care.

The chief problem with the Kefauver-Harris Amendment, and the FDA, is a faulty interpretation of the meaning of "effective."

Ask any American citizen if they want a law protecting them from ineffective drugs, and their answer will be a resounding "Yes!"

To the average lay person — and possibly many Congressmen who were in favor of the Kefauver-Harris Amendment — "effective" means "it works!"

To the pharmaceutical companies, and to the FDA, "effective" means that it supresses a symptom.

Consider a no-brainer: "This cold medicine, SniffleSnaffle, will dry up your cold like magic. No more sniffling, sneezing, coughing or lethargy. One tablet will last for 12 hours."

By the standards of the Kefauver-Harris Amendment, all that SniffleSnaffle need do is halt those <u>symptoms</u> of colds, not cure your cold.

"Effectiveness," to most of us lay folks means, "it works," that is, "it cures the cold."

"Effectiveness" to drug companies and the FDA means that it accurately depicts a symptom reliever, and that side-effects can be tolerable under certain specified conditions.

The lower bar, of course, leads to billions of dollars expended for symptom relievers and virtually nothing for cures.

We call this medical progress?

Symptom Relievers are Everywhere!

So there you have it!

Lawyers knowingly or unknowingly avoid legal-source causation and seek symptomatic relief for medical practitioners who've been denied their constitutional rights.

Pharmaceutical companies spend exhorbitant amounts of money and research seeking a patented symptom reliever.

The FDA's standard of effectiveness seeks only to show that a marketed substance buries a symptom temporarily.

Most health practitioners are taught, and practice, the art of treating and suppressing symptoms.

It's no wonder that those complementary/alternative health professionals who've become "due process" endangered under color-of-law, end up with lawyers who seek to follow benign (to the offending bureaurocrat) judicial remedies.

Violation of due process rights, under color of law, properly belongs in Federal Courts, not State Courts, even though State Courts may permit their entry.

Go to the law library and explore for yourself the multitude of case histories bound together under U.S.Code Title 42, Section 1983!

And remember — there's nothing at all like making officialdom responsible for their own actions!!

Holding decision-makers responsible for their decisions will, more than any other remedy, halt the offensive destruction of those alternative/complementary health professionals who seek patient wellness rather than symptomatic relief!

Disclosure

The author of this article is neither a licensed health practitioner nor a licensed attorney.

He has no vested interest in State or Federal courts, nor in seeking Plaintiffs.

Advice provided is merely to point toward what seems to be a proper direction and solution to an outstanding 21st Century problem — that of suppression of constructive medical practices — and is not to be taken as either medical or legal advice.

But —

The author thinks you're very, very foolish if you don't at least explore U.S.Code Title 42, Section 1983 before you begin your time-consuming, costly expense of defending yourself from violations, under color of law, of your constitutionally guaranteed American civil rights, such accusations most likely triggered through uncaring or unknowing State officialdom by the ramblings of faulty quack, quack busters who are themselves incapable of rational reasoning!

References

1. *Handbook of Section 1983 Litigation* is a must for any lawyer who prosecutes or defends a Section 1983 case. If you need the short answer to a Section 1983 question, and you can't afford to waste time running down the wrong research path, turn to the *Handbook of Section 1983 Litigation*, 2006 Edition. This essential guide is designed as the practitioner's desk book. It provides quick and concise answers to issues that frequently arise in Section 1983 cases, from police misconduct to affirmative actions to gender and race discrimination. It is organized to help you quickly find the specific information you need whether you're counsel for the plaintiff or defendant. You will find a clear, concise statement of the law governing every aspect of a Section 1983 claim, extensive citation to legal authority, every major Supreme Court ruling on Section 1983, as well as key opinions in every circuit, and a detailed overview of case law.

George S. Corbyn, Jr. says: "The handbook is a new publication which is the product of over twenty years of work by its author, Oklahoma City attorney David Lee. Lee has a rare combination of attributes to author this book. He is an exceptional trial lawyer who has been litigating Section 1983 claims for years. He is also a nationally recognized scholar and expert on all aspects of Section 1983 law. Simply put, Lee knows Section 1983 law as well as anyone in the country, and he knows what trial lawyers need in a book to properly handle a Section 1983 claim."

In April, 2005, Aspen Publishers, Inc., 1185 Avenue of the Americas, 37th Fl., New York, NY 10036, published the fifth edition. The book is available through Aspen's website at www.aspenpublishers.com.

2. Anthony di Fabio, *How to Spot and Handle Suppression in Medicine: Identical Medical and Religious Patterns of Suppression in the Late Twentieth Century*, unpublished, 1996; free download; P.J. Lisa, *The Assault on Medical Freedom,* Hampton Roads Publishing, Inc., Norfolk, VA 1994; James P. Carter, M.D., Dr. P.H., Racketeering in Medicine: *The Suppression of Alternatives, Hampton Roads Publishing Co.,* 1992, 1993.

3. Greg Seely, Attorney, "Current Legal Challenges — Patient and Physicians Rights!" Sixth International Conference on Bio-Oxidative Medicine, March 7, 1995.

4. "American Preventive Medical Association Director's Report," *Townsend Letter for Doctors & Patients*, 911 Tyler St., Port Townsend, WA , 98368-6541, July 1995, p. 12.

5. Removed.

6. Jonathon Emord, *What to Do when the FDA Shows UP: A Practitioner's Guide to surviving an FDA Raid and Protecting Constitutional Rights*, American Preventive Medical Association.

7. On May 26, 2006, the U.S. Food and Drug Administration granted accelerated approval for thalidomide in combination with dexamethasone for treatment of newly diagnosed multiple myeloma. This approval came seven years after first reports of efficacy in the medical literature, according to internet's *Wikipedia.*

8. *Black's Law Dictionary,* 6th Edition, West Publishing Co., St. Paul, Mn. 1990.

9. "Reassessing the law of preemption" *Georgetown Law Journal,* Jul 2000 by Dinh, Viet D.

10. The author has personal knowledge of this case.

11. Chapdelaine was exceedingly grateful for the legal representation provided by attorney James D. Petersen of Franklin, TN, when, after canvassing numerous others, no other attorney would take the case. Further, without having filed a Pauper's Oath, this case could not have been fought the distance. Health professional's cannot file a Pauper's Oath until the state finishes with them, and makes them paupers, perhaps the main reason so many good alternative/complementary practitioners cave before adjudication of their constitutional rights.

www.ingramcontent.com/pod-product-compliance
Lightning Source LLC
Chambersburg PA
CBHW051850170526
45168CB00001B/50